# Breast Elastography

**Richard G. Barr, MD, PhD, FACR, FSRU**
Professor of Radiology
Northeastern Ohio Medical University
Rootstown, Ohio
Staff Radiologist
Northside Medical Center and Southwoods Imaging
Youngstown, Ohio

Thieme
New York • Stuttgart • Delhi • Rio de Janeiro

Thieme Medical Publishers, Inc.
333 Seventh Ave.
New York, NY 10001

Executive Editor: William Lamsback
Managing Editor: J. Owen Zurhellen, IV
Editorial Assistant: Kate Barron
Senior Vice President, Editorial and Electronic Product Development:
  Cornelia Schulze
Production Editor: Sean Woznicki
International Production Director: Andreas Schabert
International Marketing Director: Fiona Henderson
Director of Sales, North America: Mike Roseman
International Sales Director: Louisa Turrell
Vice President, Finance and Accounts: Sarah Vanderbilt
President: Brian D. Scanlan
Printer: Sheridan Books

**Library of Congress Cataloging-in-Publication Data**

Barr, Richard G., author.
  Breast elastography / Richard G. Barr.
    p. ; cm.
  ISBN 978-1-60406-852-8 (hardcover) – ISBN 978-1-60406-853-5
(ebook)
  I. Title.
    [DNLM: 1. Breast Neoplasms–ultrasonography–Case Reports.
2. Elasticity Imaging Techniques–Case Reports. 3. Breast Neoplasms–pathology–Case Reports.  WP 870]
  RC280.B8
  616.99'449075–dc23
                        2014034707

Copyright © 2015 by Thieme Medical Publishers, Inc.
Thieme Publishers New York
333 Seventh Avenue, New York, NY 10001 USA
+1 800 782 3488, customerservice@thieme.com

Thieme Publishers Stuttgart
Rüdigerstrasse 14, 70469 Stuttgart, Germany
+49 [0]711 8931 421, customerservice@thieme.de

Thieme Publishers Delhi
A-12, Second Floor, Sector-2, Noida-201301
Uttar Pradesh, India
+91 120 45 566 00, customerservice@thieme.in

Thieme Publishers Rio, Thieme Publicações Ltda.
Argentina Building 16th floor, Ala A, 228 Praia do Botafogo
Rio de Janeiro 22250-040 Brazil
+55 21 3736-3631

Printed in the United States of America            5 4 3 2 1

ISBN 978-1-60406-852-8

Also available as an e-book:
eISBN 978-1-60406-853-5

**Important note:** Medicine is an ever-changing science undergoing continual development. Research and clinical experience are continually expanding our knowledge, in particular our knowledge of proper treatment and drug therapy. Insofar as this book mentions any dosage or application, readers may rest assured that the authors, editors, and publishers have made every effort to ensure that such references are in accordance with **the state of knowledge at the time of production of the book.**

Nevertheless, this does not involve, imply, or express any guarantee or responsibility on the part of the publishers in respect to any dosage instructions and forms of applications stated in the book. **Every user is requested to examine carefully** the manufacturers' leaflets accompanying each drug and to check, if necessary in consultation with a physician or specialist, whether the dosage schedules mentioned therein or the contraindications stated by the manufacturers differ from the statements made in the present book. Such examination is particularly important with drugs that are either rarely used or have been newly released on the market. Every dosage schedule or every form of application used is entirely at the user's own risk and responsibility. The authors and publishers request every user to report to the publishers any discrepancies or inaccuracies noticed. If errors in this work are found after publication, errata will be posted at www.thieme.com on the product description page.

Some of the product names, patents, and registered designs referred to in this book are in fact registered trademarks or proprietary names even though specific reference to this fact is not always made in the text. Therefore, the appearance of a name without designation as proprietary is not to be construed as a representation by the publisher that it is in the public domain.

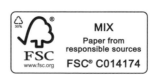

To my family, friends, and co-workers.

# Contents

# Foreword

The increasing usage of ultrasound elastography in many clinical applications, especially in the breast, makes this elegant and practical book particularly welcome. Seemingly simple to perform and of undoubted incremental diagnostic value for classifying breast masses, obtaining elastograms of diagnostic value is difficult. Handling the transducer correctly and optimizing setting up the scanner require training and dedicated practice. Recognizing when adequate elastograms have been obtained and the numerous potential artefacts, both friendly and inimical, require dedicated study and repetition. Richard Barr's fluid writing style and his elegant and germane diagrams form a powerful aid to the would-be practitioner and will speed their learning process.

Dr. Barr's achievements emanate from a wide clinical practice, remarkable for his productivity from a non-academic radiology practice. Thus, the advice and recommen-dations given are based on his practice and extensive clinical experience. This is evidenced in the numerous case studies, which are copiously illustrated. They supplement the introduction to the principles of elastography and form a guide to interpretation that will be immensely useful. Usefully, they have been performed on a wide variety of scanners from different vendors, so as to inform all users.

Overall this is an outstandingly practical book that breast sonographers and sonologists will want to keep in their scanning room and refer to frequently.

*David Cosgrove, MA, MSc, FRCP, FRCR*
*Emeritus Professor of Clinical Ultrasound*
*Imperial and King's Colleges*
*London, United Kingdom*

# Preface

This book is designed primarily for sonographers and radiologists involved in breast imaging. This is a comprehensive review of breast elastography with emphasis on clinical applications. The techniques needed to optimize each form of elastography are discussed in detail with pitfalls clearly called out. A review of all artifacts and how to avoid them is included. Some artifacts provide significant clinical information, and these are discussed in detail. The book is designed to be useful both for the beginner as well as for the experienced imager.

This book is a compilation of our experience with elastography over 10 years, from proof of concept systems to equipment now available for routine clinical use. An attempt has been made to include all of the available techniques for each clinical case to compare and contrast the different techniques. Enough information is included for each technique so those with access to only one technique will be able to optimize the clinical utility of their system. For those with multiple techniques available on different equipment a discussion of the various techniques is available to help determine which patients are best suited for each technique. Strain and shear wave imaging are complementary techniques. We find the use of both techniques on each patient provides increased confidence in the findings.

Clinical cases have been selected to demonstrate a wide range of pathology. Within a given disease state cases have been selected to demonstrate the range of elastography findings for that pathology. Cases where elastography can yield false-positive or false-negative results are highlighted and discussed in detail, with tips on how to recognize which findings may be inaccurate.

Our lab has used breast elastography for all of our breast ultrasound cases for several years. We find it an invaluable tool with which to characterize breast lesions. Since we have used elastography our biopsy rate has decreased by over 50%, whereas our positive biopsy rate has increased significantly. Further clinical work is needed to determine how to incorporate ultrasound elastography into the Breast Imagng–Reporting and Data System (BI-RADS). With a negative predictive value of approximately 99% with some techniques, it may be possible to downgrade BI-RADS scores by more than one level.

We wish to express our appreciation to the hundreds of patients that participated in our research studies, which have allowed this technology to reach routine clinical use. We also wish to thank the engineers we have worked with in the development of all these technologies for their help in optimizing these techniques for clinical use. A special thanks to the staff at Southwoods Imaging for their help in facilitating our studies and for the excellent patient care they provide that makes patients excited about participating in research studies.

# Acknowledgments

Many people have been associated with and supported our research on the development of breast elastography. The engineering and application staffs of Siemens Ultrasound, Philips Ultrasound, and Supersonics Imagine have worked together with us to make breast elastography an extremely valuable part of breast imaging. The number of our vendor collaborators is too large to name individually and all deserve acknowledgments. The staff at Southwoods Imaging have worked hard and made significant contributions to our research efforts.

A special thanks to Margaret Drummond whose diligent work and advice helped start our research efforts in our private practice setting.

Finally, I wish to thank the thousands of patients who have volunteered for our research studies that allowed the progress we made.

# Abbreviations / Terminology

**ARFI:** Acoustic Radiation Force Impulse

**EI:** Elasticity Imaging, Siemens strain imaging using manual displacement now eSie Touch

**Elasticity score:** a scoring system to characterize lesions on strain elastography. Also known as the 5-point color scale, Tsukuba score, or strain pattern.

**ElaXto:** Esaote's strain imaging

**eSie:** eSie Touch, Siemens strain imaging using manual displacement

**Five-point color scale:** a scoring system to characterize lesions on strain elastography. Also known as Tsukuba core, elasticity score, or strain pattern.

**FLR:** fat to lesion ratio, a method of semi-quantitating strain results. It determines the relative stiffness of a lesion compared to the stiffness of fat.

**FOV:** Field of View

**Length ratio:** the length of the lesion measured on strain imaging compared to the length of the lesion on B-mode imaging also known as E/B ratio

**Manual displacement method:** the use of the transducer or patient breathing and/or heart beat to generate the compression/release force needed to generate a strain elastogram.

**RTE:** Real-Time Elastography, Hitachi's strain imaging

**ROI:** Region of Interest

**SE:** Strain Elastography, generic term for all strain elastography

**SSI:** SuperSonic Imagine

**Strain ratio:** lesion to fat ratio, the ratio of the stiffness of a lesion to the stiffness of fat

**SWE:** Shear Wave Elastography, generic term for shear wave imaging

**Strain pattern:** a scoring system to characterize lesions on strain elastography. Also known as the 5-point color scale, Tsukuba score, or elasticity score.

**Tsukuba score:** a scoring system to characterize lesions on strain elastography. Also known as 5-point color scale, elasticity score, or strain pattern.

**VTi:** Virtual Touch Imaging, Siemens strain imaging using ARFI

**VTiq:** Virtual Touch Imaging quantification, Siemens shear wave imaging

**VTq:** Virtual Touch Quantification, Siemens shear wave point quantification

**Vs:** Shear Wave Velocity (expressed in meters per second (m/s))

**Width ratio:** comparison of the size of a lesion measured on strain imaging compared to the size measured on B-mode imaging

# 1 Introduction to Breast Elastography

Ultrasound evaluation of the breast was initially used to determine if a lesion was cystic or solid.[1,2] With the criteria set forth by Stavros et al,[3] ultrasound has since had a more important role in breast lesion characterization. These criteria have been incorporated into the ultrasound Breast Imaging–Reporting and Data System (BI-RADS) lexicon[4] and can be used to distinguish between benign and malignant breast lesions.

Elastography is a new ultrasound technique that can provide additional information which was previously not available. Elastography or elasticity imaging (EI) is an imaging modality based on tissue stiffness, rather than anatomy. These images show the relative difference in stiffness among tissue. For thousands of years physicians have used palpation for diagnosis of breast cancer,[5] realizing that stiffer masses on palpation were more likely malignancies. Ultrasound elastography has the potential to quantify the stiffness of a lesion, which was previously judged only subjectively by physical exam.[6–8] Krouskop et al determined that in vivo there is significant elastographic contrast between cancerous and noncancerous breast lesions.[9] This suggests that elastography should be an excellent technique for characterizing breast lesions as benign or malignant.

There are two types of elastography: strain elastography (SE) and shear wave elastography (SWE). Strain elastography produces an image based on the displacement of the tissue from a compression/release force applied by an external force (transducer or acoustic radiation force impulse [ARFI]) or a patient source (breathing and/or heartbeat). This allows for a qualitative assessment of the lesion, that is, a relative assessment of the stiffness compared with other tissues in the field of view. The exact stiffness of the lesion is not obtained. SWE applies a special "push pulse," ARFI, which results in shear wave propagation that can be measured as a velocity. Because the velocity of the shear wave through tissues is dependent on the "stiffness" of the tissue, a quantitative value of the stiffness can be obtained; that is, a measurement of lesion stiffness is obtained and expressed as a numerical value. With the addition of elastography we now have three ultrasound modes (▶ Table 1.1).

Early work in this field was complicated by the fact that B-mode imaging was performed on a conventional ultrasound machine, whereas the elastography imaging was performed on a research elastography system. With the advent of real-time dual display systems that presented both the conventional B-mode image and the elastogram this technique became clinically useful. Using the real-time dual display strain elastography system, Hall et al[10] demonstrated that there was potential to use this technique to characterize breast lesions as benign or malignant. It was also noted that on strain elastography benign lesions appear smaller in size than the corresponding B-mode image, whereas malignancies appear larger in size than the corresponding B-mode image. They proposed using the ratio of the elastography size of a lesion to the B-mode size of a lesion as a diagnostic criterion for benign or malignant.

Although current modalities of breast imaging, including magnetic resonance imaging (MRI), ultrasound, and mammography, have high sensitivities for detecting breast lesions, they do not have high specificities.[11,12] This has resulted in close monitoring or unnecessary biopsies of many benign lesions. An imaging modality with a high specificity for detecting malignant lesions could significantly decrease the amount of unnecessary biopsies.

Continued improvement in image quality, technique, and image interpretation has occurred. This book discusses the state-of-the art use of elastography of the breast at this time, emphasizing the appropriate technique and interpretation needed to obtain consistent, accurate results.

Initially introduced in 2003, elastography technology has since improved with advances in diagnostic ultrasound systems. Some form of breast elastography is available on most commercially available ultrasound systems today. Current elastography systems provide images that can not only differentiate between benign and malignant tissue but also evaluate histological information by depicting the distribution of tissue stiffness. This may have the potential to evaluate the therapeutic effect of treatment with anticancer agents. Elastography allows for diagnosis and evaluation of not only masses but also non-mass lesions.

Systems with various methods that apply strain have recently become available. They include not only systems with strain elastography, which involve a manual compression/release cycle or vibration, but also systems equipped with ARFI and SWE technology. These methods share the concept of bringing quantitative diagnostic capability (stiffness) into the field of ultrasonography, but differ in terms of theory, technique, and interpretation. Moreover, there are various methods and terms related to diagnostic assessment, such as the ratio of the lesion length on elastography to the lesion length on B-mode imaging, the E/B ratio (width ratio, length ratio), 5-point color scale (elasticity score, Tsukuba score, strain pattern), strain ratio (lesion to fat ratio [LFR]), and shear wave measurements (kPa or m/s), which often lead to confusion when one is learning elastography techniques.

In this book the principles of elastography are presented in a form easily understood by clinical sonographers and sonologists. More detailed principles of elastography can be found elsewhere.[13] The techniques required to obtain optimal images with the various methods are discussed with an emphasis on avoiding pitfalls. The interpretation of the images using the various techniques is discussed as well as how they relate to each other. A review of the literature and references to other sources of information are provided.

Elastography should be performed in conjunction with the conventional breast ultrasound. It is an additional imaging mode, like color Doppler, to evaluate a breast lesion or nonmass lesions. At this time elastography cannot be used as a screening technique, but it is an excellent diagnostic technique with

Table 1.1 Comparison of different modes of medical ultrasonography

| Mode | What is measured: | What is displayed: |
| --- | --- | --- |
| B-mode | Acoustic impedance | Anatomy |
| Doppler | Motion | Vascular flow |
| Elastography | Mechanical properties | Tissue stiffness |

which to characterize a lesion as benign or malignant. Elastography in some form is now available on most ultrasound systems. Both SE and SWE are cleared by the Food and Drug Administration (FDA) for determining if a lesion is soft or stiff. Both SE and SWE have been shown to improve characterization of breast abnormalities. The choice of which to use is a personal preference and is often influenced by experience or equipment availability. Both techniques, SE and SWE, can be performed on an abnormality within a few minutes and can increase confidence of the results if both techniques are used and are concordant. If the results are not concordant it can be an alert that the lesion is atypical, and additional evaluation may be necessary to further characterize the lesion.

Elastography can also be helpful in characterizing isoechoic lesions. If a palpable lesion is not identified on B-mode imaging, the use of elastography can often identify the lesion based on its stiffness. It is not uncommon to have an isoechoic "lesion," which is difficult to determine if the area in question is truly an abnormality or a fat lobule.

It has been suggested that the main advantage of elastography could be improved characterization of BI-RADS category 3 and BI-RADS category 4A lesions. Elastography could be used to upgrade or downgrade these lesions by one BI-RADS score. As elastography continues to improve and more clinical experience is obtained a better understanding of how elastography could be incorporated in the BI-RADS classification. Guidelines have been recommended by several organizations.[14–16]

We have used elastography on all our diagnostic breast ultrasound cases for several years and as a research tool for over 10 years. In our experience we have significantly decreased our biopsy rate while increasing our positive biopsy rate. We find elastography helpful in all BI-RADS category lesions. The bull's-eye artifact (see Chapter 3) has been extremely helpful in increasing confidence when a lesion is a benign complicated cyst and short-term follow-up or biopsy is not required. However, we recommend that a site confirm their technique and results before canceling a biopsy. Correlation of elastography with pathology has added an additional check for adequacy of our image-guided biopsies.

There are many methods of displaying the elastography data. Several color scales have been used. In this book we will use the convention of black is stiff and white is soft for SE and red is stiff and blue is soft for SWE. We use the color scale in SWE because it depicts the quantitative value of the stiffness; therefore, any lesion that is stiff enough to color code above our cutoff value is easy to identify. We use a gray scale in SE because we believe we can identify the changes in relative stiffness more accurately than with use of a color scale where a small change in relative stiffness may be depicted as an abrupt color change. We also believe we are able to measure a lesion more accurately on the elastogram using the gray scale. On strain imaging the mapping onto the gray scale or color scale is a postprocessing function, and most systems allow changing the map on a frozen image. Regardless of the map used the information in the elastogram is identical, only the display is changed. In this book we will use the convention that SE refers to strain imaging using a manual compression/release technique (not using an ARFI technique) unless stated. Tips and tricks are included and highlighted when appropriate.

Terminology in elastography has been confusing, with multiple terms used to describe the same ideas or techniques. In this book we use the terminology suggested by the World Federation for Ultrasound in Medicine and Biology (WFUMB) guidelines.[16] Other terminology is included in parentheses.

Although several studies have been published evaluating elastography for characterization of lesions as benign or malignant, at the time of writing this book few studies have been performed to evaluate elastography in specific breast pathologies. Where available these are referenced in the case studies. The case studies are the author's experience with the use of elastography in characterization of breast pathologies.

# 2 Principles of Elastography

## 2.1 Overview

Elastography is a recently developed technique in ultrasound that can provide clinically useful information about tissue stiffness not previously available. Elastography, or elasticity imaging, is an imaging modality based on tissue stiffness rather than anatomy. Palpation has been used to assess stiffness to evaluate for malignancies for over a thousand years.[17] Ultrasound elastography can be considered the imaging equivalent of clinical palpation because it can quantify the stiffness of a lesion, which was previously judged only subjectively by physical exam.

There are two types of elastography: strain elastography (SE) and shear wave imaging (SWE).[18] SE produces an image based on how tissues respond to a displacement force from an external (transducer or acoustic radiation force impulse [ARFI]) or patient source (breathing and/or heartbeat). This allows for a qualitative assessment of the lesion in terms of how stiff the tissue is compared with surrounding tissues in the field of view (FOV). In other words, with SE the "exact" stiffness is not known, only how stiff one tissue is in comparison with other types of tissue in the FOV. SWE uses ARFI imaging, or in lay terms a "push pulse," which acts as the compressing force. A natural sequel to this push pulse is the production of shear waves, which, when their velocities are measured, allow quantification of stiffness.

## 2.2 Strain Elastography

SE determines the *relative* strain or elasticity of tissue within an FOV.[18] The more an object deforms when a force is applied the higher the strain and the softer the lesion. To determine the strain of a tissue or lesion one must evaluate how the lesion deforms when an external force is applied. For example, if we had an almond in a bowl of gelatin (▶ Fig. 2.1a) and pushed down on the gelatin (▶ Fig. 2.1b), the gelatin would deform, indicating it has high strain and is therefore soft. However, the almond, having low strain, would not deform and is therefore stiff.

SE is performed on standard ultrasound equipment using specific software that evaluates the frame-to-frame differences in deformation in tissue when a force (stress) is applied. The force can be from patient movement (such as breathing, heartbeat) or external compression with rhythmic motion of the ultrasound transducer or acoustic radiation force impulse (ARFI) as the source of the movement.[18] In SE the absolute strain (Young) modulus value (a numerical value quantifying the stiffness) cannot be calculated because the amount of the force cannot be accurately measured. The real-time SE image is displayed with a scale based on the *relative* strain (or stiffness) of the tissues within the FOV. Therefore, if the types of tissue in the FOV are different, a different scale may be used for the display map.

▶ Fig. 2.2 demonstrates a simplified explanation of how the mapping of SE data is performed on most systems. The boxes on the left represent tissue identified on B-mode imaging before the addition of any force. The boxes in the middle represent the size of the tissue on B-mode imaging after the compressive force. The tissues that do not change shape are very stiff, whereas those that are soft change size based on their relative

stiffness. The strain elastography algorithm evaluates the relative changes in size of the tissues and assigns a color (or shade of gray) based on the distribution of the size changes. In our example in ▶ Fig. 2.2a, the tissue that does not change shape at all is color coded black because it is the stiffest of all the tissue being evaluated. The lower box changes the most and is therefore the softest and is color coded white. The tissue in between these extremes is given a shade of gray corresponding to the amount of change in the tissue; darker gray if stiffer and lighter gray if softer. However, if we did not include the stiffest tissue in ▶ Fig. 2.2a, different color coding of the other tissues would

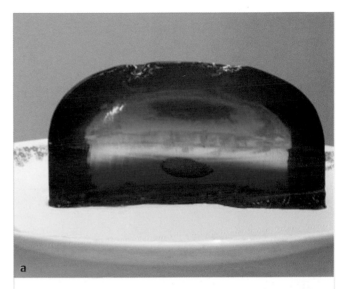

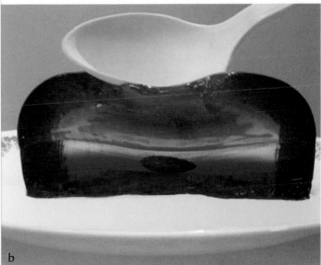

**Fig. 2.1** (a,b) A simplistic model of the principal of strain elastography is to consider an almond in gelatin. If we apply a stress such as compressing the gelatin with a spoon, the gelatin changes shape because it is soft (more strain), whereas the almond does not change shape because it is stiff (less strain). The ultrasound strain system compares the frame-to-frame changes of tissue when the tissue is compressed/released. Tissues that deform the most are considered soft, whereas those that deform the least are considered stiff.

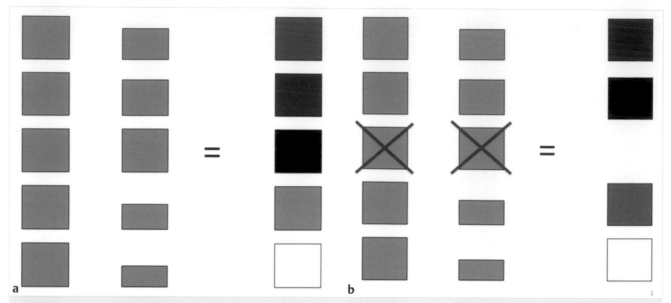

**Fig. 2.2** The color-coding of the pixels in the elastogram is based on the changes that occur with the compression/release cycle. In the diagrams the boxes on the left depict different tissues within the field of view (FOV). When the compression is applied the boxes change shape based on their stiffness (center vertical column). The box that changes shape the most is color coded white, whereas the box that changes the least is color coded black. The boxes that change between these two extremes are color coded shades of gray based on the amount of change they experience (a). If the FOV is different and the stiffest tissue in (b) is not included the color mapping changes with the second box now the stiffest and therefore being color coded black. The dynamic range of the color coding is changed and the first and fourth tissues are now color coded with darker shades of gray.

occur as in ▶ Fig. 2.2b. Note that the coloring of the first three tissues has changed because the second tissue is now the stiffest and therefore coded black. Thus the "dynamic range" of stiffness values changes depending on the tissues present in the FOV.

Therefore if similar stiff tissues and soft tissues are included in each image acquisition a relatively constant color display will be obtained. In breast strain elastography, if a portion of the pectoralis muscle and some fat are included in the FOV, a more consistent color depiction of tissues between images will be obtained. The fat will be the softest tissue coding white and the pectoralis muscle will be the stiffest tissue (if a cancer is not present) coding black. The color scale (or dynamic range of stiffness values) will be fairly constant because the stiffness of fat and muscle are very constant between patients and within a patient. However, if a breast cancer is present within the FOV it will be the stiffest tissue and be color coded black with most other tissues being displayed as white or light gray.

The technique required to obtain the optimal images varies with the algorithm used by the manufacturer of the system.[18] For SE the amount of external displacement needed varies depending on the algorithm used. With some systems very little if any manual compression/release is needed, with others a rhythmic compression/release cycle is required. With experience and practice the optimum compression/release technique for a specific system to obtain optimal image quality can be learned. Applying too large a compression/release cycle will result in image noise, whereas not applying enough will result in no image being obtained. Learning the "sweet spot" for the equipment being used is critical for optimal images and is discussed in detail in Chapter 3.

The algorithm used in SE requires that the strain changes be measured in a lesion that remains within the imaging plane. The same slice of the lesion needs to remain in the imaging plane during the entire compression/release cycle. Monitoring of the B-mode image to confirm the lesion is displaced only in depth (not in and out of plane) during scanning and moving only axially in the FOV will allow for optimal images. An organ cannot be surveyed with the displacement SE technique; scanning must be done in one stationary position.

Results can be displayed in gray scale or with various color displays; preference is often determined by the user's exposure to elastography and preference in interpretation. The display map preference is a postprocessing function, and on most equipment the map can be changed when the image is frozen. The default on many systems has the elastogram displayed over the gray scale B-mode image. Most systems display in a dual mode with a separate B-mode image also displayed. This helps in determining the location of the elastographic findings. However, if a gray scale map is chosen the background B-mode image in the elastogram should be turned off because the two superimposed gray scale images are difficult to interpret. This book uses a gray scale map with soft coded white and hard coded black without a superimposed B-mode image unless otherwise stated. It is important to remember that, even when using the color-coded SE a *relative* scale is displayed, which should not be confused with SWE where an absolute stiffness value is obtained and color coded on a per pixel basis. On SWE a lesion will have the same color (assuming the same color scale is used) regardless of the other tissues present in the FOV. On SE the lesion may appear a different color if the other tissues in the FOV are different.

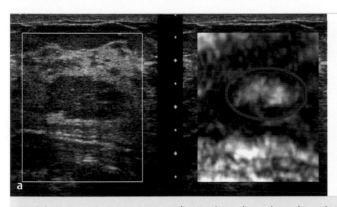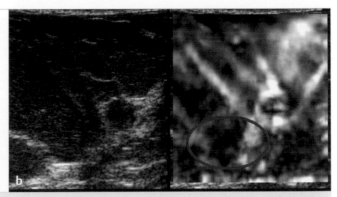

Fig. 2.3 Because strain imaging is qualitative the scale used to color code the image is relative to the tissues within the field of view. For example, fat within an image with dense breast tissue will code as white because it is the softest tissue within the field of view (a, circle). However, if an image contains only fat some of the fat will be coded dark because it is the stiffest tissue (stiffest of the fat in the image) in the field of view (b, circle). Therefore a given tissue or mass may be color coded differently on various frames if the tissues within the field of view are different. To help minimize the difference it is advisable to include a similar variety of tissues (fat, dense breast tissue, and pectoralis muscle) in all images. (Reprinted with permission from Barr RG. Sonographic breast elastography: a primer. J Ultrasound Med 2012;31(5):773–783)

Because SE is a relative technique, a lesion may appear a different shade of gray (or color) depending on the other tissues in the FOV. For example, in a patient with normal dense breast tissue and fat, the fat will appear white (soft) because it is the softest tissue in the FOV. However, if only fat is in the FOV some of the fat will appear black (stiff) because it is the stiffest tissue in the FOV (▶ Fig. 2.3). This can cause difficulty in interpretation. Therefore, a large FOV with multiple tissue types of varying stiffness is helpful in image interpretation. The color scale can be relatively constant in SE by including fat as the softest tissue and pectoralis muscle as the stiffest tissue. These tissues do not vary in stiffness from patient to patient and therefore can fix the dynamic range of stiffness if only benign tissue is present. When a malignancy is present it will be stiffer than pectoralis muscle and will reset the dynamic range so it is the stiffest tissue.

A critical factor in generating a diagnostic elastogram is the amount of pressure applied with the probe during scanning.[19] This is called precompression or preload. This is different than the amount of displacement (compression/release) used in generating the elastogram. Scanning with a "heavy hand" compresses the tissues and changes their elastic properties. This precompression markedly changes the image quality and can significantly affect results (▶ Fig. 2.4).[19] This is confirmed with SWE where the velocity of the shear wave (Vs) can change by a factor of 10 with precompression (▶ Fig. 2.5). As precompression increases, the differences in shear wave speed between tissues decrease, leading to less conspicuity between tissues on the strain elastogram. If enough precompression is applied all tissues will have similar stiffness, and the SE elastogram will be mostly noise, whereas the SWE will have high shear wave speeds thoughout the image.

▶ Fig. 2.5 is a diagram summarizing the Vs of the different tissue types in breast at various amounts of precompression that we used for the results and discussion that follow. The amount of precompression is classified into 4 categories: Zone A, minimal precompression 0–10%, Zone B, mild precompression 10–25%, Zone C moderate precompression 25–40%, and Zone D marked precompression > 40%.

## 2.2.1 How Can Precompression Affect Strain Elastography Images?

In SE, images are based on the *relative* stiffness of the lesions within an image. It is qualitative (how stiff relative to other tissues in the FOV) but not quantitative (an absolute value). The imaging scale used is relative and based on tissues within the image plane. In the case where both soft tissues (fat, fibroglandular tissue) and a very stiff lesion (malignancy) are present in Zones A, B, and C, the difference in elasticity (Vs values measured in m/s) between the soft tissues and malignancies are adequate to generate an accurate elastogram. However, in Zone D the elasticity of both soft tissues and malignancies are similar; hence the elastogram is not diagnostic and represents only noise.

However, the results are different in the case where the area of interest contains only "soft" tissues (fat, fibroglandular, soft fibroadenoma, fibrocystic change). In Zone A the elasticity differences between the tissues allows for a diagnostic elastogram. In Zone B the elastogram is borderline for diagnostic value, with some frames of good diagnostic quality and some with poor diagnostic value. This is due to precompression creating a smaller difference of stiffness between tissues. Based on the author's experience this appears to depend on whether the frame was taken in a compression or in a release phase of the cycle. This may be due to the increased precompression on the compression phase of the cycle. In Zones C and D, the elasticity properties of the soft tissues are very similar due to the precompression, and the elastogram is mostly noise and is nondiagnostic.

A technique to apply a minimal amount of precompression reproducibly has been described.[19] In this technique a structure in the far field is identified such as a rib or Cooper ligament. The transducer is lifted slowly while the structure is watched. As the probe is lifted the object will move deeper in the image. The elastogram is obtained with the structure as deep in the image as possible while adequate probe contact is maintained. The use of ample coupling gel is helpful. Another method is to make a standoff pad with coupling gel, making sure some coupling gel is present between the transducer and the patient

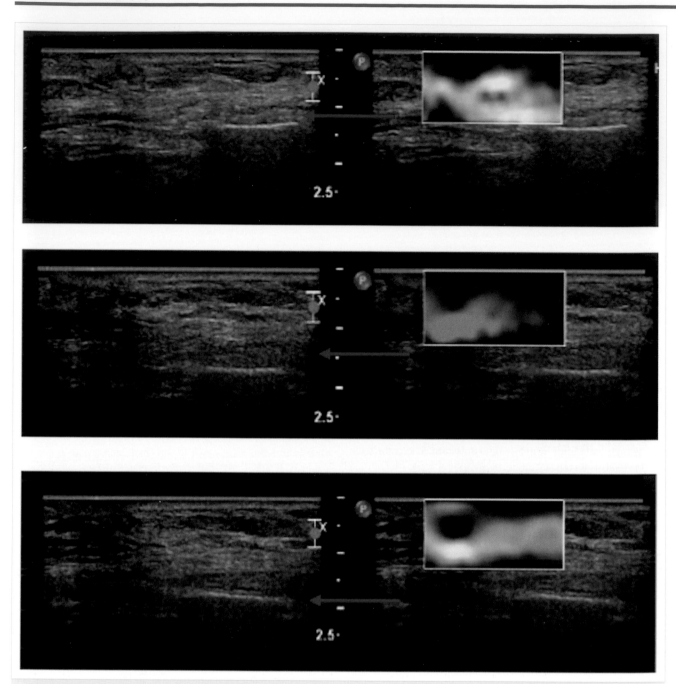

**Fig. 2.4** When precompression (applying pressure with the transducer) is applied it can significantly affect the elastogram. When minimal compression is applied optimal elastograms are obtained (a) as in this example of an epidermal cyst. When mild precompression is applied the frames obtained on the release phase are often good however, those on the compression phase are of poor quality (b). This leads to a video clip were the lesion is adequately visualized on a few frames. When a significant amount of precompression is applied the elastogram is only noise and is not interpretable (c). A method to limit the amount of precompression is to identify a structure in the far field of the image (red arrows pointing out a rib in this case). As the transducer is lifted the structure will move deeper in the image. When the structure is as deep in the far field as possible and adequate contact with the transducer is maintained minimal precompression is applied and an optimal elastogram will be obtained. (Reprinted with permission from Barr RG, Zhang Z. Effects of precompression on elasticity imaging of the breast: development of a clinically useful semiquantitative method of precompression assessment. J Ultrasound Med 2012;31(6):895–902)

when obtaining the elastogram. Usually a small amount (10–20%) of precompression is used to obtain B-mode images because it improves B-mode image quality. The "quality factor" or "compression bar" used in some equipment does not assess the amount of precompression being applied. It only evaluates the amount of displacement of tissues during the compression/release cycle. This is discussed in Chapter 3. Even when significant precompression is applied leading to a poor elastogram the quality factor or compression bar can suggest a good elastogram.

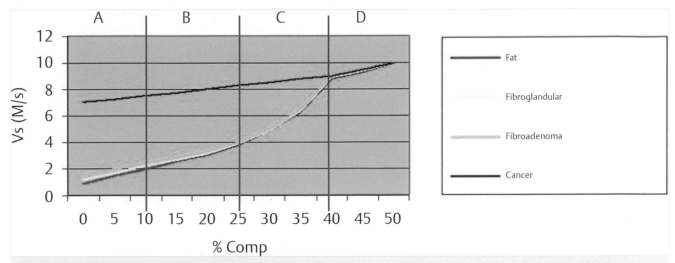

**Fig. 2.5** The stiffness of tissues when precompression is applied can be measured with shear wave elastography. Shear wave velocity (Vs) increases with increasing tissue stiffness. The Vs of various breast tissues and pathologies at varying amounts or precompression are presented in this figure. As precompression is applied the difference of stiffness between tissues and pathology is decreased. Above 40% compression all tissues have the same stiffness. At this amount of precompression strain elastograms will depict only noise, and shear wave elastograms will suggest all tissues are malignant. Maintaining precompression in the 0 to 10% range optimal results will be obtained. Between 10 and 40% precompression strain elastography (SE) images that do not contain a malignancy are of poor quality because the stiffness differences of all benign tissues are similar. If a malignancy is present, an adequate elastogram will be obtained because there remains a large difference in stiffness between the malignancy and the benign tissues. At above 25% precompression all tissues will have Vs suggestive of a malignancy on shear wave imaging. (Reprinted with permission from Barr RG, Zhang Z. Effects of precompression on elasticity imaging of the breast: development of a clinically useful semiquantitative method of precompression assessment. J Ultrasound Med 2012;31(6):895–902)

## 2.2.2 Strain Elastography Using Acoustic Radiation Force Impulse

An ultrasound pulse can be reflected, absorbed (attenuated), or create momentum transfer (pushes). The transfer of energy causes tissue to move. Increased energy in the ultrasound beam creates increased force and hence movement. The movement of the tissue has two consequences for elastography: (1) the measurement of the movement directly: strain elastography; or (2) tissue movement generates a lateral transverse (shear) wave, the speed of which through the tissue can be measured: shear wave elastography (▶ Fig. 2.6).

ARFI is the use of a low-frequency ultrasound pulse that is tailored to optimize the momentum transfer to tissue.[20–22] An SE image can be obtained by using ARFI to create the displacement of tissue and analyzing the displacement changes with a similar strain algorithm. The ARFI pulse replaces the patient or probe movement to generate the stress on the tissues. This technique may be less user dependent than the manual compression technique. This push pulse generates both axial displacement and shear waves. When the axial displacement is measured the technique is similar to SE called Virtual Touch Imaging (VTI, Siemens Medical Solutions USA, Inc., Mountain View, CA). Note that this is different than SWE where the Vs generated from the ARFI pulse is measured. The former is qualitative (gives only relative differences in tissue stiffness in the FOV), whereas the latter is quantitative (provides a numerical value of the stiffness). The ARFI push pulse power is limited by guidelines of the amount of energy that can be input into the body, thus limiting the depth of tissue displacement and therefore the depth of the SE elastogram. This is usually not a problem when a manual displacement technique is used because it

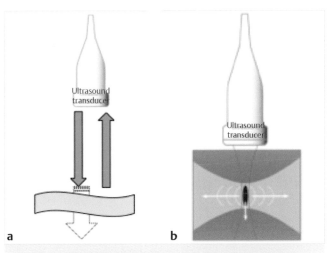

**Fig. 2.6** An ultrasound pulse can be reflected (a, blue arrows) or absorbed (attenuated) (a, white arrow) or can transfer momentum (pushes) to tissue. A low-frequency strong ultrasound pulse can be used to optimize momentum transfer to tissue (b). This is called acoustic radiation force impulse (ARFI). The movement of the tissue can be measured directly (strain imaging), or a lateral transverse shear wave can be generated and its speed through the tissue measured (shear wave imaging).

can be adjusted to have appropriate displacement at any depth in breast imaging.

There are several differences between SE and VTI. One important difference is that radiation force in ARFI imaging is maximized at the point of focus, whereas in SE, strain is more uniform laterally in the image based on transducer compression and the amount of stress applied locally and changes with depth. Therefore a strain ratio for VTI should not be used as a semiquantitative method. A quantitative value of stiffness cannot be obtained using VTI.

If an ARFI push pulse is used to generate the tissue displacement, no manual displacement (transducer compression/release) should be used. The probe should be held steady and the patient asked to suspend respiration and remain motionless during the acquisition. The algorithm used to generate the elastogram is similar to SE on the same system. The color-mapping algorithm is slightly different than in the manual compression technique, and some differences in the appearance of the elastogram between the two techniques can be seen. In general the ARFI push pulse is limited in producing displacement deeper than 4 to 5 cm with most breast imaging transducers.

## 2.3 Shear Wave Elastography

A second technique with which to determine the elastic properties of a tissue is SWE. In this technique an initial ultrasound pulse (push pulse) or ARFI pulse is applied to the tissue that induces a shear wave perpendicular to the ultrasound beam. This is similar to dropping a stone (the push pulse) into a pond of water. The ripples generated correspond to the shear waves. Conventional B-mode ultrasound sampling techniques are used to calculate the velocity of the shear wave generated through the tissues by monitoring the tissue displacement caused by the shear waves. This is diagramed in ▶ Fig. 2.7. The strain modulus (Young's modulus) can be estimated from the velocity of the shear wave through the tissues. The velocities of the shear waves are directly correlated with higher velocities representing stiffness and vice versa. The stiffness of a lesion can be displayed as the Vs in m/s through the tissue, or derived and displayed as the strain modulus in kilopascals (kPa). The strain modulus (or Young's modulus) is calculated by making some assumptions (density of tissue is 1 g/cm$^3$ and Poisson ratio is 0.5) regarding the tissue and using the following equation:

$$(kPa) = 3Vs^2$$

With SWE a quantitative measure of the lesion stiffness is obtained either in point of interest (point quantification) or in a larger FOV with pixel-by-pixel color coding of the Vs (shear wave imaging). ▶ Table 2.1 lists the conversion of the two scales at various measurements. Most systems allow the user to select which scale they prefer.

Two shear wave imaging systems are presently available for breast applications. In the ACUSON S2000/S3000 ultrasound system (Siemens, Mountain View, CA), a measurement in a small region of interest (ROI) can be obtained (Virtual Touch tissue quantification [VTq]) as well as a pixel by pixel evaluation (shear wave imaging) of a larger FOV using a color map (Virtual Touch IQ [VTIQ]). In VTIQ, after the initial push pulse, tracking signal vectors are used to detect the tissue displacement as the shear wave passes and thus reconstruct its velocity in a region of interest, which can be displayed as a qualitative image of elasticity or a quantitative image displayed as shear wave speed. A single image is obtained, and a few seconds are required before imaging can be resumed. This use of tracking vectors with focused transmit results in less noisy and more stable shear wave signal detection.

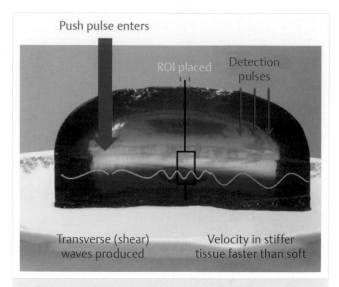

Fig. 2.7 A simplified model of shear wave imaging using our almond in gelatin example is presented in this figure. The acoustic radiation force impulse (ARFI) (push) pulse (wide red arrow) is applied generating shear waves (green waves). The shear waves travel through the tissues and change speed depending on the stiffness of the tissue. Conventional B-mode pulses are used to identify the shear waves and calculate their speed.

Table 2.1 Conversion of shear wave velocity to the Young modulus (kPa)

| kPa | m/s |
| --- | --- |
| 180 | 7.7 |
| 150 | 7.1 |
| 125 | 6.5 |
| 100 | 5.8 |
| 90 | 5.5 |
| 80 | 5.2 |
| 70 | 4.8 |
| 60 | 4.5 |
| 50 | 4.1 |
| 40 | 3.7 |
| 30 | 3.2 |
| 25 | 2.9 |
| 20 | 2.6 |
| 15 | 2.2 |
| 10 | 1.8 |

In the Aixplorer (SuperSonic Imagine [SSI], Aux en Provence, France), the effect of the push pulses is amplified by sending a series of pulses successively focused at increasing depths faster than the shear wave's velocity, so that a mach cone front is generated. A high imaging frame rate is achieved by transmitting a plane wave that insonates the entire field of view in a single burst. The result is that the shear wave velocity can be

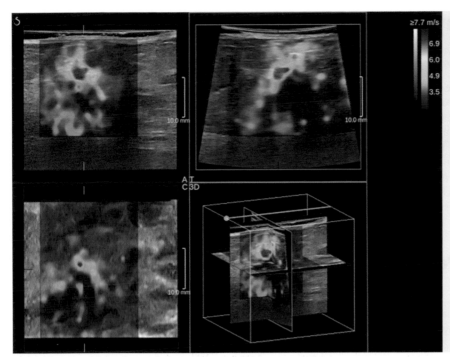

**Fig. 2.8** Shear wave imaging can be performed using a three-dimensional (3D) probe allowing evaluation of an entire lesion with one data collection. In this example of an invasive ductal cancer the image in the upper right is the shear wave elastogram from the imaging plane. The image in the upper left is the image perpendicular to the acquisition plane, whereas the lower left image is the C plane (coronal image). The bottom right image is the 3D depiction. In this case the pixels with high shear wave velocity (suggestive of a malignancy) are color coded red.

measured and displayed (in m/s or kPa) as a quantitative color overlay image at a frame rate of around one frame per second. However, to obtain accurate measurements the several frames need to be obtained in a stationary position.

The principles of scanning using SE also pertain to SWE. Precompression can change results, and it is recommended the same technique to limit precompression already discussed be used to acquire shear wave images.

### 2.3.1 How Can Precompression Affect Shear Wave Elastography Images?

As one applies precompression, Vs in the tissue increases, regardless if the tissue is "soft" or "hard" (► Fig. 2.5). In general, for tissues present in breast, the rate of change in Vs with increasing precompression is greater with soft tissues and less with hard tissues. Thus the velocity of the shear wave (Vs) or the Young modulus (kPa) increases in all tissue types as the amount of precompression is applied. At 10% precompression the shear wave velocity of most "soft" tissues approximately doubles. With amounts of precompression in Zones A and B benign lesion Vs will remain within the range suggestive of benign lesions. However, in Zones C and D a benign lesion may have Vs suggestive of a malignant lesion. This is discussed in more detail in Chapter 4.

On some systems SWE can be performed in real time; however, optimal images are obtained by remaining in the same plane for several seconds to make accurate measurements. Shear wave propagation by an ARFI pulse is depth limited. If a shear wave is not generated a value will not be obtained in the point quantification method (represented by x.xx), and there is no color coding of the area in the shear wave imaging method. Repositioning the patient to make the lesion closer to the skin surface can help in these cases. A 3D probe is now available that allows for volumetric SWE elastograms (► Fig. 2.8).

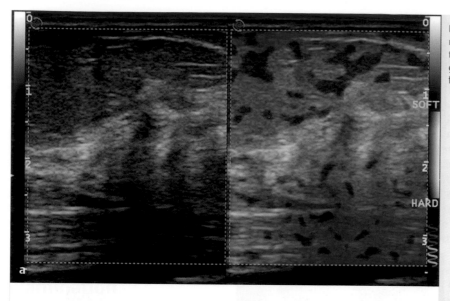

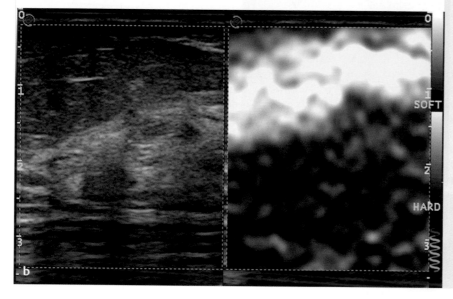

Fig. 3.3 The strain elastography appearance of normal glandular tissue and fat is presented using the color scale with blue as stiff (a) and with the gray scale map (b). Note that the image contains fat, glandular tissue, and the pectoralis muscle.

compression, minimal compression or vibration, and moderate compression. The amount of compression may vary with the size of the breast or the depth of the lesion. With experience and practice one can learn the optimal compression/release needed for an optimal quality elastogram for a given system.[18] The B-mode image is useful to access the amount of tissue displacement. ▶ Table 3.1 lists the various available systems and the techniques they require.

## No Manual Compression Systems

Place the probe vertically on the skin without consciously applying any vibration/compression (▶ Fig. 3.2). Keep the probe lightly touching the skin and try not to apply pressure. It is important to keep the transducer perpendicular with no pressure (minimal precompression) and without movement on the skin above a target. A technique to consistently apply minimal precompression has been described[19] and is discussed in detail in Chapter 3.2.3.

This method gets the compression/decompression cycle from vibration caused by involuntary muscle contraction in the hand and vibration caused by muscle contraction, breathing, and heartbeat of the patient. There is minimal tissue movement, so extremely fine image display is possible. However, in some cases with large breasts or deep lesions minimal compression/release movement with the transducer or transducer vibration may be required to obtain the optimal elastogram. In patients with small breasts the motion may still be too great and having the patient hold her breath may be helpful in obtaining optimal elastograms.

## Minimal Compression/Vibration Systems

Place the probe vertically on the skin and apply very mild vibration (compression/release cycle). Ensure that you *do not push too hard*. The compression/release stroke should be no more than 1 mm. Keep the probe lightly touching the skin, and apply extremely fine vibration with a fast cycle, as if lifting up the

**Table 3.1** List of the available elastography systems for the various techniques

| Technique | Product name | Vendor |
| --- | --- | --- |
| No manual compression | eSie Touch | Siemens (Mountain View, CA) |
| | Elastography | Philips (Bothell, WA) |
| Minimal compression | ElaXto | Esaote (Indianapolis, IN) |
| | Real-time tissue elastography (RTE) | Hitachi Aloka (Wallingford, CT) |
| | Elastography | Toshiba (Minato, Tokyo, Japan) |
| Moderate compression | Elastography | GE (Fairfield, CT) |
| | Real-time tissue elastography (RTE) | Hitachi Aloka (Wallingford, CT) |
| | Elastography | Zonare/Mindray (Shenzhen, China) |

skin with the probe. This method can be used for relatively shallow lesions to moderately deep lesions, and it allows elastography imaging of fine targets several millimeters in size such as nonmass abnormalities. It is also possible to depict in detail the distribution of soft areas (areas with significant strain), and it provides a great deal of diagnostic information.[23] The frequency and degree of displacement of the compression/release cycle can be varied to identify the optimal technique. For learning the technique it is recommended that the scanner vary the degree of compression/release cycle as well as the frequency of the compression/release cycle and observe the changes in the elastogram. With the appropriate technique there should be minimal changes in the appearance of the elastogram.

## Moderate Displacement Systems

Place the probe vertically on the skin, and apply fairly moderate compression/release (about 1–2 mm) similar to the minimal displacement technique except for applying more probe displacement. This method was recommended on older systems, but some newer systems now require much less motion. On the systems that require no displacement, the use of this moderate displacement technique will generate an elastogram composed of noise. This technique requires more skill to avoid precompression and thereby maintain scanning in the same location of the lesion (out-of-plane movement of the lesion).

## 3.2.2 Degree of Displacement Measuring Tools

Some devices have a display bar or number to confirm that you are applying the appropriate amount of displacement (compression/release cycle) to generate the elastogram (▶ Fig. 3.4). When the appropriate amount of displacement is being applied, the number display or the color bar has the maximum value. If the displacement is either too great or too small the number display or color bar shows a lower value. When learning how to perform SE with the manual displacement method, it is helpful to practice varying the amount of displacement and frequency of displacement while watching the display bar or number. You can identify the appropriate technique required by experimenting with your displacement technique and using the color bar or number to identify the optimal technique for your system.

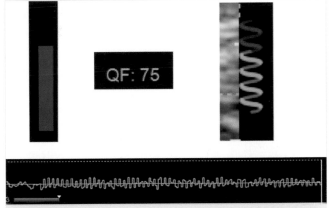

**Fig. 3.4** Various numerical or visual scales are used to optimize the amount of the compression/release cycle. Several of them are presented in this image. When the appropriate amount of compression/release is applied the scales are maximized. If the compression/release cycle is either too great or too small the scale will be minimized.

When the appropriate technique is used the elastogram should be similar on all frames. Some systems provide a visual scale on the frequency and amount of displacement you are generating. This real-time feedback bar or number only evaluates the amount of lesion displacement (tissue deformation). Other factors are important in obtaining optimal images so a high quality factor does not guarantee you will have optimal images.

## 3.2.3 Precompression

A critical factor in generating a diagnostic elastogram is the amount of pressure you apply when scanning. This is called precompression (▶ Fig. 3.5). This is different than the amount of displacement (compression/release) you are applying. If you scan with a "heavy hand" you compress the tissues and change their elastic properties. For example, if you have a balloon filled with air and lightly touch the balloon you create a moderate displacement of the balloon. However, if you compress the balloon between two heavy books and use the same amount of pressure you will create a much smaller displacement because the compression caused by the books increases the air pressure

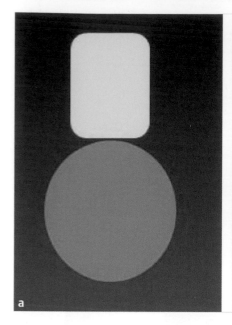 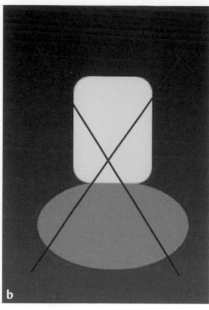

**Fig. 3.5** Precompression should not be applied to the breast when obtaining an elastogram. (a) Minimal precompression applied to the breast. (b) Precompression applied to the breast. Note the dimpling of the breast caused by the pressure of the transducer.

in the balloon. This precompression markedly changes the image quality and can significantly affect results (see ▶ Fig. 2.4). This is confirmed with shear wave technology where the shear wave velocity can change by a factor of 10 based on precompression (▶ Fig. 3.6). In ▶ Fig. 2.5 graphs the effects of precompression for various tissues that occur in the breast. Note that as precompression increases the *differences* in shear wave velocity between tissue types decrease, leading to less conspicuity between tissues. If enough precompression is applied all tissues are similar, and the elastogram changes are mostly noise. Chapter 2 provides a detailed discussion of the effects of precompression on both SE and SWE.

The following technique has been suggested to apply only a minimal amount of precompression reproducibly.[19] In general some amount of precompression is applied to obtain the B-mode image because it improves B-mode image quality (▶ Fig. 3.7). When obtaining the elastogram focus on an object in the FOV (e.g., a rib). Lift the transducer, watching the object in B-mode. As the transducer is lifted (decreasing the precompression) the object moves deeper in the image. When the object is as deep in the image as possible and adequate probe contact is maintained, the elastogram is obtained. This technique has been shown to be highly reproducible both intraoperator and interoperator.[19] This is a similar technique used for color Doppler imaging because precompression can occlude blood vessels. The use of a large amount of coupling gel is helpful. The "quality factor" or "compression bar" used in some manufacturers' equipment *does not* assess the amount of precompression being applied.

Better-quality elastograms can be obtained if the patient raises the ipsilateral hand above the head, the patient is positioned so the transducer is perpendicular to the floor (▶ Fig. 3.2), lesion motion with respiration moves the lesion within the imaging plane, and the patient refrains from talking during data acquisition.

The center of the lesion does not have to be used to obtain the elastogram. In fact it is better if a lesion position is chosen where the lesion measures between 1 and 1.5 cm. This allows

for other tissues to be included in the FOV and accounts for size changes that occur in cancers in elastography. A malignant lesion may appear more than three times the size of the B-mode image. Therefore, if you have a 2 cm malignancy on B-mode it may appear as 6 cm on the elastogram, filling the entire FOV, and may not be appreciated. The size changes are discussed in detail in the interpretation section of this chapter.

Results can be displayed in gray scale or with various color displays; preference is often determined by the user's exposure to elastography and preference in interpretation. If a color map is used care must be taken because a standard has not been established, and a color map using red as stiff or the opposite color map with blue as stiff can be used. The color scale should always be included on the image for accurate interpretation. It is important to remember that in SE a *relative* scale is displayed and should not be confused with SWE where an absolute stiffness value is obtained and color coded on a per pixel basis. In SWE, all vendors use the standard of red as stiff and blue as soft. Remember SE is a relative technique, and a lesion may appear a different shade of gray or color depending on the other tissues in the FOV (see ▶ Fig. 2.2). For example, in a patient with normal glandular breast tissue and fat, the fat will appear soft because it is the softest tissue in the FOV. However, if only fat is in the FOV, some of the fat will appear hard because it is the hardest tissue in the FOV (see ▶ Fig. 2.3). This can cause difficulty in interpretation. By including some fat, normal dense breast tissue, pectoralis muscle, and the lesion in the elastogram FOV, one can minimize these changes between images. This is discussed in detail in Chapter 2. Having a soft tissue (fat) and a harder tissue (muscle) helps maintain a similar gray scale or color display (dynamic range of mapping). A large FOV is helpful in image interpretation because including more tissue will set a scale that allows for better differentiation between tissues.

If an ARFI push pulse is used to generate the tissue displacement (Virtual Touch Imaging [VTI], Siemens Ultrasound, Mountain View, CA), then no manual displacement should be used. The probe should be held steady, and the patient should remain motionless, with no breathing or talking during the acquisition.

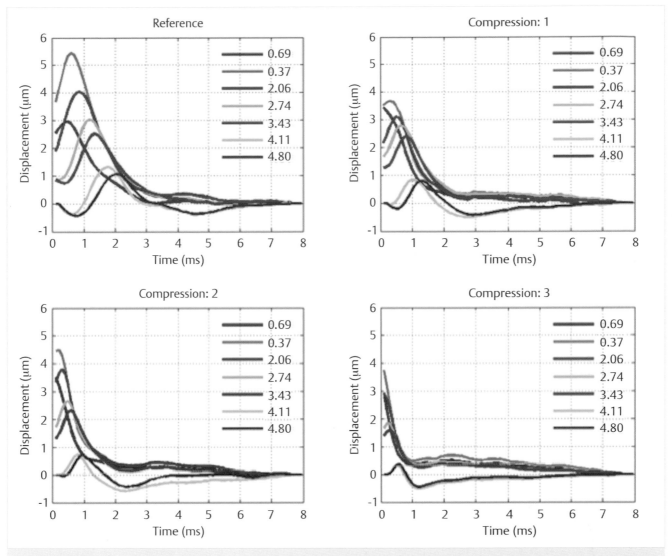

**Fig. 3.6** The effect on shear waves speed with the application of precompression on normal breast tissue is shown in this figure. The graphs display the tissue displacement at various locations from the acoustic radiation force impulse (ARFI) pulse over time. The reference image was obtained with minimal precompression, whereas the other graphs were obtained with increasing amounts of precompression. Note that as precompression is applied the tissue displacement occurs sooner (increased shear wave velocity). (Reprinted with permission from Barr RG, Zhang Z. Effects of precompression on elasticity imaging of the breast: development of a clinically useful semiquantitative method of precompression assessment. J Ultrasound Med 2012;31(6):895–902)

Because of the acoustic power of the ARFI pulse, the system will freeze for a few seconds for transducer cooling. During this period the system will not respond to knob activation. The algorithm used to generate the elastogram is similar to that for SE on the same system. In general the ARFI push pulse is limited in producing displacement deeper than 4 to 5 cm with the breast imaging transducer. If the lesion is deeper a satisfactory elastogram may not be obtained. The image displays are similar to those for SE images with the B-mode image on the left and the VTI elastogram on the right. When using an ARFI pulse to generate a strain image a region of interest (ROI) box is placed at the site of the lesion. The ARFI pulse is generated only within the ROI box, therefore only the ROI box has strain data within it on the elastogram (▶ Fig. 3.8).

### 3.2.4 Tips

- Keep the FOV large to include fat, normal breast tissue, pectoralis muscle if possible, and the lesion. This will maintain a more constant color map (consistent dynamic range of strain values) between images.
- If the lesion is large (> 2 cm) select an image plane not in the maximum diameter of the lesion, where the lesion is between 1 and 1.5 cm, to obtain the elastogram.
- Use the B-mode image to determine the amount of tissue displacement being applied.
- Maintain the transducer perpendicular to the skin and floor.
- Use the appropriate technique for your system.
- Use the B-mode image to confirm that the scan plane through the lesion remains constant.

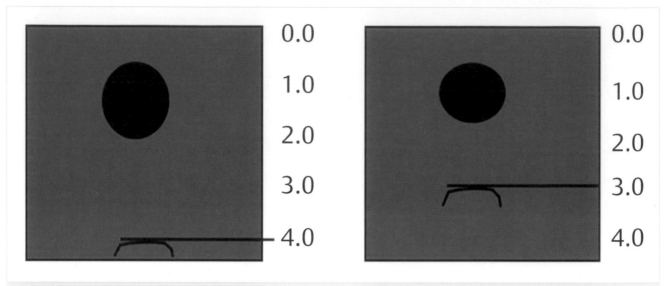

**Fig. 3.7** A technique to confirm that minimal precompression is applied has been proposed. A structure in the far field of the image is identified (i.e., rib or Cooper ligament). As the transducer is lifted the structure will move deeper in the image. When the structure is as deep in the far field as possible and adequate contact with the transducer is maintained minimal precompression is applied and an optimal elastogram will be obtained. In this pictogram the rib with minimal precompression was located at 4 cm depth. If precompression is applied such that the rib is at 3 cm depth this would be considered a 25% precompression. (Reprinted with permission from Barr RG, Zhang Z. Effects of precompression on elasticity imaging of the breast: development of a clinically useful semiquantitative method of precompression assessment. J Ultrasound Med 2012;31(6):895–902)

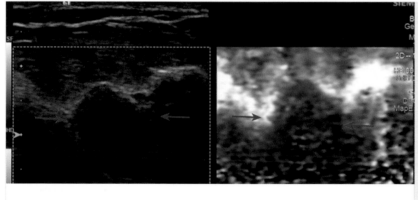

**Fig. 3.8** Example of Virtual Touch Imaging (VTI, Siemens Ultrasound) (strain image using acoustic radiation force impulse [ARFI]). This is an example of an invasive ductal carcinoma (arrows). As opposed to strain elastography (SE) using the manual compression technique the field of view (FOV) has a maximum allowable size. The FOV is placed to include the lesion. A very light touch is used with the transducer on the breast. The patient is asked to remain still and not to talk, and the update button is pressed to activate the ARFI pulse. The system will freeze for a few seconds, and the VTI image will be displayed. The gray scale map is used here with black as stiff and white as soft. The lesion is significantly stiffer than the surrounding breast tissue.

- Position the patient so the displacement motion is in the plane of the transducer.
- Do not apply precompression with the transducer.
- Compare the lesion stiffness to other tissues (fat, normal breast tissue).
- Have the patient hold still and maintain uniform shallow breathing with no talking during data acquisition.
- Turn off background B-mode on the elastography image if a gray scale map is used for the elastogram.
- Remain in a stationary plane when acquiring data (do not survey).

## 3.3 Interpretation/Clinical Results

Three methods of interpreting strain images have been proposed, evaluating the size change between the B-mode image and the elastogram (E/B-mode ratio), a 5-point color scale (Tsukuba score, elasticity score), and the ratio of the lesion stiffness to fat (strain ratio, lesion to fat ratio [LFR]). The relative stiffness (i.e., whether the lesion is stiff or soft compared with other breast tissues) can also be helpful clinically in interpreting images.

### 3.3.1 Elastography Length: B-Mode Length (E/B Ratio)

Using a real-time dual strain elastography system, Hall et al[10] demonstrated that there was potential to use this technique to characterize breast lesions as benign or malignant. It was noted on SE that benign lesions measure smaller in size than the corresponding B-mode image, whereas malignant lesions measured larger (▶ Fig. 3.9 and ▶ Fig. 3.10). They proposed using the ratio of the lesion size on elastography to the B-mode size (E/B ratio) as a diagnostic criterion for benign or malignant. They used an E/B ratio of > 1.2 for a lesion to be malignant based on

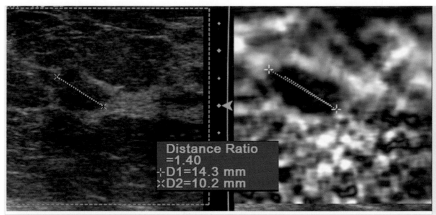

Fig. 3.9 Strain elastogram of an invasive ductal carcinoma. The image on the left of the dual display is the conventional B-mode image. The image on the right is the elastogram. A black and white color scale is used, with black corresponding to the stiffest tissue. In this example the lesion measures 10.2 mm on the B-mode image and measures 14.3 mm on the elastogram, resulting in an E/B ratio of 1.4, suggestive of a malignancy. A copy or shadow function is used to "duplicate" the measurement on the B-mode image onto the same location on the elastogram (yellow lines). This function is helpful to confirm the location of a lesion in the elastogram or vice versa.

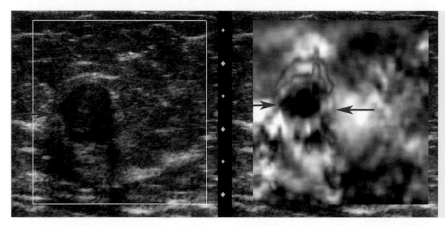

Fig. 3.10 Strain elastogram of a biopsy-proven benign fibroadenoma (red arrows). The lesion is well circumscribed with lobulations and taller than wider in the B-mode image, classifying the lesion as a Breast Imaging–Reporting and Data System 4B (BI-RADS 4B) lesion. The lesion is significantly smaller on the elastogram, suggestive of a benign lesion.

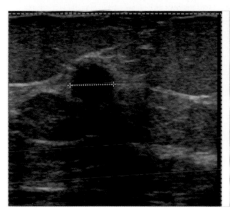
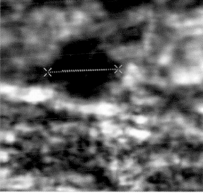

Fig. 3.11 The use of a "copy" or "shadow" function can help in confirming the location of a lesion noted on one image but not well seen on the other. This function allows one to measure a lesion and have the measurement placed in the identical position in the other image. In this example the yellow measurement was done on the B-mode image. The yellow line was copied to the elastogram, and a separate measurement of the lesion was performed to obtain the E/B ratio (green line).

the Receiver Operating Characteristics (ROC) curve of a small data set. With these criteria they found a sensitivity of 100% and a specificity of 75.4%. Barr[24] in a single-center unblinded trial of 123 biopsy-proven cases using an E/B ratio of < 1 as benign and ≥ 1 as malignant had a sensitivity of 100% and a specificity of 95% in distinguishing benign from malignant breast lesions. A large multicenter, unblinded trial evaluating 635 biopsy-proven cases using Barr's criteria had a sensitivity of 99% and a specificity of 87% in characterizing breast lesions as benign or malignant.[25] In a single-center trial of 230 lesions a 99% sensitivity, 91.5% specificity, Positive Predictive Value (PPV) of 90%, and a Negative Predictive Value (NPV) of 99.2% using the E/B ratio.[26]

The location of the elastogram within the lesion does not affect results.[18] Either the lesion length ratio or a lesion area ratio can be used. Measuring the length measurements is usually easier and faster to perform and can limit the time of the examination. The lesion is measured in the same position on both the elastogram and the B-mode image. The use of a copy, shadow, or mirror function in the measurement technique is helpful. These software keys allow one to measure the lesion on either the B-mode image or the elastogram image in a dual mode display and have the length measurement depicted on the opposite image in the exact same position (▶ Fig. 3.11). This allows one to determine if the ratio is greater or less than 1 visually. One can then correct the copied or mirrored image

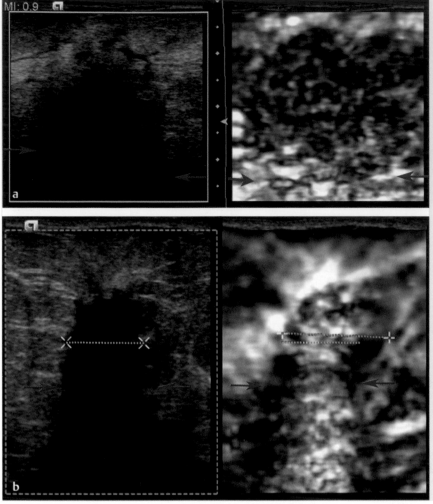

**Fig. 3.12** The B-mode image of this invasive ductal carcinoma (IDC) has shadowing, which prohibits identification of the posterior border of the lesion. The strain elastogram clearly identifies the posterior border of the lesion (a). If the shadowing is marked the elastogram will demonstrate a white/black artifact pattern in the area of the shadowing, and the posterior border of the lesion will not be identified (b). The yellow line measures the lesion on B-mode while the green line measures the lesion on SE. The E/B ratio in this case is > 1, consistent wit this malignancy.

measurement to obtain the ratio. This method of interpretation requires that the lesion be visualized well enough to get an accurate measurement on both the B-mode image and the elastogram image. Because cases of ductal carcinoma in situ (DCIS) and invasive lobular carcinoma are often poorly visualized on B-mode imaging, this technique should not be used unless they are defined masses that can be measured with true distinguishable borders. Difficulty can occur when measuring the lesion size on the elastogram when a fibroadenoma or fibrocystic lesion is present in dense breast tissue. The strain properties of the fibrocystic change or fibroadenoma are similar to the background dense breast tissue. Therefore, one may visualize the combination of the lesion and normal dense breast tissue as one lesion, creating a false-positive.[18] This problem can be avoided by comparing the stiffness of the lesion to surrounding tissue; if it is similar to fibroglandular tissue it is most likely benign (to be discussed in detail).

Using the color scale or lesion to fat ratio methods (discussion follows) may help eliminate this problem. In the multicenter trial[25] this accounted for a large number of the false-positives decreasing the specificity. Strain images obtained using the ARFI technique can be interpreted using this technique.

Shadowing, which can be seen with some cancers on B-mode, is not seen on the accompanying elastogram. Therefore, the inferior border of the cancer can often be identified on the

elastogram.[18] As long as there is some B-mode signal identified in the shadowing, the algorithm will be able to determine the strain in those pixels. However, if the shadowing is extreme and no returning signal is identified there is no correlation identified, and the pixels will be coded as white or blocks of alternating white and black (► Fig. 3.12).[27]

In addition to using the E/B ratio to determine if a lesion is more likely benign or malignant, asking if the lesion is soft or hard or visible on SE is clinically helpful in some situations. It is sometimes difficult to determine if a lobular hypoechoic lesion is a fat lobule on conventional ultrasound. If the lesion is a fat lobule it will appear very soft on the elastogram and similar to the other fat in the image (► Fig. 3.13). Lesions can be isoechoic to background tissue on B-mode imaging and not recognized as a lesion. These lesions may have different strain properties compared with the background and can be clearly visualized on SE. This is very common with complicated cysts (► Fig. 3.14). Evaluation of the EI pattern can also define where to best biopsy a lesion (► Fig. 3.15), selecting the hardest location to target the biopsy. The SE pattern can help characterize a complex lesion (► Fig. 3.16).

Previous studies have demonstrated that the sensitivity of this technique is quite high (> 98%).[24–26] ► Fig. 3.17 is a box plot of the results. In a large, multicenter trial there were 3 cancers out of 222 that had a ratio of less than 1. In retrospect, one

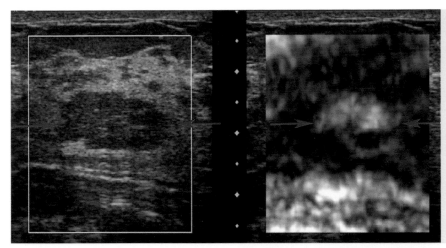

**Fig. 3.13** It is often difficult to determine if an isoechoic lesion surrounded by dense breast tissue is a fat lobule or an isoechoic mass. Elastography can be used to determine if the lesion is a fat lobule. As demonstrated in this case of a fat lobule in dense breast tissue the fat lobule is white (arrows), confirming it is softer than fibroglandular tissue and is a fat lobule. (Reprinted with permission from Barr RG. Sonographic breast elastography: a primer. J Ultrasound Med 2012;31(5):773–783)

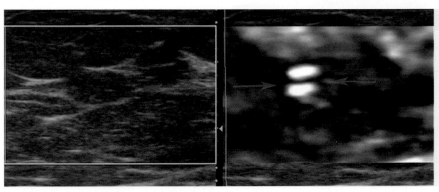

**Fig. 3.14** Elastography can be used when a palpable mass is present but is not identified on B-mode imaging. In this example, a palpable mass in a 42-year-old was not identified on mammography or B-mode ultrasound (left image). By placing the probe over the palpable abnormality and activating strain elastography a bull's-eye artifact (red arrows on elastogram, right image) is obtained, confirming the oval lesion centrally in the B-mode image (red arrows B-mode) is an isoechoic, complicated cyst.

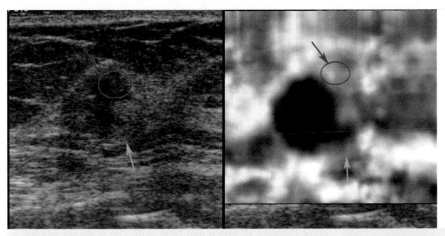

**Fig. 3.15** Elastography can be helpful in determining the best location to perform a biopsy. In this example a mass lesion is identified on B-mode imaging that has a "head" (red circle), a body, and a tail (green arrow). On the elastogram the body and tail of the lesion increase in size and are very stiff. The head of the lesion is soft and blends into the background breast tissue. On biopsy the body and tail of the lesion were invasive ductal carcinoma, whereas the head was a benign fibroadenoma. Careful evaluation of the elastogram should be undertaken because it is not uncommon for two adjacent lesions to appear as one on the B-mode image but be clearly distinguishable on elastography. The reverse can also be true. It is common for fibrocystic change or a fibroadenoma to be similar in stiffness to surrounding fibroglandular tissue and not be identified on the elastogram but be clearly different on the B-mode image. (Reprinted with permission from Barr RG. Sonographic breast elastography: a primer. J Ultrasound Med 2012;31 (5):773–783)

lesion was measured incorrectly on B-mode. The second "lesion" may have been two adjacent lesions, one benign and one malignant, confounding the measurements. The third increased in size in anterior to posterior dimension but got smaller in width. Because cases of DCIS and invasive lobular carcinoma are often poorly visualized on B-mode, imaging with this technique

should not be used in them unless they are defined masses that can be measured accurately. Another difficulty that occurs is measuring the lesion size on the elastogram when a fibroadenoma or fibrocystic lesion is present in dense breast tissue. The strain properties of the fibrocystic change or fibroadenoma are similar to the background dense breast tissue. Therefore one

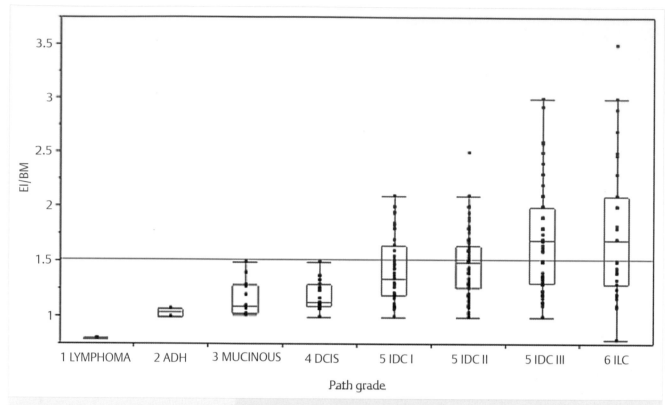

**Fig. 3.20** The E/B ratio has been reported related to tumor grade, with more aggressive tumors having a higher E/B ratio. This figure is a box whisker plot of the E/B ratio for various types of tumors. Note that as the tumor grade increases the E/B ratio also tends to increase, although there is a wide range of variability. (Used with permission from Grajo JRB, Barr RG. Strain elastography in the prediction of breast cancer tumor grade. J Ultrasound Med 2014;33(1):129–134)

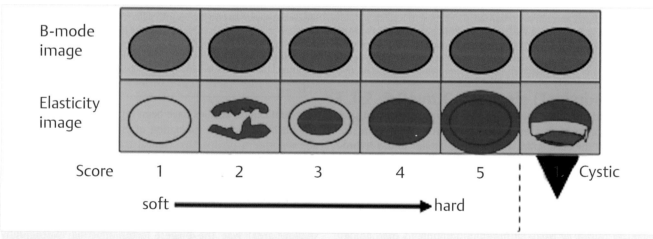

**Fig. 3.21** A 5-point color scale has been proposed as a method of characterizing breast masses as benign or malignant. In this example of the scale stiff lesions are coded blue, and soft lesions are coded green and red. If a lesion is entirely soft it is given a score of 1. If the lesion has both soft and stiff components it is given a score of 2. If the lesion is stiff but smaller than the lesion on B-mode imaging it is scored as 3. If the lesion is stiff and the same size as on the B-mode image it is given a score of 4, and if it is stiff and larger than on the B-mode image it is given a score of 5. A score of 1, 2, or 3 is suggestive of a benign lesion, whereas a score of 4 or 5 is suggestive of a malignant lesion. (Used with permission from Ueno EIA. Diagnosis of breast cancer by elasticity imaging. Eizo Joho Medical 2004;36:2–6)

### 3.3.3 Strain Ratio (Lesion to Fat Ratio)

In an attempt to semiquantify the measurements, the ratio of lesion stiffness to fat has been suggested. This technique has been called the lesion to fat ratio, strain ratio, or LFR. This ratio was based on the knowledge that the properties of fat are fairly constant, whereas the properties of other surrounding tissues and lesions are variable. This diagnostic approach was advocated by Ueno et al[42] as a semiquantitative method of evaluating stiffness. It is the ratio of the strain in a mass to the strain in

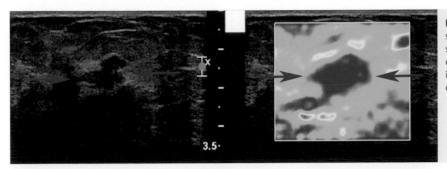

Fig. 3.22 An example of a breast mass with a score of 5 on the 5-point color scale. The lesion is stiff (blue, arrows) and appears larger on the elastogram than on the corresponding B-mode image. The lesion was a grade 1 invasive ductal cancer on surgical pathology.

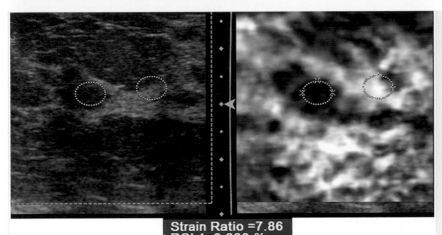

Strain Ratio =7.86
ROI 1=0.330 %
ROI 2=0.042 %

Fig. 3.23 Although strain imaging is qualitative, an estimate of the stiffness (semiquantitative) can be determined by comparing the relative stiffness of the lesion to fat, the strain ratio. Fat has a relatively constant stiffness between patients. In this technique a region of interest (ROI) is placed within the lesion (left circle in each image) and an ROI is placed in fat (right circle in each image). The system can then compare the relative stiffness of the two ROIs and calculate a strain ratio. In this example the strain ratio is 7.9. A ratio of greater than 4.5 is suggestive of a malignancy. On biopsy this lesion was an invasive ductal carcinoma. (Used with permission from Ueno EUT, Bando H, Tohno E, Waki K, Matsumura T. New quantitative method in breast elastography: lesion to fat ratio (LFR). Paper presented at: Radiological Society of North America 93rd Scientific Assembly and Annual Meeting; November 25–30, 2007; Chicago, IL)

subcutaneous fat, and it can be thought of as a semiquantitative method for numerically evaluating how many times stiffer a target mass is compared with subcutaneous fat. The target ROI for the tumor should not protrude from the interior of the tumor in B-mode. The target ROI for subcutaneous fat should be a circle of sufficient size and be limited to skin and fat that does not contain breast tissue. The ROIs should be taken at the same depth if possible to limit errors from compression, especially if using the moderate displacement technique. When applying the compression/release cycle tissues at different depths experience different amounts of compression that change the stiffness of the tissue. Care should be taken not to use the very soft signal sometimes seen adjacent to lesions because this is an artifact (see Artifacts later in chapter) and will artificially elevate the lesion to fat ratio (strain ratio).

Because it is possible to evaluate the stiffness of one specific part of a mass by setting the target ROI, not only is it possible to measure very large tumors, it is also possible to evaluate the stiffness of nonmass abnormalities. This stiffness of a tumor is an approximation. It is easy to perform, and the results of clinical studies using this diagnostic approach have already been reported.

Initial studies[42–44] have found this technique valuable in determining if a lesion was benign or malignant (▶ Fig. 3.23). Care must be taken with these measurements because precompression can significantly change the strain value of fat.[19] As precompression is applied the stiffness of all tissues increases.

However, the stiffness of fat changes more than that of normal breast tissue and lesions. Therefore with precompression the ratio of lesion to fat will decrease. Care must also be taken that the FOV for the fat measurement contains only fat. The measurement should be taken at the same depth in the image as the degree of tissue compression varies with depth. This ratio is based on the knowledge that the properties of fat are fairly constant, whereas the properties of other surrounding tissues and lesions are variable. Lesions with densities similar to fat therefore have smaller ratios.

In addition to performing a single measurement comparing the lesion strain to fat strain ratio, one vendor offers parametric imaging. In this technique an ROI is placed in an area of fat, and the entire FOV is color-coded based on the ratio of each pixel stiffness to the stiffness of fat (▶ Fig. 3.24). A color-coded semiquantitative image is obtained over a large FOV. The area with the highest lesion to fat ratio can then be identified visually and a point measurement obtained.

Thomas et al[43] compared B-mode BI-RADS category score, the 5-point color scale, and the lesion to fat ratio in 227 breast lesions. Based on the ROC curve they selected a cutoff of 2.455 to distinguish benign from malignant lesions using the lesion to fat ratio (strain ratio, LFR). The mean ratio for malignant lesions was 5.1 +/- 4.2 while for benign 1.6 +/- 1 ($p < 0.001$). They found a sensitivity and specificity of 96% and 56% for B-mode imaging, 81% and 89% for the 5-point color scale, and 90% and 89% for the lesion to fat ratio.

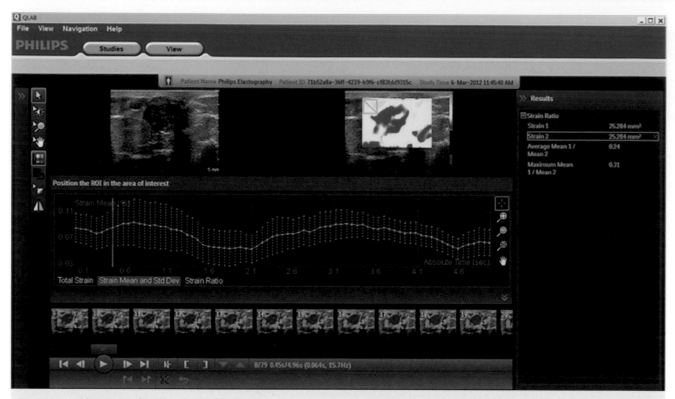

**Fig. 3.24** In addition to performing a single measurement of the ratio of the lesion stiffness to fat stiffness (strain ratio or lesion to fat ratio), parametric imaging can be performed. A region of interest (ROI) is placed to demarcate fat, and the entire image is color coded to the strain ratio. In this example the green box is the ROI placed on fat for the reference. The image is then color coded, with red being higher strain ratios.

Zhi et al[45] in a similar study compared the strain ratio and the 5-point color scale in 559 breast lesions. They found the strain ratio of benign lesions was 1.83 +/- 1.22, whereas malignant lesions were 8.38 +/- 7.65. These were significantly different ($p$ < 0.00001). Based on their ROC curves they selected a cutoff point of 3.05. The area under the curve for the 5-point color system was 0.885, whereas that of the strain ratio was 0.944 ($P$ < 0.05). In a different study of 408 lesions[42] a lesion to fat strain ratio with a cutoff of 4.8 found a sensitivity of 76.6% and a specificity of 76.8%.

Farrokh et al[44] reported sensitivity of 94.4% and specificity of 87.3% with a cutoff above 2.9 in a prospective study using strain ratio (LFR). Alhabshi et al[46] reported that width ratio and strain ratio were the most useful methods of lesion characterization, with a cutoff value of 1.1 for width ratio and a cutoff value of 5.6 for strain ratio, in a study using B-mode, strain pattern (elasticity score), width ratio, and strain ratio. Using an iU22 xMATRIX ultrasound system (Philips Healthcare, Bothell WA), Stachs et al[47] demonstrated the LFR utility in 224 breast masses in 215, reporting that the strain ratio was predominantly higher in malignant tumors (i.e., 3.04 ± 0.9 (mean ± standard deviation [SD]) for malignant tumors versus 1.91 ± 0.75 for benign tumors.

The appropriate cutoff for this technique varies greatly between studies. Using quantitative ARFI we have been able to change the speed of sound through fatty tissue by a factor of 10 with precompression.[19] As precompression is applied the stiffness of all tissues increases. However, the stiffness of fat changes more than that of normal breast tissue and lesions; therefore, with precompression the ratio of lesion to fat will decrease. Care must also be taken that the FOV for the fat measurement contain only fat. The measurements should be taken at the same depth in the image as the degree of compression varies with depth. These factors were not controlled in the studies and may account for the variability of the results. When using this technique the appropriate cutoff should be determined in your lab with your technique and equipment.

### 3.3.4 Lesion Relative Stiffness (Is the Lesion Hard or Soft?)

In addition to using the interpretation methods previously discussed to determine if a lesion is benign or malignant, the information as to whether the lesion is soft or hard or visible on EI is helpful in some clinical situations.

It is sometimes difficult to determine if a lobular hypoechoic lesion is a fat lobule on conventional ultrasound. If the lesion is a fat lobule it will appear very soft on the elastogram and similar to the other fat in the image (▶ Fig. 3.13). If a lesion is difficult to accurately measure to utilize the E/B ratio comparing the elasticity of the lesion to dense breast tissue can be helpful. If the elasticity is similar to dense breast tissue it is probably benign, whereas if it is stiffer than dense breast tissue it is most likely malignant.

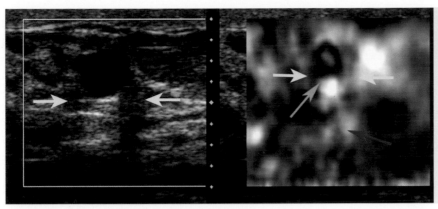

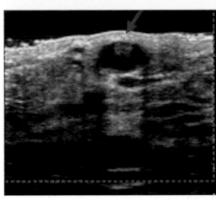

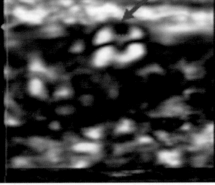

Fig. 3.25 On some systems an artifact is identified with benign simple and complicated cysts. This bull's-eye artifact is characterized with the lesion black (yellow arrows) with a bright central spot (green arrow) and a bright spot behind the cyst (red arrow). This artifact has been shown to have a very high sensitivity and specificity for characterization of benign cystic lesions. (Used with permission from Barr RG, Lackey AE. The utility of the "bull's-eye" artifact on breast elasticity imaging in reducing breast lesion biopsy rate. Ultrasound Q 2011;27(3):151–155)

Fig. 3.26 If a cystic lesion has a solid component (i.e., a complex cystic mass) the solid component will appear as a stiff defect in the bull's-eye pattern. In this example of a benign papillary lesion the solid component (red arrow) appears as a stiff defect in the bull's-eye pattern. (Courtesy of Carmel Smith, Brisbane, Australia)

## 3.3.5 Limitations

Accuracy can differ between shallow sites and deep sites due to problems associated with variable displacement at different depths. Further improvement of applications and adjustments to imaging methods are needed to overcome these problems. It is possible to use all of the three interpretation techniques to increase confidence in lesion characterization. If a lesion cannot be measured accurately or is a nonmass lesion for the E/B ratio to be accurately calculated, the other two techniques can be used to characterize the lesion.

At present, reports related to strain ratio (lesion to fat ratio, LFR) have used significantly different cutoff values. This is due to different techniques and no consistent method of ROI position in calculating the ratio. A prospective multicenter study with well-defined acquisition parameters is needed to determine the appropriate cutoff value.

## 3.4 Artifacts

There are several artifacts that can be encountered with SE. Some occur when technique is suboptimal, whereas some contain diagnostic information.

### 3.4.1 Bull's-Eye Artifact

A unique artifact, called the bull's-eye artifact, is identified within cystic lesions in some systems (▶ Fig. 3.25). This artifact is characterized by a white central signal within a black outer signal and a bright spot posterior to the lesion.[48] This artifact is

caused because the fluid is moving and there is de-correlation between images. This artifact has been described in detail.[48] This artifact has a high predictive value for the lesion being a benign simple or complicated cyst. If there is a solid component in the cyst it will appear as a solid lesion within the pattern (▶ Fig. 3.26). This artifact is not seen in mucinous or colloid cancers due to their high viscosity (▶ Fig. 3.27).

The bull's-eye cyst pattern can be seen with lesions that appear solid and suspicious on B-mode imaging. These lesions have been shown to be complicated cysts.[48] These lesions can be aspirated to confirm that the lesion resolves after aspiration. If core biopsies are performed notifying the pathologist the lesion is a complicated cyst as opposed to a solid mass will lead to better pathology imaging correlation. If the pathologist is told the lesion is solid, the report may not mention that a cyst wall is present, which may suggest that the suspected solid lesion is not in the specimen, leading to stress on the radiologist and the patient. Note that this artifact is seen with Siemens and Philips equipment and may not be seen in other manufacturers' equipment. With other systems cysts may give a layering color pattern blue/ green/ red (BGR artifact to be discussed).

This artifact can be used to decrease the number of biopsies performed.[48] In one series 10% of complicated cysts appeared solid on B-mode and were identified with this technique.[48] If core biopsies are performed, notifying the pathologist the lesion is a complicated cyst as opposed to a solid mass will lead to better pathology/imaging correlation. The pathologist, when told the lesion is solid, may not mention that a cyst wall is present and suggest the suspected solid lesion is not in the specimen, leading to a nonspecific diagnosis.

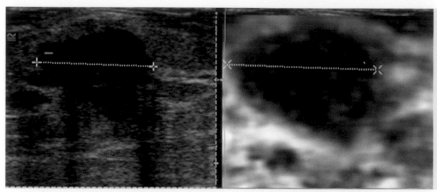

**Fig. 3.27** The bull's-eye artifact occurs because of de-correlation of the fluid components of a cystic lesion. If the material within the lesion is very viscous such as a hematoma or mucin the bull's-eye artifact will not occur. This is an example of a mucinous malignancy that does not demonstrate the bull's-eye pattern (dotted line).

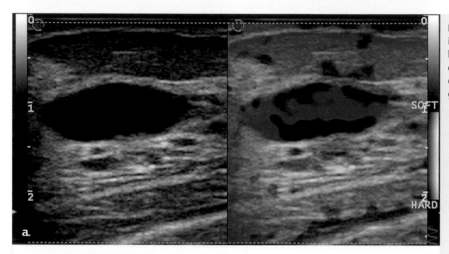

**Fig. 3.28** In some systems the bull's-eye pattern is not observed for cystic lesions, but a blue, breen, red (BGR) pattern is observed. This is an example of this artifact in a simple cyst using the color map of blue to indicate stiff (a) and on a gray scale (b).

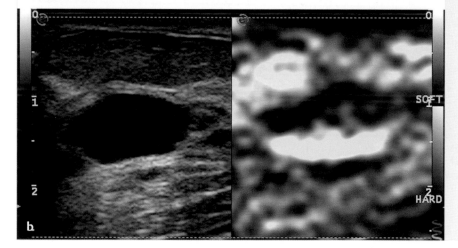

## 3.4.2 Blue/Green/Red (BGR) Artifact

Some systems have a different artifact that occurs in cysts (▶ Fig. 3.28). There is a 3-color-layering pattern of blue, green, red (BGR) identified in cystic lesions.[18,29,30] A detailed study evaluating the sensitivity and specificity of this artifact has not been performed.

## 3.4.3 Sliding Artifact

A white ring or group of wavelike artifacts around a lesion on the elastogram indicates the lesion is moving in and out of the imaging plane while the elastogram is being obtained (▶ Fig. 3.29). This has been named the sliding artifact.[18] Having the lesion remain within the imaging plane during the acquisition can eliminate the artifact. Repositioning the patient, using less compression, or having the patient hold her breath may help keep the lesion in the scanning plane. This artifact suggests the lesion is freely moveable within the adjacent tissues and is most likely benign. This artifact can be seen with fibroadenomas or lipomas. This has been proposed as a method to determine if there is an invasive component to an intraductal malignancy.[49]

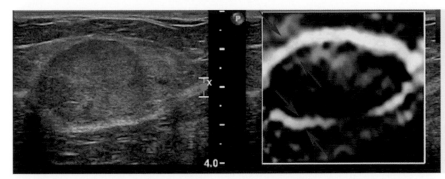

**Fig. 3.29** When a lesion is moving in and out of the plane during the elastogram acquisition a sliding artifact occurs. The artifact is characterized by a white ring or series of rings surrounding the lesion on the elastogram. This example of the sliding artifact is a lipoma. The artifact (red arrows) signifies that the lesion is not attached to adjacent tissue and is therefore unlikely to be a malignancy. (Used with permission from Barr RG. Sonographic breast elastography: a primer. J Ultrasound Med 2012;31(5):773–783)

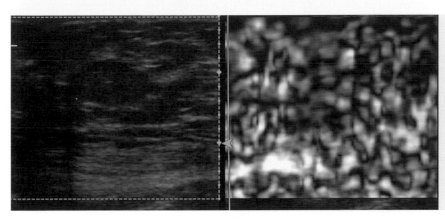

**Fig. 3.30** When there is very little variability of the tissues within the strain elastogram field of view, only noise is obtained. The pattern is one of varying white and black areas within the entire field of view as seen in this example. This artifact can be seen when significant precompression is used.

## 3.4.4 Worm Pattern

If there is very little variability in the elastic properties of the tissues within the FOV or when significant precompression is applied, a pattern of varying signal is noted representing noise (▶ Fig. 3.30). This has been named the worm pattern.[18] There is no clinical information in these images. This artifact can be eliminated by the use of minimal precompression and including various tissues within the FOV.

## 3.4.5 Shadowing Artifact

The returning B-mode signal is used to determine the degree of tissue deformation required to generate the strain elastogram. In cases where there is B-mode shadowing the returning signal is decreased in areas of shadowing. If the shadowing is not severe a strain elastogram is obtained in the area of shadowing (▶ Fig. 3.12a). However, if the shadowing is severe and minimal or no signal is returned an accurate strain value is not obtained, and a pattern of white/black blotches is obtained (▶ Fig. 3.12b). This artifact can also occur in areas of marked refractive shadowing.

# 4 Shear Wave Elastography

## 4.1 Overview

A second technique to determine the elastic properties of a tissue is shear wave velocity measurement.[5,20,21,22,50,51,52,53] In this technique an initial ultrasound pulse (push pulse) applied to the tissue induces a shear wave perpendicular to the ultrasound beam. The velocity of the shear wave generated through the tissues may be calculated using standard B-mode ultrasound sampling techniques (▶ Fig. 4.1). From the velocity of the shear wave through the tissues the strain (Young) modulus can be estimated. The velocity of the shear wave is proportional to the tissue stiffness. The stiffness of a lesion can be displayed as the shear wave velocity (Vs in m/s) or the strain modulus (expressed in kPa).

With shear wave elastography (SWE) a quantitative measure of the lesion stiffness is obtained either in a region of interest (ROI), point quantification SWE (pSWE) or pixel-by-pixel using a color map, 2-D SWE. Examples of a benign and malignant lesion are presented in ▶ Fig. 4.2 and ▶ Fig. 4.3.

Precompression can markedly change values.[19] ▶ Fig. 4.4 and ▶ Fig. 4.5 demonstrate the effect of precompression on both a benign and a malignant lesion. Note that with precompression

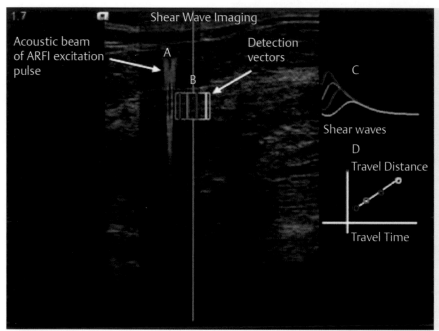

**Fig. 4.1** The shear wave velocity is calculated using B-mode scanning to monitor the shear wave movement through tissue. This diagram depicts the process. (A) The acoustic radiation force impulse (ARFI) that generates the shear wave. (B) The area that is monitored by B-mode imaging to monitor the tissue movement caused by the shear wave. (C) The curves that are identified by plotting the tissue displacement at a given location over time. (D) The slope of the line by plotting the time of the maximum tissue displacement at the different locations from the ARFI pulse is the shear wave velocity.

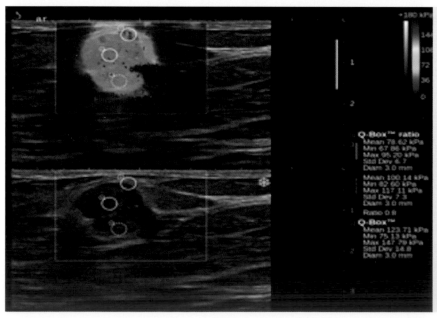

**Fig. 4.2** Shear wave elastography images use a color overlay on the B-mode image to provide the shear wave velocity (Vs) in m/s (or estimated Young modulus in kPa) for each pixel in the field of view. Some systems also provide a B-mode image in a dual display. In this case the elastogram overlaid on B-mode image is the upper image, whereas the B-mode image is the lower image. The white square is the region of interest (ROI) where shear wave imaging was performed. Opposed to strain imaging, the color coding here corresponds to quantitative measurements that can be used to characterize a breast lesion. In this case of an invasive ductal carcinoma the Vs values are elevated in the malignancy to a maximum Vs of 6.3 m/s (118 kPa) and 2.2 m/s (15kPa) suggestive of a malignancy. When an ROI is placed over the area of interest the maximum, minimum, mean, and standard deviation of the pixels in the ROI is displayed.

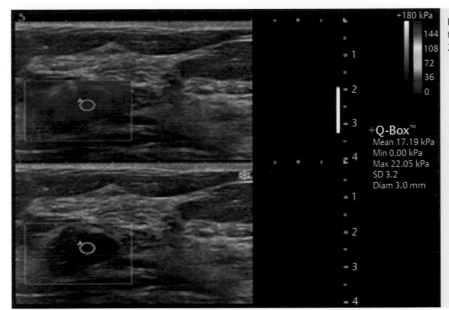

**Fig. 4.3** In this case of a benign fibroadenoma the lesion color codes soft with a maximum Vs of 2.7 m/s (22 kPa) suggestive of a benign lesion.

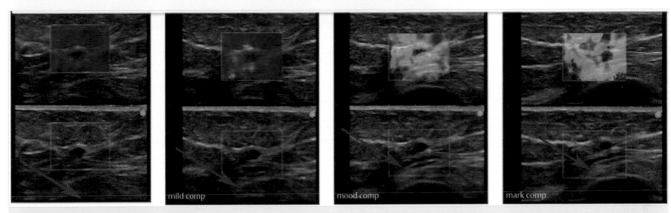

**Fig. 4.4** The effect of increased precompression can significantly change the shear wave elastography (SWE) results. In this figure the SWE of a simple cyst is presented with increasing amounts of precompression. Note that rib (arrow) in the far field is located closer to the transducer as precompression is added. With moderate precompression a benign lesion can have Vs values suggestive of a malignancy. (Reprinted with permission from Barr RG, Zhang Z. Effects of precompression on elasticity imaging of the breast: development of a clinically useful semiquantitative method of precompression assessment. J Ultrasound Med 2012;31(6):895–902)

even a benign lesion can have high Vs suggestive of a malignant lesion. Precompression will also increase the Vs surrounding a malignant lesion. The technique to apply only minimal precompression described in Chapter 3 is recommended to limit this effect.[19]

## 4.2 Technique/How to Perform an Examination

In SWE an initial ultrasound pulse (push pulse, also referred to as the acoustic radiation force impulse [ARFI]) is applied to the tissue that induces a shear waves perpendicular to the ultrasound pulse. Shear waves are similar to dropping a stone in a pond (analogous to a push pulse) and ripples will occur (analo-

gous to shear waves). Using ultrasound B-mode sampling techniques, the velocity of the shear wave generated through the tissues can be calculated. From the velocity of the shear wave in the tissue, the Young modulus can be estimated using some assumptions (see Chapter 2). The velocity of the shear waves is proportional to the stiffness. The stiffness of a lesion can be displayed as the shear wave velocity (Vs) in m/s through the tissue, the shear modulus, or the Young modulus in kilopascals (kPa). Both systems allow you to obtain either measurement or convert from one to the other on the system.

The principles of scanning technique using strain elastography (SE) also pertain to SWE. Maintaining the same location of the lesion with no movement is important to obtain accurate results. After the ARFI pulse is applied data acquisition occurs for a short period of time. During the data acquisition period

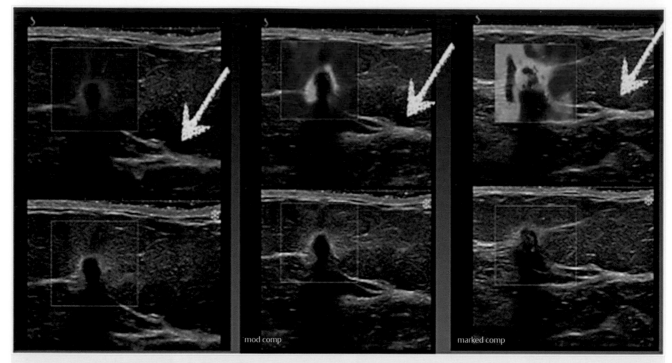

**Fig. 4.5** The same effects of precompression can be seen with a malignant lesion. This figure demonstrates the effect of increasing precompression on an invasive ductal cancer. The arrow points to a ligament. Notice that as precompression is added the ligament is located closer to the transducer. Note that as precompression is added a ring of high Vs is created at the lesion/normal tissue interface. (Reprinted with permission from Barr RG, Zhang Z. Effects of precompression on elasticity imaging of the breast: development of a clinically useful semiquantitative method of precompression assessment. J Ultrasound Med 2012;31(6):895–902)

the movement of the shear wave is monitored by B-mode imaging. If there is tissue movement caused by movement of the transducer or the patient the system will interpret this non–shear wave movement in the calculation of Vs. For more accurate measurements, patients must hold still and hold their breath.

Precompression can change results, and we recommend the same technique discussed in Chapter 3 be used to acquire images using shear wave technology. As previously discussed the shear wave speed of fat in the breast can be changed by a factor of 10 with precompression, therefore it is important not to compress the tissue with the transducer. SWE on one system can be performed in real time; however, to obtain adequate measurements and optimal images one must remain in the same plane for several seconds. Shear wave generation is depth limited, and, depending on tissue density, if a lesion is deeper than 4 to 5 cm a result may not be obtained. It may help to reposition the patient and bring the ROI closer to the transducer. If there is no shear wave generation, no color coding will occur in this area. With SWE a quantitative measure of the lesion stiffness can be obtained either in a small fixed ROI (point quantification) or pixel by pixel in a field of view (FOV) using a color map (shear wave imaging). The results are color coded, usually with a convention of red as hard and blue as soft.

Two shear wave systems are presently available. In the S2000 and S3000 system (Siemens Ultrasound, Mountain View, CA), either a measurement in a small ROI can be obtained (Virtual Touch tissue quantification [VTq]) or a pixel-by-pixel evaluation can be made of a larger FOV using a color map (Virtual Touch IQ [VTIQ]). In VTIQ after the initial push pulse, tracking signal vectors are used to detect the tissue displacement as the shear wave passes and thus reconstruct its velocity in a region of interest, which can be displayed as a quantitative image displayed as shear wave velocity. With this technique a single image is obtained. The tracking vectors with focused transmit results in less noisy and more stable shear wave signal detection. This system obtains one image and the system is frozen for a few seconds do to the power output.

The second shear wave system, the Aixplorer (SuperSonic Imagine [SSI], Aix en Provence, France) uses rapid sequence of ARFI pulses that generates a mach wave and measures the sear wave velocity over a wide FOV. The system operates in real-time, but the probe needs to be held steady over a lesion for several seconds to get an accurate shear wave measurement. The system color codes the pixels within the FOV with the shear wave velocities or kPa. Multiple ROIs can be placed in FOV to measure the shear wave velocities at various locations.

With shear wave imaging the color scale can be changed. Red always codes to the stiff tissues and blue to the soft tissues. However, the stiffness where the color changes occur can be changed. For breast tissues a scale with a maximum of 7.7 m/s (180 kPa) is usually the default. With this scale, lesions coded green, yellow, and red are stiff within the range of malignancies. When evaluating tissue with only benign tissue, decreasing the maximum value of the color scale (e.g. 3.7 m/s [40 kPa]) will allow for greater color differentiation of the stiffness of benign tissues. However, red will no longer code for a stiffness value suggestive of a malignancy.

Three-dimensional (3D) shear wave imaging is available. No studies with the use of 3D SWE have been published. It is unknown if the volumetric data using the 3D technique will provide additional information or allow for breast screening.

### 4.2.1 Tips

- Keep the FOV slightly larger than the lesion to evaluate the surrounding tissue.
- Maintain the transducer perpendicular to the skin.
- Hold the transducer still and ask patients to hold their breath during measurements.
- Do not apply precompression with the transducer.
- When using real-time shear wave imaging allow several seconds for the image to stabilize before taking a measurement.

## 4.3 Interpretation/Clinical Results

### 4.3.1 Shear Wave Imaging

With shear wave imaging the elasticity results are calculated as either the velocity of the shear wave through the tissue (Vs expressed in m/s) or the Young modulus (expressed in kPa). The results are color coded with red as stiff and blue as soft. Tissue measurements in an ROI can be displayed in velocities (m/s) or in pressure/elasticity (kPa). The measurement of stiffness should be obtained from the area of highest stiffness within the lesion or the surrounding tissue. This can be performed by placing a large ROI over the entire lesion or evaluating the color map and placing a small ROI in the area of highest stiffness determined by the color mapping. The latter is preferred. Multiple measurements can be performed in the same image.

Examples of a benign and malignant lesion are presented in ► Fig. 4.2 and ► Fig. 4.3. One system S2000/S3000 (Siemens Ultrasound, Mountain View, CA) provides a color-coded velocity map as well as three other maps—a quality measure map, a time map, and a displacement map. The quality map is discussed later in this chapter. The time map displays the "time to maximum displacement," which is another method of displacing the shear wave velocity data. The displacement map displays the amount of tissue displacement caused by the ARFI pulse. The time and displacement maps are useful for research purposes and are not required to interpret the results in a clinical setting. The velocity and quality maps are used in routine clinical practice to interpret the results.

The other system Aixplorer (SuperSonic Imagine [SSI], Aix en Provence, France) provides both the B-mode image and the velocity map. When placing an ROI on this system the ROI is displayed on both the B-mode image and the elastogram. This system incorporates the quality map onto the velocity map by not color coding areas where an accurate shear wave velocity cannot be calculated.

Measurements of the Vs are obtained by placing an ROI in the area of concern. Most studies have used the Vs maximum (max) as the criterion to determine if a lesion is benign or ma-

lignant. Both SWE systems provide the max, mean, and minimum (min) pixel value within the ROI as well as the standard deviation of the values within the ROI. By visual inspection of the color map the area of maximum Vs is usually easily identified. The ROI can then be placed in this area. The adjacent tissue can also be measured. A measurement of fatty tissue is helpful to confirm that precompression is not applied.

Shear waves will not propagate through simple cysts, and they will not be color coded. The shear wave is detected by B-mode echo signal. Therefore, when areas in the B-mode image show extremely low signal, the echo signal is too low for successful detection of the tissue displacement caused by the shear wave. These areas are not color coded. This will also occur with marked shadowing such as is seen with ribs, tumors with significant shadowing, and areas with macrocalcification.[18]

Chang et al[54] in a study of 158 consecutive patients found the mean elasticity values were significantly higher in malignant masses (153 kPa +/- 58) than in benign masses (46 kPa +/- 43) ($P < 0.0001$). They determined an optimal cutoff value of 80 kPa, which resulted in a sensitivity and specificity of 88.8% and 84.9%. The area under the receiver operating characteristics (ROC) curve was 0.898 for conventional ultrasound; 0.932 for SWE; and 0.982 for the combined data. In a study of 48 breast lesions, Athanasiou et al[55] found similar results with similar stiffness values for benign lesions (45 +/- 41 kPa) and malignant lesions (147 kPa +/- 40) ($P < 0.001$). Their results suggest the addition of SWE to conventional ultrasound could be used to decrease the number of biopsies performed in benign lesions.

In a small series Evans et al[56] found the sensitivity and specificity for SWE (97% and 83%) to be greater than those for B-mode alone (87% and 78%). In their series they used a cutoff value of 50 kPa. They also confirmed that the technique is highly reproducible.

In a series of 161 masses including 43 malignancies, using a shear wave speed cutoff of 3.6 m/s (38 kPa), a sensitivity of 91% and a specificity of 80.6% were achieved.[57]

Based on a recent large multicenter study (BE1), a cutoff value of 80 kPa (5.2 m/s) was determined to distinguish benign from malignant lesions.[58] This large multicenter trial demonstrated that, when added to Breast Imaging–Reporting and Data System (BI-RADS) classification in B-mode imaging, SWE increased diagnostic accuracy.[58] They found that the evaluation of SWE signal homogeneity and lesion to fat ratios were the best differentiators of benign and malignant lesions. The addition of SWE increased the characterization of lesions over BI-RADS alone, with a sensitivity and specificity of 93.1% and 59.4% in BI-RADS and 92.1% and 7.4% with the addition of SWE. The authors comment that the major value of the addition of SWE is in BI-RADS 3 and 4a lesions where the SWE results are used to upgrade or downgrade the lesion.[58,59] The SSI technique (Aixplorer, SuperSonic Imagine [SSI], Aix-en-Provence, FR) has been shown to be highly qualitatively reproducible based on shape, homogeneity, and color distribution, with only 1.6% of cases being very dissimilar.[60] Lesion size measurements were highly reproducible (> 0.9). Interobserver reliability for maximum and mean elasticity values was also highly reproducible (> 0.8).[60]

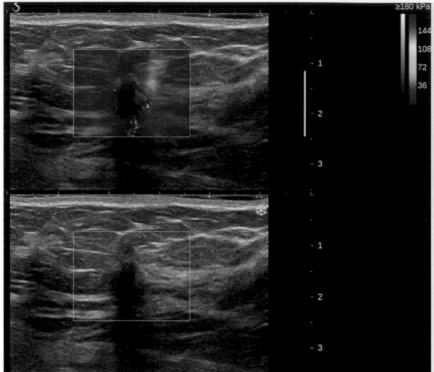

**Fig. 4.6** If the shear wave velocity cannot be determined at a location the pixel is not color coded (arrow). This can occur if the lesion is too deep and the acoustic radiation force impulse (ARFI) is attenuated and no longer strong enough to generate a measureable shear wave, the tissue does not support generation of shear waves (e.g., simple cysts), or there is significant noise in the displacement results and an accurate shear wave speed cannot be calculated. A unique feature of breast cancers is that some do not allow for adequate shear waves for accurate measurement. In these cases the tumor will also not be coded as in this figure.

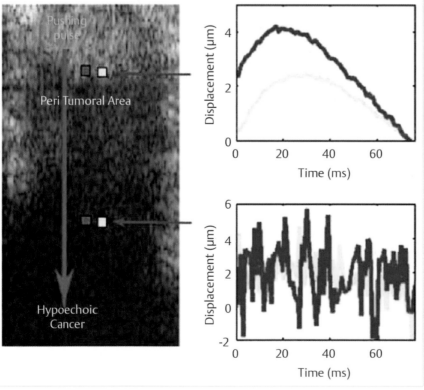

**Fig. 4.7** The observation that some malignancies code as soft in shear wave elastography but code as hard in strain elastography has been reported. It has been suggested that this may be due to significant noise in the shear wave tissue displacement, which is color coded as soft as opposed to black (accurate shear wave speed cannot be calculated). This figure shows a soft (blue) cancer with some high signals surrounding the lesion. When the shear wave displacements are evaluated the area color coded as blue shows high displacements with marked noise leading to inaccurate shear wave speed estimation. In the peritumoral location there is slight noise in the tissue displacement curves, but an accurate estimation of the shear wave speed can be calculated. (Reprinted with permission from Barr RG. Shear wave imaging of the breast: still on the learning curve. J Ultrasound Med 2012;31 (3):347–350)

See the box for a summary of the BE1 study rules.

## Summary of BE1 Study Rules

1. Any of the features analyzed in SWE were able to globally improve the diagnostic performance according to the areas under the curve (AUCs) of the BI-RADS scoring system. This means that SWE features have to be combined with the B-mode features in order to complement the BI-RADS classification and should not be used alone in comparison with the BI-RADS classification.

2. The best performing SWE features were the "quantification" of the maximum stiffness of the lesion (inside or on periphery), as E max measurement (Q Box) or visual color assessment (five-level color scale).

3. The publication came out with suggested aggressive and conservative rules (i.e., using different stiffness thresholds) to help assess the level of suspicion of the breast masses, depending on their initial BI-RADS score. In the studied population:

   a) All BI-RADS 3 masses with high stiffness (E max > 160 kPa (7.3 m/s) or E color = red with SWE scale at 180 kPa (7.7 m/s) could have been upgraded to biopsy. This would have enabled the early management of 4 breast cancers.

   b) BI-RADS 4a masses with low stiffness could have been downgraded to follow-up. This would have increased the specificity and Positive Predictive Value (PPV) for biopsy of the ultrasound diagnosis.

      • Aggressive rule: low stiffness would be considered with E max below 80 kPa (5.2 m/s) or E color light blue or below with SWE scale set at 180 kPa (7.7 m/s).

      • Conservative rule: low stiffness would be considered with E max below 30 kPa (3.2 m/s) or E color dark blue or below with SWE scale set at 180 kPa (7.7 m/s).

      • The aggressive rule would have enabled a higher improvement in specificity; however, four cancers would have been downgraded to follow-up. With the conservative rule, all cancers would have remained in the initial biopsy group, still with a significant increase in specificity.

3D shear wave elastography is available on one system.[61,62] This allows for visualizing of the SWE findings over a volume. No studies have been performed to determine if 3D has an advantage compared with two-dimensional (2D) SWE.

## 4.3.2 Point Quantification Shear Wave Measurement

When using Virtual Touch quantification (VTq, Siemens Ultrasound, Mountain View, CA), where a single measurement is obtained from a small fixed ROI, it is not possible to determine where the area of highest stiffness is located on the B-mode image. The ROI is placed on the B-mode image. The ARFI pulse is then applied and a single numerical value obtained of the shear wave velocity. Multiple measurements within the lesion

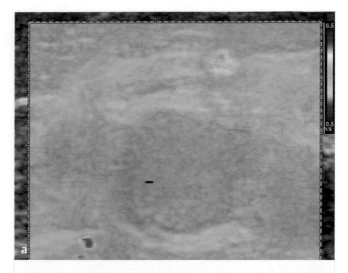

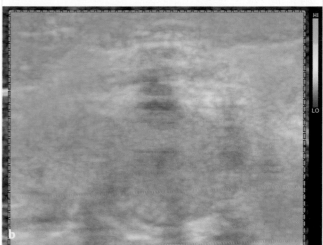

**Fig. 4.8** One method of improving the accuracy of the color coding is to provide a quality map that provides improved assessment of the shear wave quality. This map uses a "stop light" pattern; green (go) for high quality shear waves and yellow (caution) and red (stop). If the shear wave quality is not adequate for accurate measurement. Future improvements in the algorithms may allow for improved shear wave assessment on the initial map having areas of poor quality shear waves not color coded. The velocity map of a shear wave elastography image from an invasive ductal cancer (red arrow) is presented in (a). The Vs is suggested of a benign lesion. The quality map from the same case is presented in (b). The area of the tumor is color coded yellow and red, documenting that the shear waves results are not accurate and should not be used in interpretation. Other vendors do not color code the areas that have inadequate shear waves for analysis.

and surrounding tissue must be obtained to acquire optimal measurements. The measurement within the tumor often results in "x.xx" signifying that adequate shear waves for evaluation were not obtained.[63] This corresponds to a poor quality map (to be discussed) or no color coding on the shear wave imaging systems. Bai et al[64] reported that if a lesion is solid and x.xx is obtained the lesion is most likely a malignancy. With this assumption they obtained a sensitivity and specificity of 63.4% and 100%.

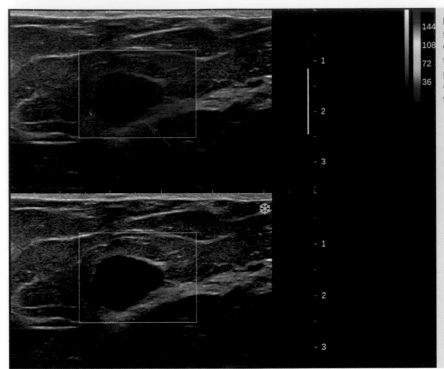

**Fig. 4.9** Shear waves do not propagate in simple fluid such as a simple cyst. In these cases the cyst will not be color coded (arrow). Occasionally there is some bleeding of color in the proximal portion of the cyst. If the cyst is complicated, it can support shear wave propagation and the cyst will be color coded.

### 4.3.3 Quality Factor

In very hard lesions such as invasive cancers, the shear wave may not propagate in an orderly fashion. No results are therefore obtained, and the area with no results is not color coded (▶ Fig. 4.6). In these areas interpretation is not possible. However, in general the periphery of the tumor will be hard surrounding the tumor and appear as hard halo surrounding the lesion. Even if the entire mass is not coded as hard, heterogeneity of the SWE is part of the criteria for a suspicious lesion. Care must be taken with precompression because this can also create the same appearance in a benign lesion.[19]

In a large number of malignant lesions, the area identified on B-mode as the hypoechoic mass often does not code on SWE because a shear wave is not identified or may code with a low Vs. Bai et al found that 63% of breast malignancies have this finding.[64] Preliminary work in the evaluation of this phenomenon suggests that shear waves may not propagate as expected in some malignant lesions (▶ Fig. 4.7).[63] Evaluation of the shear waves in these malignant lesions demonstrates significant noise that may be incorrectly interpreted by the algorithm as a low shear wave velocity.

The addition of a quality measure that evaluates the shear waves generated and determines if they are adequate for an accurate Vs (or kPa) measurement will help in eliminating possible false-negative cases (▶ Fig. 4.8).[65] On the Siemens systems a Quality Map has been added. The "traffic light" display aids in a visual assessment of the shear wave quality. A region color-coded green has high quality shear waves and an accurate estimation of Vs is possible. In regions color-coded yellow or red there is significant signal to noise (SNR) or there is minimal displacement by the shear waves and an accurate assessment of the Vs is not possible. On the SSI system the shear wave quality is incorporated into the velocity map by not color coding the areas with poor shear wave quality. This phenomenon of poor shear wave generation appears to be mostly a problem with breast cancers. As more knowledge of this phenomenon is learned better algorithms are being developed that will decrease the possibility of false-negative breast cancers on SWE. The areas of poor shear waves will be marked (quality mape or no color-coding) so that erroneous low Vs coding will be recognized and not interpreted as a false negative.

In a recent study[65] the addition of a quality measure (QM) in shear wave imaging of the breast can limit false-negative findings (sensitivity without QM 22/46 [48%, 95% CI 33–63%], with QM 42/46 [91%, 95% CI 79–98%], $P < 0.0001$).

### 4.3.4 Limitations

Shear waves will not propagate though fluids with low viscosity and will not be color-coded. The shear wave is detected by standard B-mode ultrasound. Therefore, when areas in the B-mode image show extremely low signal (anechoic), the echo signal is too low for successful shear wave detection. These areas are not color coded. This will occur with marked shadowing such as seen with ribs, tumors with significant shadowing, and areas with macrocalcification.[18] The possibility of a false-negative result with certain breast cancers can occur as already discussed. Algorithms are being improved to limit this phenomenon; however, this miscoding, due to poor quality shear waves, usually occurs in masses that are BI-RADS category 4 or 5 lesions, which should be worked-up appropriately based on their BI-RADS category score.

## 4.4 Artifacts

There are several artifacts that you can encounter. Some of these tell the operator the technique is suboptimal, and several contain diagnostic information.

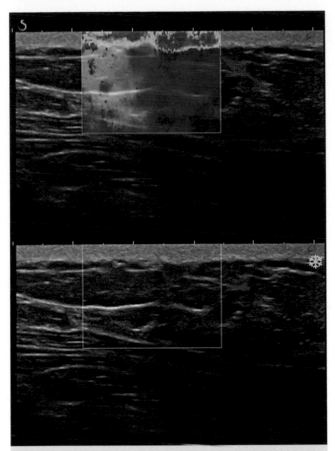

**Fig. 4.10** If too much pressure is applied with the transducer (precompression) the near field in shear wave elastography will appear stiff (red) as in this case (arrow). This can be corrected by decreasing the pressure being applied by the transducer.

### 4.4.1 No Color Coding (Lack of Shear Wave Signal)

Shear waves will not propagate through simple cysts, and they too will not be color coded (▶ Fig. 4.9). The shear wave is detected by ultrasonic echo signal. Therefore, when areas in B-mode image show extremely low signal, it indicates the echo signal is too low for successful detection. These areas are not color coded. This will occur in areas with marked shadowing, such as ribs, tumor with significant shadowing, and areas with calcification.[18]

The ARFI push pulse is attenuated as it travels through tissue and reaches a point where adequate shear waves are not generated for a measurement of Vs. These areas are also not color-coded. For most breast SWE systems this occurs greater than 4.5 cm depth.

In very hard lesions, such as invasive cancers, the shear wave may not propagate. No results are therefore obtained, and the area with no results is not color coded (▶ Fig. 4.6). This is discussed in detail earlier in the chapter.

### 4.4.2 Bang Artifact

If one uses precompression there will be a pattern of red in the near field (▶ Fig. 4.10).[18,19] This can be corrected by using minimal pressure from the transducer on the patient.

# 5 Combination of Shear Wave and Strain Elastography

There is a trend for systems to offer both strain elastography (SE) and shear wave elastography (SWE) for breast elastography evaluation. The advantages and disadvantages of SE and SWE are complementary. ▶ Table 5.1 summarizes the advantages and disadvantages of the two complementary techniques. There may be situations where one technique will provide accurate results, whereas the other has limitations. For example, an adequate shear wave may not be measured in deep lesion due to attenuation of the ARFI pulse, however an adequate SE can be obtained. In cases where a benign lesion is adjacent to glandular tissue and the stain values are similar for both SE may be difficult to interpret where the quantitative nature of SWE will provide accurate results. Having the appropriate elastographic tool for a given patient may increase the accuracy of elastography in characterization of breast lesions.

The combination of SE and SWE can be helpful in increasing confidence of a result if both are concordant. Both techniques are measuring the stiffness of the tissue so similar results are

Table 5.1 Comparison of the properties of strain and shear wave elastography

| Property | Strain elastography | Shear wave elastography |
|---|---|---|
| Imaging at depth | ++++ | + |
| Effect of precompression | +++ | +++ |
| Sensitivity (Is a lesion malignant?) | ++++ | ++ |
| Specificity (Is a lesion benign?) | ++ | ++++ |
| Quantitative | + | ++++ |
| Cyst characterization | ++++ | ++ |

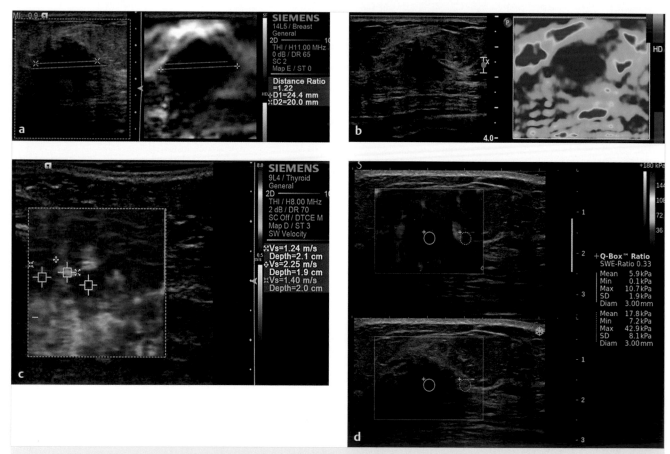

Fig. 5.1 The discrepancy between strain elastography (SE) and shear wave elastography (SWE) with some malignancies is not vendor specific. In this case of an invasive ductal carcinoma in a 37-year-old presenting with a right breast mass, both SE systems (a, Siemens, Mountain View, CA) and (b, Philips Ultrasound, Bothell, WA) have an E/B ratio of > 1 accurately predicting a malignancy. However both SWE systems (c, Siemens, Mountain View, CA) and (d, SuperSonic Imagin, Aix-en-Provence, France) code the malignancy with a Vs suggestive of a benign lesion.

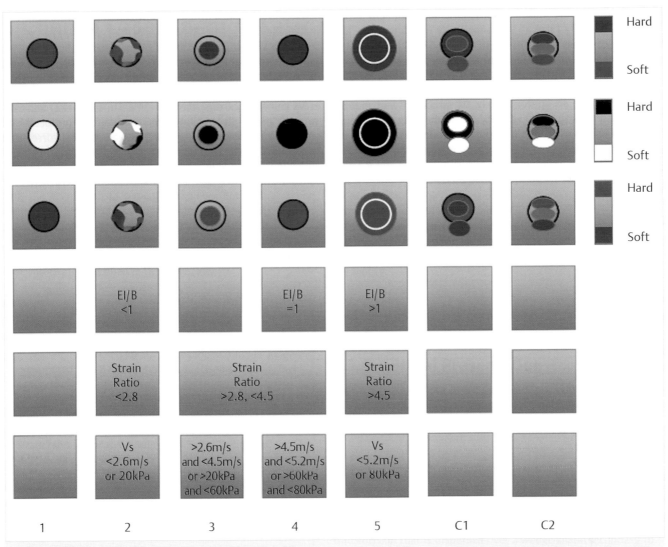

| 1 | 2 | 3 | 4 | 5 | C1 | C2 |
|---|---|---|---|---|----|----|

Fig. 5.2 This illustration summarizes the results of published studies on strain elastography and shear wave elastography and lists the parameters for each based on the Breast Imaging–Reporting and Data system (BI-RADS) classification probability of malignancy. (See Chapter 3 and 4 for discussion.) (Used with permission from ACR, ACR, American College of Radiology Breast–Imaging Reporting and Data System (BI-RADS) Ultrasound. 4th ed. 1st ed. Reston VA: American College of Radiology; 2003.)

expected. Discordant results require further evaluation of the findings. If a reason for the discordant results is not apparent the possibility of two adjacent lesions appearing as one on B-mode should be considered. If a reason for the discordant results is not identified, the more suspicious finding should be acted on.

An example of discordant results is presented in ▶ Fig. 5.1. Both SWE systems demonstrate the lesion to have shear wave velocity (Vs) values suggestive of a benign lesion; however, two SE systems have an E/B ratio of > 1, suggestive of a malignant lesion. This is an example of poor shear wave generation with the invasive ductal cancer leading to a false-negative finding. This phenomenon is secondary to the properties of the breast cancer. With the addition of a quality measure and improved SWE algorithms this problem will be overcome. With improved algorithms that have improved assessment of shear wave quality, these "soft" cancers will be accurately identified and not color coded.

One study has compared the results of SE and SWE with the addition of a quality measure.[65] Both strain (sensitivity 53/55 [96%, 95% CI, 87–99.6%], specificity 94/107 [88%, 95% CI, 80–93%]) and shear wave with quality measure (QM) (sensitivity 42/46 [91%, 95% CI, 79–98%], specificity 82/94 [87%, 95% CI, 79–93%]) elastography have high sensitivities and specificities in characterization of breast masses as benign or malignant. Additional improvements in algorithms will continue to improve the accuracy of both SE and SWE.

▶ Fig. 5.2 summarizes all of the literature on the various techniques. The results are placed on a Breast Imaging–Reporting and Data System (BI-RADS) classification based on the probability of a malignancy corresponding to those of the BI-RADS classification. The first three lines are the 5-point color scale (Tsubuka score, strain score) provided with different color maps, red as hard, black as hard, blue as hard. It is important to remember that the color map is a postprocessing function, and there is no difference in the information

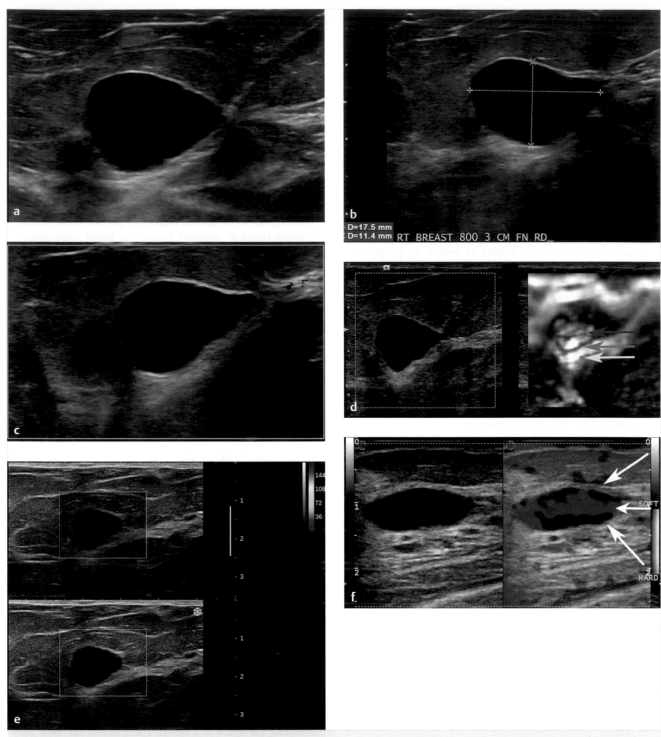

**Fig. 6.1** (a) B-mode image of a mass identified on computed tomography. The mass is anechoic, has a thin wall, through transmission, and no internal echoic, thus meeting all criteria for a benign cyst. (b) The simple cyst noted in (a) measures 17 × 11 mm. (c) On power Doppler imaging the cyst does not have internal or peripheral blood flow. (d) The strain elastogram of the lesion; the left image is the corresponding B-mode image and the image on the right is the strain elastogram. There is a bull's-eye artifact on the elastogram characterized by the central white area (red arrow), black surrounding rim (green arrow) and a distal white spot (yellow arrow). (e) The shear wave elastogram of the lesion. The lower image is the corresponding B-mode image, whereas the upper image is the shear wave elastogram. Note that the majority of the cyst does not color code. Simple cysts do not support shear waves so none are detected and therefore not color coded. There is some "bleeding" of blue color in the anterior portion of the cyst that can sometimes occur. (f) The strain elastogram of a *different* simple cyst using the Esaote system (Esaote North America, Inc., Indianapolis, IN). This system does not produce the bull's-eye artifact, but instead the blue, green, red (BGR) artifact. The three arrows point out the three colored layers.

### 6.1.4 Discussion

Cysts meeting all the criteria for simple cysts (thin walled, anechoic, no internal blood flow, and through transmission) can be confidently classified as BI-RADS category 2 lesions (benign). In these cases elastography is not required to confirm the diagnosis. Occasionally, a solid homogeneous lesion may simulate a benign cyst, particularly if the ultrasound settings are not properly set. In these cases strain elastography is helpful in determining if the lesion is cystic or solid.

In SE the bull's-eye artifact occurs when the contents are freely movable. If a lesion is solid or has a very high viscosity the artifact will not occur. If there is a solid component within the cyst it will cause a stiff defect in the artifact (see Cases 6.6 and 6.7). The bull's-eye artifact is characterized by (1) an outer rim of black (stiff) signal, with (2) a centrally located white (soft) area, and (3) a white (soft) area distal to the lesion. All three components are required for a confident diagnosis that the lesion is a benign cystic lesion.[48] The use of the bull's-eye artifact has been shown to decrease the biopsy rate and increase the positive biopsy rate.[48] The bull's-eye artifact occurs with equipment from both Philips and Siemens. When using the Philips equipment an elasticity imaging (EI) setting of 2 is required to obtain the bull's-eye artifact. When an EI setting of 1 is used the central white area is not present. Because of the possibility of a stiff lesion being just anterior to a soft lesion that can simulate a cyst with EI setting 1, an EI setting of 2 is suggested for use in evaluation of cystic lesions. Another technique using this artifact is anechoic imaging (AI) available on Philips systems. AI codes the areas of freely moveable fluid as yellow and areas with nonmoveable tissue as blue. Equipment from other vendors identifies a blue, green, red (BGR) tricolor pattern (▶ Fig. 6.1f). This artifact has not been studied in detail to determine its sensitivity and specificity for benign cystic lesions. The appearance or nonappearance of the BGR sign in complex cystic lesions has not been studied.

A simple cyst does not support shear wave generation and therefore will not be color coded. Color coding will also not occur when adequate shear waves are not generated within the tissue. This can occur if a lesion is deep (usually > 4 cm) or if the lesion is very stiff as in some cancers. However, if there is debris in the cyst or if it has viscosity increased over simple fluid it will generate a shear wave and will be color coded with low (benign) Vs. In the presented case shear waves are not generated (color coded black) confirming the lesion is a simple benign cyst. As in this case, there is often bleeding of color from the adjacent soft tissue into the proximal portion of the cyst. If a cyst is complicated, shear waves will be generated, and the lesion will be color coded blue (soft). The appearance of a complicated cyst and fibroadenoma will be identical on shear wave imaging. Both of these lesions will be color coding as soft lesions with a low Vs value (blue). Note that with strain imaging the distinction between a cystic lesion and fibroadenoma can be made.

Based on the proposed BI-RADS like elastography classification system presented in Chapter 5, this would be considered to have an approximately 0% change of malignancy.

## 6.2 Case 2: Cystic Lesion—Complicated Cyst

### 6.2.1 Clinical Presentation

A 51-year-old woman presented with a palpable mass in her left breast. Prior mammograms were classified as BI-RADS category 1 with heterogeneously dense breasts. A mammogram was not performed at the time of presentation.

### 6.2.2 Ultrasound Findings

B-mode ultrasound (▶ Fig. 6.2a) shows a 1.8 cm oval lobulated cystic lesion with internal echoes that did not change on repositioning of the patient. On color Doppler imaging (▶ Fig. 6.2b) there is some blood flow in surrounding tissue but no blood flow within the lesion. The lesion was characterized as BI-RADS category 3.

On strain elastography (▶ Fig. 6.2c) a bull's-eye artifact is identified in the cystic area without internal echoes. The echoes within the cyst are stiff and are color coded black. The shadow or copy function was used here to correlate the finding on elastography with the B-mode image. On VTI (strain imaging using ARFI) (▶ Fig. 6.2d) the majority of the lesion color codes as soft (white). When using VTI as opposed to manual displacement strain imaging (e.g., eSie Touch, Siemens) the bull's-eye artifact may not occur. On shear wave imaging (▶ Fig. 6.2e) the color coding at the lesion's center is not consistent with coding for simple fluid. The walls of the lesion color code softer than the surrounding glandular tissue. The use of three-dimensional (3D) SWE is helpful to confirm that there are not stiff areas within or adjacent to the lesion. The 3D results can be displayed as slices in a selected plane (▶ Fig. 6.2f).

### 6.2.3 Diagnosis

Complicated cyst. The lesion was aspirated with a 20-gauge needle under ultrasound guidance. The lesion completely resolved on aspiration. Pathology was cyst contents with no evidence of malignancy.

### 6.2.4 Discussion

Cystic lesions of the breast may be present in women of any age but are most common between 30 and 50 years of age. They may be detected incidentally on screening examinations (mammography, ultrasound, or magnetic resonance imaging [MRI]) or present as a palpable mass or nipple discharge. Complex cysts accounted for 41% of BI-RADS category 3 lesions in the ACRIN 6666 study.[66] BI-RADS category 3 lesions are common and although the recommendation is a short-term interval follow-up, many lesions are aspirated or biopsied (17% in the ACRIN 6666 study) with a low positive biopsy rate.[66] A technique that can improve confidence that a BI-RADS category 3 lesion is benign (or even downgrade the lesion to BI-RADS category 2) could decrease the need for biopsy or short-term follow-up.

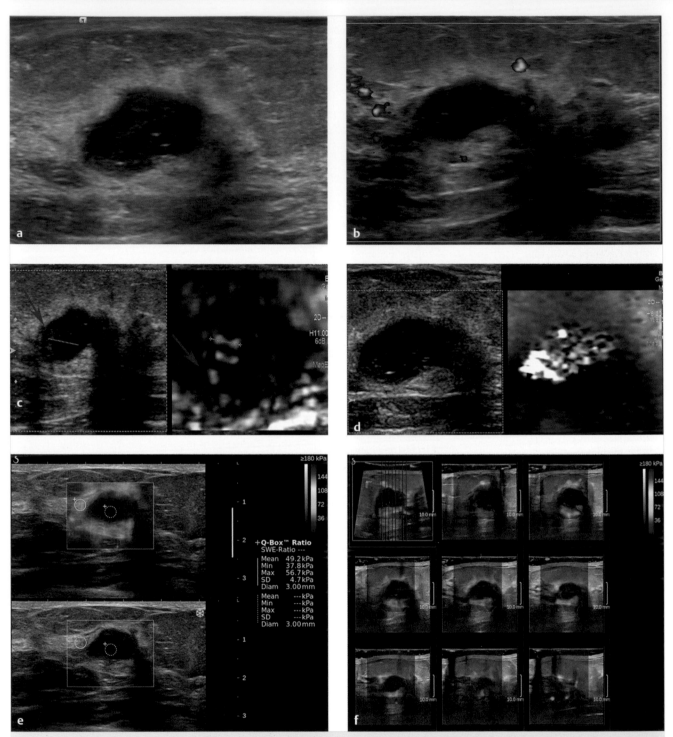

**Fig. 6.2** (a) B-mode image of the palpable mass. The mass is lobular, well circumscribed, and contains multiple internal echoes. There is through transmission. (b) Power Doppler image of the lesion demonstrates there is no internal blood flow but some peripheral blood flow. (c) Strain elastogram of the lesion demonstrates a bull's-eye artifact in a portion of the lesion (dotted line). The area with increased echoes along the wall (arrow) is coded soft (white) on the elastogram. This implies the material is not freely moving but is soft. (d) The Virtual Touch Image (VTI, Siemens) displays the complicated cyst as a soft lesion (white). VTI uses an acoustic radiation force impulse (ARFI) push pulse to generate the displacement used to calculate a strain image. The bull's-eye artifact does not always occur with VTI because a different algorithm is used. (e) Shear wave elastography (SWE) of the lesion demonstrates the area with the bull's-eye artifact is not color coded, consistent with simple fluid (dotted circle). The areas with increased echoes along the wall are color coded blue, suggesting they are viscous enough to support shear wave propagation. The surrounding glandular tissue has a Vs of 4.1 m/s (49 kPa) consistent with dense glandular benign tissue. (f) Results of a three-dimensional (3D) shear wave elastogram where the 3D volume is sliced as demonstrated in the upper left image, and each individual slice is displayed. Similar to the 2D strain image a portion of the complicated cyst is not color coded, the periphery of the lesion is color coded blue, and the surrounding glandular tissue is color coded teal, demonstrating the glandular tissue is stiffer than the viscous portion of the complicated cyst.

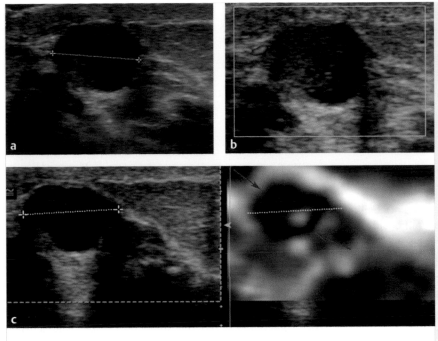

**Fig. 6.3** (a) B-mode imaging of the asymmetric density noted on mammography identifies a 1.2 cm well circumscribed cystic lesion with some internal echoes. (b) Power Doppler imaging of the lesion demonstrates more internal echoes with in the lesion with the appearance of an acorn cyst. There is some peripheral blood flow, but no internal blood flow. (c) On the strain elastogram the anechoic portion of the lesion has a bull's-eye artifact (dotted arrow), whereas the portion of the lesion with internal echoes has a stiff appearance (solid arrow). This implies that the echogenic portion is not freely moveable. It does not necessary mean that it is "solid." Viscous debris within the cyst can give the same appearance as a solid mass. This appearance on strain elastography raises the concern that the lesion could be a complex cystic mass; however, it does not confirm it. In this case the "solid" component is coded black, meaning it is stiffer than the surrounding tissue. In this case all of the surrounding tissue is fat; therefore we can't determine if this lesion is stiff enough to be suspicious for a malignancy. The lesion to fat ratio (not done in this case) could be helpful in characterizing the solid component as benign or malignant. The use of shear wave imaging (not performed in this case) would also help in determining the stiffness of the solid component.

Complicated cysts are usually well-defined cysts with low-level internal echoes or intracystic debris. The debris may layer and shift with changes in patient position. The homogeneous internal echoes within some complicated cysts may produce an appearance identical to that of a circumscribed solid mass. Complicated cysts should be distinguished from complex cystic lesions that have solid components within the cyst, thickened walls, or thick septa. The elastographic appearance of complex cystic lesions is discussed in Case 6.6.

The bull's-eye artifact has been shown to have a very high sensitivity and specificity for diagnosis of a lesion as benign simple or complicated cysts.[48] The use of this artifact to downgrade the BI-RADS category 3 cystic lesions needs further evaluation. The bull's-eye artifact occurs on Philips and Siemens ultrasound systems. In other systems the BGR artifact occurs. This is discussed in Chapter 3. The BGR artifact has not been evaluated in detail to determine the sensitivity and specificity of this artifact in characterization of benign cystic lesions.

In the present case the complicated cyst does not have a classic appearance on conventional ultrasound. The lesion does not have a thin, well-defined wall and has the appearance of a complicated cystic mass with a solid component. Until further research is done to determine if downgrading a BI-RADS category 4A or higher lesion is evaluated, canceling a biopsy based on the bull's-eye artifact is not recommended. However, it is important to alert the pathologist that the lesion may be a complicated cyst and not a solid mass for improved imaging–pathology correlation of the lesion. At this time it may be appropriate to downgrade a BI-RADS category 3 lesion to a BI-RADS category 2 if a bull's-eye artifact is present. Downgrading a BI-RADS category 4A lesion to short-term follow-up may also be appropriate. Limited work by the author suggests that downgrading a

BI-RADS category 4A lesion to a BI-RADS category 2 lesion when a bull's-eye artifact is present may be appropriate (RG Barr, personal observation, October, 1, 2013).

Based on the proposed elastography classification system (similar to the BI-RADS classification) presented in Chapter 5 we would consider this an elastography result with an approximately 0% chance of malignancy.

## 6.3 Case 3: Cystic Lesion—Complicated Cyst

### 6.3.1 Clinical Presentation

The patient is a 72-year-old woman with the development of a 1 cm asymmetric density in the left breast on screening mammography, new from the prior exam. The mammogram was classified as BI-RADS category 0, and an ultrasound was advised for further workup.

### 6.3.2 Ultrasound Findings

B-mode imaging (▶ Fig. 6.3a) shows a 1.2 cm well circumscribed cystic lesion with some internal echoes. On power Doppler imaging (▶ Fig. 6.3b) there is a small amount of peripheral blood flow. No internal blood flow was identified. On power Doppler the internal echoes within the cyst are better appreciated.

On strain imaging (▶ Fig. 6.3c) the bull's-eye artifact is identified in the anechoic portion of the cystic lesion. The area with echoes color codes stiffer than surrounding glandular tissue. The E/B ratio of the stiff component is 0.9.

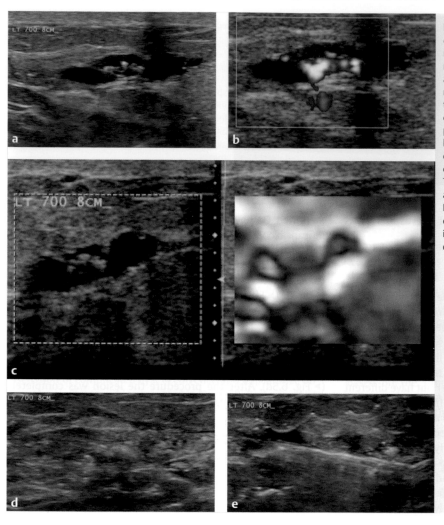

Fig. 6.5 (a) On B-mode imaging the lesion has a complex appearance with both cystic and solid nodular components. There is no through transmission identified. (b) On power Doppler evaluation there is significant blood flow in the solid nodular components of the lesion, suggesting this is a complex cystic lesion and not a complicated cyst. (c) On the elastogram the peripheral cystic areas both have well identified bull's-eye artifacts (arrows). The central portion of the lesion that has both cystic and solid components is a light gray on the elastogram. This is partially due to overlapping bull's-eye artifacts in the small cysts in this region. (d) Image from the vacuum-assisted 12-gauge needle biopsy removal of the lesion. (e) B-mode image of the area confirming complete removal of the lesion at biopsy.

## 6.6 Case 6: Cystic Lesion—Complex Cystic Lesion

### 6.6.1 Clinical Presentation

An 85-year-old woman presents with a new palpable mass in the left breast. Mammography confirms the presence of a 2 cm relatively well circumscribed lesion. The mammogram was classified as BI-RADS category 0, and an ultrasound was advised for further workup.

### 6.6.2 Ultrasound Findings

B-mode imaging (▶ Fig. 6.6a, b) demonstrates a 2.1 cm oval mass with some indistinct borders and some septated cystic components. There is refractive shadowing noted as well as through transmission. The "solid" components do not change on repositioning of the patient. There is significant blood flow in the solid components and in the periphery of the lesion on color Doppler imaging (▶ Fig. 6.6c). The lesion was classified as a BI-RADS category 4B lesion.

On SE (▶ Fig. 6.6d, e) there is a complex pattern of overlapping bull's-eye artifacts from the cystic components. The solid components are stiff, confirming they are fixed and not mobile. Because of the irregular shape and intervening cystic compo-

nents calculation of an E/B ratio or strain ratio is difficult. We calculated an E/B ratio of 1 based on selecting one area of the stiff component. With blood flow noted on power Doppler within the "solid" components we know that the stiff area is a solid lesion and not adherent debris or an area of increased viscosity. This lesion is therefore a complex cystic lesion and not a complicated cyst. On shear wave elastography (▶ Fig. 6.6f) the cystic components have low Vs values (1.3–1.8 m/s; 5–10 kPa), whereas the solid components have high Vs values of up to 6 m/ s. On a different shear wave system (▶ Fig. 6.6g) the solid components have elevated Vs of up to 4.5 m/s (60 kPa), and the cystic components have Vs values of 1.2 to 1.8 m/s (4–10 kPa).

### 6.6.3 Diagnosis

Large duct papilloma. The cystic components were aspirated with a 20-gauge needle under ultrasound guidance. The solid components were then biopsied using 12-gauge vacuum-assisted needle under ultrasound guidance. Pathology was a large duct papilloma without atypia.

### 6.6.4 Discussion

Complex cystic lesions have mixed cystic and solid components, a thick wall or thick septations, or an intracystic mass. These

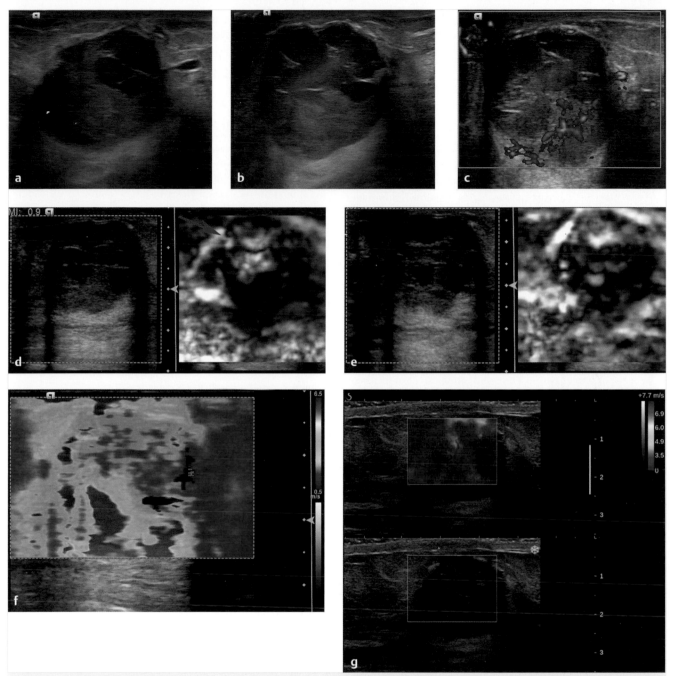

**Fig. 6.6** (a) B-mode image of the palpable mass demonstrates a mass with some ill-defined borders, solid and cystic components, refractive shadowing, and through transmission. (b) B-mode at another location demonstrates more cystic components with fine septations. The solid portion of the lesion accounts for greater than 50% of the lesion. (c) Power Doppler imaging confirms the presence of blood flow in a portion of the solid component and within the wall of the lesion. Some of the "solid"-appearing components on the B-mode images are more hypoechoic than the solid component with blood flow (solid arrow) and may represent internal echoes from debris and not a solid component (dotted arrow). (d) Strain elastogram confirms the presence of a bull's-eye artifact (arrow) in the anechoic portions of the lesion. The remainder of the lesion color codes stiffer than the surrounding tissue. (e) Strain elastogram in a different location has similar findings with multiple bull's-eye artifacts noted (arrows). The solid avascular areas noted on power Doppler do not have bull's-eye artifacts, suggesting they are either very viscous or solid. (f) Shear wave imaging of the lesion has high Vs in the solid components of the lesion (solid arrow) and low Vs in the cystic portions of the lesion (dotted arrow). (g) Real-time shear wave imaging demonstrates similar findings with the solid components color coding teal. The cystic components code dark blue, suggesting they are not simple fluid but have some debris within them.

lesions merit biopsy with a 23% malignant rate in the series of Berg et al.[68] Complex cysts are associated with a variety of benign, atypical, and malignant diagnoses. Common benign causes of complex cystic masses include fibrocystic changes, intraductal or intracystic papilloma without atypia, and fibroadenoma. Atypical findings include atypical ductal hyperplasia, lobular neoplasia, and atypical papilloma. Malignant findings include DCIS, infiltrating ductal carcinoma, and infiltrating lobular carcinoma.[69] Because of the significant chance of malignancy, image-guided or surgical biopsy is usually indicated.

At ultrasound breast cysts are categorized as simple, complicated, or complex.[4,68] By using the criteria adapted from Berg et al,[68] complex cystic breast masses can be categorized into four classes on the basis of their ultrasound features: type 1 masses have a thick outer wall, thick internal septa, or both; type 2 masses contain one or more intracystic masses; type 3 masses contain mixed cystic and solid components and are at least 50% cystic; and type 4 masses are predominantly (at least 50%) solid with eccentric cystic foci.[69] The method of biopsy for these lesions is described elsewhere.[69]

It is important to determine if a lesion is a complicated cyst or a complex cystic mass. If the internal echoes are movable on B-mode imaging without stationary components the diagnosis of a complicated cyst can be made. If blood flow is noted on color or power Doppler within the "solid" component of the lesion the diagnosis of a complex cystic lesion can be made. However, there are many lesions that have characteristics between these two presentations. Internal debris can be stationary, such as in an acorn cyst, and solid components in a lesion may not have perceivable blood flow on color or power Doppler.

SE can be extremely helpful in distinguishing these two cases. When a solid component is present it will appear stiffer than the adjacent components in the lesion. If the internal echoes are freely moveable they will not affect the bull's-eye artifact, and a diagnosis of a complicated cyst can be made. If the viscosity of the cystic component is very high, a bull's-eye artifact will not occur, but it will code as soft. If there is a solid component, the E/B ratio or strain ratio can be used to determine if the lesion is benign or malignant.

However, with shear wave imaging both complicated cysts and benign complex cystic lesions will color code as soft (blue). If the solid component is a malignancy it will code as stiff enough to suggest a malignancy. Therefore strain imaging is helpful in characterizing a cystic lesion as a complicated cyst or a complex cystic lesion, and, if a complex cystic lesion, whether it is benign or malignant. Shear wave imaging is helpful in determining if the lesion is benign or malignant. ▶ Table 6.1 lists the elastographic appearance of cystic lesions.

In the present case we have a mass with greater than 50% solid components and a cystic area with septations, a type 4 lesion. On power Doppler imaging blood flow is noted confirming this lesion is a complex cystic lesion and not a complicated cyst. Strain imaging demonstrates a bull's-eye artifact in the cystic component, whereas the solid component is stiff. In this case the E/B ratio is 1 and should therefore be considered as possible for malignancy. The shear wave imaging on both systems has some increased peripheral Vs and should be considered a possible malignancy and requires biopsy.

Based on the proposed elastography classification system (similar to the BI-RADS classification) presented in Chapter 5 we would consider the elastography findings as having a greater than 95% chance of malignancy (2–95% on SE, and > 95% on SWE).

## 6.7 Case 7: Cystic Lesion—Complex Cystic Lesion

### 6.7.1 Clinical Presentation

The patient is a 68-year-old woman who presents with a right breast bloody discharge and palpable mass in the right breast. A diagnostic mammogram demonstrates a 4 cm lobular mass. The mammogram was classified as BI-RADS 0, and an ultrasound was advised for further workup.

### 6.7.2 Ultrasound Findings

On B-mode imaging (▶ Fig. 6.7a) a complex 4.5 cm complex, well-defined lobular mass is identified. A panoramic view (▶ Fig. 6.7b) of the lesion demonstrates two components—a medial portion with a fluid-fluid level and a lateral portion with a lobular mass within a cystic area. Medial to the lesion extending to the nipple is a tubular structure (▶ Fig. 6.7c). Power Doppler evaluation (▶ Fig. 6.7d) demonstrates peripheral blood flow extending into the solid component of the lesion. The lesion was classified as BI-RADS category 4B.

On strain imaging (▶ Fig. 6.7e) the medial portion of the image is very soft, whereas the lateral portion of the mass is stiffer than surrounding breast tissue. The lateral lesion has an E/B ratio of 0.9, suggestive of a benign lesion. On the 5-point color scale the lesion would have a score of 2. Shear wave imaging is not available for this case.

### 6.7.3 Diagnosis

Large duct papilloma. The medial portion of the lesion was aspirated using a 20-gauge needle under ultrasound guidance and had the appearance of old blood. The lateral portion of the lesion was biopsied with a 12-gauge vacuum-assisted core needle under ultrasound guidance. On pathology the lateral solid lesion was large duct papilloma, whereas the aspirated fluid contained old blood products.

### 6.7.4 Discussion

A discussion of complex cystic lesion is presented in Case 6.2.

It is important to determine if a lesion is a complicated cyst or a complex cystic mass. If the internal echoes are movable on B-mode imaging without stationary components the diagnosis of a complicated cyst can be made. If blood flow is noted on color or power Doppler within the "solid" component of the lesion the diagnosis of a complex cystic lesion can be made. However, there are many lesions that have characteristics between these two presentations. Internal debris can be stationary, such as in an acorn cyst, and solid components in a lesion may not have perceivable blood flow on color or power Doppler.

SE can be extremely helpful in distinguishing these two cases. When a solid component is present it will appear stiffer than the adjacent components in the lesion. If the internal echoes are freely moveable they will not affect the bull's-eye artifact, and a diagnosis of a complicated cyst can be made. If the

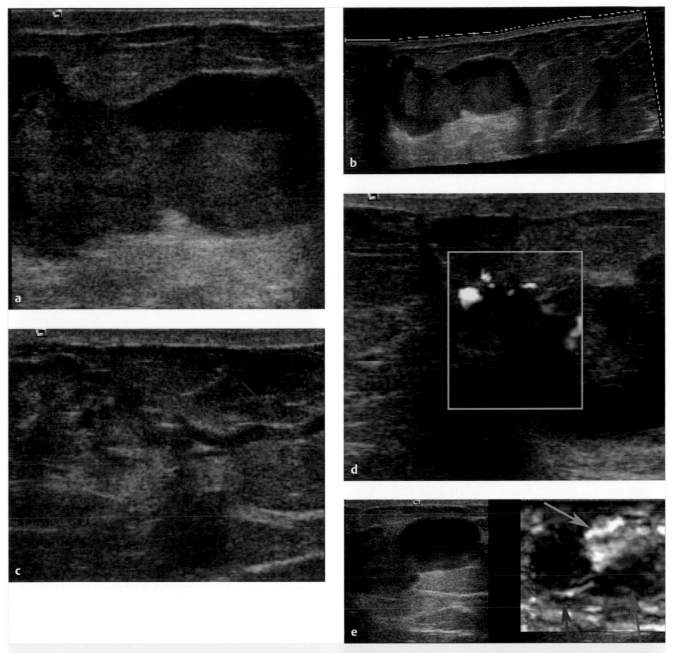

**Fig. 6.7** (a) B-mode image of a large complex lesion. The lesion has a dumbbell appearance with cystic and solid-appearing components in each portion. (b) A panoramic B-mode image of the lesion demonstrates the lesion is well circumscribed, has through transmission on both components, and appears to have a fluid-debris level in the medial component (arrow). (c) On B-mode imaging there is a ductal structure extending from the lesion to the nipple (arrow). (d) On power Doppler imaging there is internal blood flow noted in the lateral component but not in the medical component (not shown). (e) On strain elastography the lateral component codes stiffer (black) than surrounding tissue and has an E/B ratio of 0.9 (red arrow). The medical component of the lesion color-codes softer (white) than surrounding tissue (green arrow). A bull's-eye artifact is not identified. Close inspection demonstrates the debris in the medial component color codes stiffer than the remainder of the component (blue arrow). In this case the medial component was old blood products that have enough viscosity to not allow formation of the bull's-eye artifact. The lateral component codes stiff with an EI/B ratio of < 1, suggesting it is a benign solid component.

viscosity of the cystic component is very high, a bull's-eye artifact will not occur, but it will code as soft. If there is a solid component the E/B ratio or strain ratio can be used to determine if the lesion is benign or malignant.

However, with shear wave imaging both complicated cysts and benign complex cystic lesions will color code as soft (Vs < 4.5 m/s [ > 60 kPa]). If the solid component is a malignancy it will code as stiff (Vs > 4.5 m/s [ > 60 kPa]). Therefore strain imag-

ing is helpful in characterizing a cystic lesion as a complicated cyst or a complex cystic lesion, and, if a complex cystic lesion, whether it is benign or malignant. Shear wave imaging is helpful in determining if the lesion is benign or malignant.

In the presented case we have a lesion with both freely movable debris in one portion of the lesion and a solid component in the other. The solid component accounts for less than 50% of the lesion so this would be classified as a type 3 complex cystic lesion. On strain imaging the solid component of the lesion codes as stiff with an E/B ratio of 0.9. The other portion codes white (very soft). Because a bull's-eye artifact is not identified the fluid is viscous enough to not allow the bull's-eye artifact. Given that the patient presented with a bloody discharge the soft component is suggestive of a hematoma.

Shear wave imaging is not available in this case. We would expect that the solid component would code with a Vs suggestive of a benign lesion given that diagnosis is benign. The cystic component would color code as soft (Vs < 3 [28 kPa]).

Both Cases 6.6 and 6.7 in this chapter have the same pathological diagnosis of a large duct papilloma. In Case 6.6, the elastographic features were suggestive of a malignant lesion, whereas in Case 6.7, the elastographic features were suggestive of a benign lesion. It is not known if the elastographic features can determine the aggressiveness of the large duct papilloma (i.e., whether elastography can identify which lesions are at higher risk for conversion to a malignancy).

Based on the proposed elastography classification system (similar to the BI-RADS classification) presented in Chapter 5 we would consider this lesion to have an approximately 0% chance of malignancy.

## 6.8 Case 8: Fibrocystic Change—Lesion Blends in with Adjacent Tissue on Elastography

### 6.8.1 Clinical Presentation

A 55-year-old woman presents with a new partially obscured 1.5 cm mass in the left breast on screening mammography. Mammogram was classified as BI-RADS 0, and an ultrasound was recommended for further workup.

### 6.8.2 Ultrasound Findings

On B-mode ultrasound (▶ Fig. 6.8a,b) a heterogeneous, 1.5 cm well circumscribed hypoechoic, oval mass with internal septations is identified. Through transmission was noted. The lesion

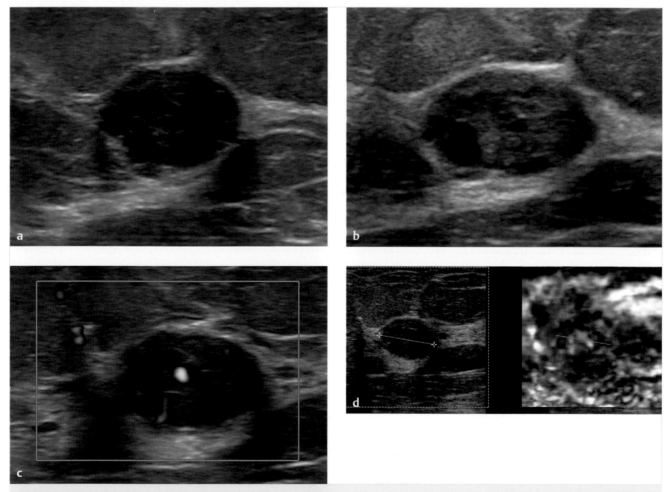

**Fig. 6.8** (a) B-mode image of the lesion corresponding to the mammographic abnormality. The mass is a heterogeneous, hypoechoic, well circumscribed lesion with internal septations. There is refractive shadowing and some through transmission. (b) Another B-mode image of the lesion demonstrating the heterogeneity of the mass with a question of small calcifications. (c) Power Doppler evaluation of the mass demonstrates significant blood flow within the mass. (d) On strain elastography the lesion is also heterogeneous, and its borders are difficult to locate. To add in locating the lesion on the elastogram, the copy or shadow function has been used. The lesion in the left B-mode image was measured and the copy function used. The system places a dotted line in the exact on the elastogram as the measurement taken in the B-mode image. It is not uncommon for benign lesions to be poorly visualized on strain elastography because their elastic properties (stiffness) are similar to those of glandular tissue. (*Continued*)

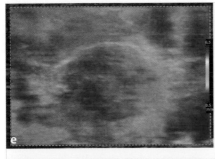

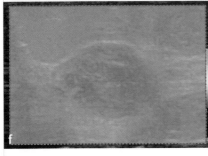

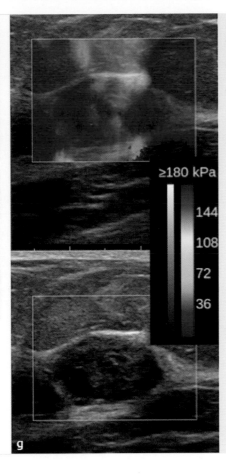

Fig. 6.8 (Continued) (e) Shear wave elastogram demonstrating that the stiffness of the lesion is similar to adjacent breast tissue and has a Vs (color-coded blue) predictive of a benign lesion. (f) The corresponding quality map to the shear wave image in (e) confirms that the shear waves are adequate for accurate measurement (green = high quality). (g) Similar findings are obtained on a real-time shear wave system. The lesion color codes with a Vs of < 4.1 m/s (< 50 kPa).

has internal blood flow with a blood vessel entering perpendicular to the capsule on color Doppler imaging (▶ Fig. 6.8c). The lesion was classified as BI-RADS 4A.

On strain elastography (▶ Fig. 6.8d) the stiffness of the lesion is heterogeneous, containing both softer and stiffer components. The lesion is softer than the adjacent fibroglandular tissue. It is difficult to determine an E/B ratio because the lesion borders are difficult to determine on the elastogram. The use of the copy or shadow function is helpful in these cases. The lesion can be measured on the B-mode image and the measurement copied onto the elastogram. The lesion would have a score of 2 on the 5-point color scale. On shear wave imaging (▶ Fig. 6.8e) it has a Vs of 1.2 to 2.2 m/s (kPa values of 7 to 15). The quality map (▶ Fig. 6.8f) confirms that good quality shear waves were generated. Findings are similar on a second shear wave system (▶ Fig. 6.8g).

### 6.8.3 Diagnosis

Fibrocystic change and focal fibroadenomoid hyperplasia. The lesion was biopsied using a 12-gauge vacuum-assisted core biopsy needle. The pathology was fibrocystic change and focal fibroadenomoid hyperplasia.

### 6.8.4 Discussion

*Fibrocystic change* is a generalized term used to describe a variety of benign changes in the breast that affect both glandular and connective tissue. Symptoms of this condition are breast swelling or pain, as well as nodules, lumpiness, or nipple discharge. At least half of all women will be affected by fibrocystic change at some point in their life. Women of childbearing age are affected most commonly, but women of all ages can develop fibrocystic changes. Most of these symptoms stop after menopause, unless hormone replacement therapy is used.

Many fibrocystic changes are a reflection of the response of breast tissue to monthly hormonal changes. Even though these changes are very common and are not life threatening, some of the symptoms are similar to those of breast cancer, so it is important to evaluate the cause of the symptoms to rule out the possibility of cancer. In addition, some fibrocystic changes may indicate that a woman has an increased risk of later developing breast cancer. A definitive diagnosis will lead to a better understanding of breast cancer risk and the appropriate screening programs for a woman to follow.

*Fibrosis* refers to the formation of fibrous tissue. Fibrous tissue is the material that composes ligaments and scar tissue. Fibrous breasts have areas that feel firm or hard to the touch. No special treatment is required for this condition. Fibrosis is not associated with an increased breast cancer risk.

Mammography cannot reliably diagnose focal fibrocystic change due to a wide variation of imaging findings. On mammography focal fibrocystic change can mimic breast cancer when it presents as a discrete mass or density.[70] In a study by Shetty and Shah[71] the sonographic findings of focal fibrocystic change appeared as a solid mass in 47% and as cysts in 13%. In

15%, heterogeneously echogenic tissue was seen, and in the remaining 25% of cases, there was no sonographically visible focal change. In their study, 46.4% of the masses were classified as sonographically indeterminate, 1% as probably malignant, and 23% of masses were sonographically benign. A significant number of cases of focal fibrocystic change appear as solid masses. The sonographic features are not specific enough to differentiate between those that have a dominant component of focal fibrosis, sclerosing adenosis, or apocrine metaplasia from fibrocystic change without a specific histologic subtype. Many of these solid masses may appear indeterminate.[71] Imaging findings on MRI are also nonspecific, with a significant number of cases having rapid enhancement and washout kinetics suggestive of a malignancy.[70]

In this case the patient presented with a mass on mammography that was a well-defined heterogeneous hypoechoic mass on ultrasound. The lesion had significant internal blood flow on power Doppler. On both SE and SWE the lesion is as soft as adjacent benign breast tissue. As is often the case with fibrocystic change the lesion is not well defined on strain elastography because the elastic properties (stiffness) of fibrocystic change are similar to glandular breast tissue. This can lead to difficulty in using the E/B ratio; however, these cases will usually color code with a score of 2 on the 5-point color scale and have a strain ratio of less than 4.5. It can be difficult to identify the lesion on the elastogram; the use of the copy, mirror, or shadow function is helpful to confirm the location of the lesion on the elastogram. On SWE the lesion borders are less critical because a quantitative measurement of the stiffness of the lesion can be obtained.

It is appropriate in BI-RADS category 4A lesions such as these that have concordant benign strain and shear wave findings to recommend a short-term interval follow-up as opposed to image-guided biopsy. Further study is needed to determine if these lesions can be classified as BI-RADS 2 if the SE and SWE findings are concordant and benign.

Based on the proposed elastography classification system (similar to the BI-RADS classification) presented in Chapter 5 we would consider this lesion to have an approximately 0% chance of malignancy.

# 6.9 Case 9: Fibrocystic Change—Fibroadenomoid Hyperplasia

## 6.9.1 Clinical Presentation

The patient is a 35-year-old woman with a strong family history of breast cancer at an early age. The patient has had yearly screening mammograms and ultrasound for 3 years. The patient's screening mammogram was unchanged from prior studies, with heterogeneous dense breasts. The mammogram was classified as BI-RADS 2. Screening ultrasound was also performed.

## 6.9.2 Ultrasound Findings

On B-mode imaging (▶ Fig. 6.9a) there is a new 0.7 cm irregular hypoechoic lesion with internal septations in the right breast.

On power Doppler imaging (▶ Fig. 6.9b) there is some internal blood flow. The lesion was classified as a BI-RADS category 4A.

On SE (▶ Fig. 6.9c) the lesion is stiffer than surrounding breast tissue and has an E/B ratio of 0.61, suggestive of a benign lesion. The strain ratio (lesion to fat ratio) is 2.7, also suggestive of a benign lesion (▶ Fig. 6.9d). On the 5-point color scale this lesion would have a score of 3. On VTI (▶ Fig. 6.9e) the lesion is stiffer than surrounding tissue and smaller on the elastogram than the B-mode image, consistent with the manual displacement strain findings. On shear wave imaging the lesion color codes soft with a Vs of 2.9 m/s (25 kPa) on one system (▶ Fig. 6.9f) and 2.6 m/s (20 kPa) on another (▶ Fig. 6.9g), both suggestive of a benign lesion.

## 6.9.3 Diagnosis

Fibroadenomoid hyperplasia. The lesion was biopsied using a 12-gauge vacuum-assisted core biopsy needle. The pathology was fibrocystic change and focal fibroadenomoid hyperplasia, negative for atypia.

## 6.9.4 Discussion

Fibroadenomatoid hyperplasia is a well described but rare benign breast lesion with composite features of fibroadenoma and fibrocystic change. This condition was previously described as sclerosing lobular hyperplasia, fibroadenomatosis, or fibroadenomatoid mastopathy.[72–74] It is characterized by a microfocal proliferation of fibrous stroma containing hyperplastic epithelial elements similar to those seen in fibroadenoma. No well circumscribed mass lesion and no apparent capsule are seen. It may be a localized or diffuse process. The mean age of presentation is in the third decade, occurring in approximately 5 to 7% of benign surgical biopsies.[73]

The findings in this case are different than those in Case 6.8. The lesion in this case is stiffer than surrounding glandular tissue and is therefore easily identified on the strain elastogram. The E/B ratio and strain ratio (lesion to fat ratio) are easily calculated. All of the strain findings are suggestive of a benign lesion. In our lab we use an EI/B ratio of < 1 as suggestive of a benign lesion and an EI/B ratio of ≥ 1 as suggestive of a malignant lesion. We use a strain ratio of < 4.5 as suggestive of a benign lesion and > 4.5 as suggestive of a malignant lesion. The shear wave finds in both systems are also suggestive of a benign lesion with Vs of < 4.5 (< 60 kPa). These cutoff values were determined from the results of several hundred biopsy-proven cases with a wide range of pathology.

When both the strain and the shear wave finds are concordant there is increased confidence in the characterization of the mass. In this case the BI-RADS category 4A finds could have been downgraded to a BI-RADS category 3 lesion. With future study it may be possible to downgrade the lesion to BI-RADS category 2 when both strain and shear wave findings are concordant.

Based on the proposed elastography classification system (similar to the BI-RADS classification) presented in Chapter 5 we would consider this lesion as having an approximately 0% chance of malignancy.

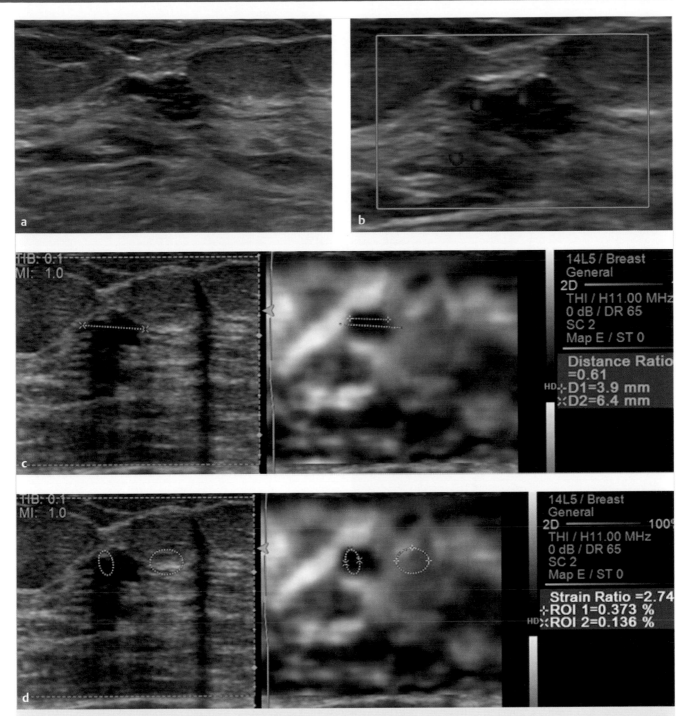

**Fig. 6.9** (a) B-mode image of a lesion identified on ultrasound screening. The lesion is a 7 mm irregular well circumscribed lesion with septations. (b) On power Doppler imaging there is internal blood flow noted in the lesion. (c) On strain elastography the lesion is stiffer than surrounding tissue and has an E/B ratio of 0.6, suggestive of a benign lesion. In this case the copy or shadow function was used to copy the measurement of B-mode onto the elastogram. The B–mode copied measurement (yellow dotted line) was changed to correspond to the elastographic measurement (green dotted line), and the system automatically calculated the E/B ratio. This case would have a score of 3 on the 5-point color scale. (d) The lesion to fat ratio was also calculated. A region of interest (ROI) was placed to contain only surrounding fat and the second ROI placed in the lesion. The system calculated a strain ratio of 2.7; that is, the lesion is 2.7 times stiffer than fat. This finding is also suggestive of a benign lesion. (*Continued*)

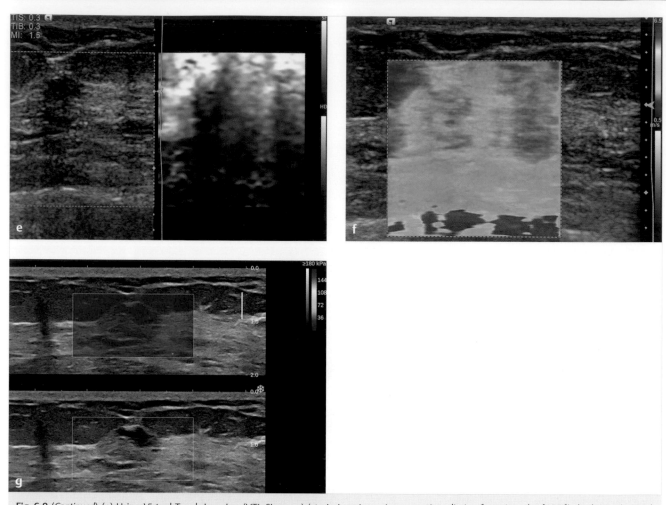

**Fig. 6.9** (*Continued*) (e) Using Virtual Touch Imaging (VTI, Siemens) (strain imaging using acoustic radiation force impulse [ARFI]) the lesion (arrows) appears stiffer than surrounding tissue and smaller than on the corresponding B-mode image. (f) On shear wave imaging the lesion codes soft with a Vs of 2.9 m/s (25 kPa), also suggestive of a benign lesion. (g) Similar findings of a benign lesion are found with a second shear wave system.

## 6.10 Case 10: Fibrocystic Change— Lesion Blends in with Adjacent Tissue on Elastography

### 6.10.1 Clinical Presentation

A 53-year-old woman presented with a new palpable mass in her right breast. A diagnostic mammogram was negative (BI-RADS category 1). The patient was referred for a diagnostic ultrasound.

### 6.10.2 Ultrasound Findings

A 1.9 × 0.4 cm hypoechoic lobular lesion with some posterior shadowing adjacent to dense glandular tissue is identified on B-mode imaging (▶ Fig. 6.10a). There is a small amount of blood flow adjacent to the lesion on color Doppler imaging (▶ Fig. 6.10b). The lesion was classified as BI-RADS category 4A.

The lesion is minimally stiffer than the adjacent fatty tissue but of similar stiffness to adjacent glandular tissue on strain elastography (▶ Fig. 6.10c). Because the lesion is of similar stiffness to the adjacent glandular tissue, the borders of the lesion are not identified, and an E/B ratio cannot be accurately calculated. But because we know the lesion's stiffness is similar to the glandular tissue we can assume the lesion has a high probability of being benign. Note that on the elastogram there are several bull's-eye artifacts, suggesting several cystic components in the lesion (▶ Fig. 6.10d). On the 5-point color scale this lesion would have a score of 2. A strain ratio (lesion to fat ratio) was not performed. In cases such as these where there are both cystic and solid components care must be taken in calculating the strain ratio because the value will be inaccurate if both cystic and solid components are included in the region of interest (ROI). On shear wave imaging (▶ Fig. 6.10e,f) the lesion has a low Vs of 1.2 m/s (7 kPa).

### 6.10.3 Diagnosis

Fibrocystic change. The lesion was biopsied using a 12-gauge vacuum-assisted core biopsy needle. The pathology was fibrocystic change.

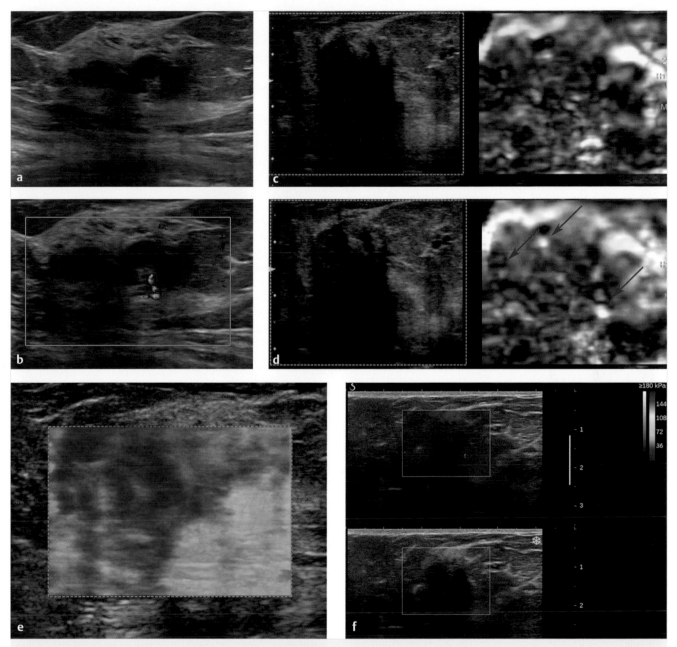

**Fig. 6.10** (a) The palpable mass corresponded to a lobular hypoechoic lesion with some posterior shadowing on B-mode imaging. Note that the lesion is surrounded by glandular tissue. (b) On color Doppler evaluation the lesion has some blood flow adjacent to the lesion but no internal blood flow. (c) On strain elastography the lesion is not identified and blends in with the adjacent glandular tissue. This lesion has a score of 2 on the 5-point color scale. The E/B ratio cannot be accurately calculated. By using the copy function to locate the lesion a strain ratio (lesion to fat ratio) can be calculated (not performed in this case). (d) The strain elastogram in a different location demonstrates several bull's-eye artifacts (arrows), suggesting there are several small cystic areas within or adjacent to the lesion. (e) On shear wave imaging the lesion has a low Vs of 2.2 m/s (15 kPa), suggestive of a benign lesion. (f) On a different shear wave system the lesion does not color code. This can be due to one of several factors: (1) the shadowing in the lesion prevented the tracking B-mode pulses from getting an accurate returned signal to calculate the Vs, (2) patient or sonologist movement may have led to poor shear waves and the system rejected the data and therefore did not color code the lesion. There is a surrounding ring of high Vs noted.

## 6.10.4 Discussion

Many breast lumps turn out to be caused by fibrosis or cysts, benign changes in breast tissue that happen in many women at some time in their lives. Fibrosis is the formation of scarlike (fibrous) tissue, and cysts are fluid-filled sacs. These changes are called fibrocystic changes, and were previously called fibrocys-

tic disease. They are most often diagnosed based on symptoms, such as breast lumps, swelling, and tenderness or pain. These symptoms tend to be worse just before a woman's menstrual period is about to begin. The patient's breasts may feel lumpy and, sometimes, a clear or slightly cloudy nipple discharge will be noticed.

These changes are most common in women of childbearing age, but they can affect women of any age. They are the most common benign condition of the breast. They may be found in different parts of the breast and in both breasts at the same time.

Many different histologic changes can be found in fibrocystic breast tissue. Most of these changes reflect the way the woman's breast tissue has responded to monthly hormone changes and have little other importance.

This case is similar to Case 6.8, where the elastographic features of the lesion are similar to those of the surrounding glandular tissue and the lesion is therefore poorly visualized on the strain elastogram. It is difficult to measure the E/B ratio in these cases. By using the copy or shadow function the lesion location can be identified on the elastogram and the strain ratio (lesion to fat ratio) calculated. A 5-point color score can also be given and is usually a score of 2 as in this case. Knowing that the stiffness of the lesion is similar to glandular tissue is suggestive of a benign lesion. The added confidence of low Vs on shear wave imaging as in this case increases confidence the lesion is benign. Elastography could have been used to downgrade this lesion from a BI-RADS category 4A to a BI-RADS category 3. Further studies are need to determine if the lesion could be downgraded to a BI-RADS category 2 lesion based on concordant strain and shear wave benign findings.

Based on the proposed elastography classification system (similar to the BI-RADS classification) presented in Chapter 5 we would consider this lesion to have an approximately 0% chance of malignancy.

# 6.11 Case 11: Fibrocystic Change—Stromal Fibrosis

## 6.11.1 Clinical Presentation

A 41-year-old woman was noted to have a new asymmetric density in her right breast on screening mammography. Spot compression views confirmed the presence of the asymmetry. The lesion was classified as BI-RADS category 0, and ultrasound was advised for further workup.

## 6.11.2 Ultrasound Findings

On B-mode imaging (▶ Fig. 6.11a) a 1.6 cm irregular, spiculated, hypoechoic mass is identified. A single vessel entering the lesion perpendicular to the lesion is identified on power Doppler imaging (▶ Fig. 6.11b). The lesion was classified as BI-RADS category 4C.

On SE (▶ Fig. 6.11c) the lesion is stiffer than adjacent normal breast tissue with an E/B mode ratio of 2.3. The lesion to fat ratio was 6.2 (▶ Fig. 6.11d). This lesion has a score of 5 on the 5-point color scale. On VTI (strain imaging using ARFI) similar findings are obtained (▶ Fig. 6.11e), a stiff lesion that is larger on the elastogram. On shear wave imaging (▶ Fig. 6.11f) the lesion does not color code, with a Vs of 1.4 m/s (9 kPa) adjacent to the lesion. The quality map (▶ Fig. 6.11g) confirms that shear waves were of poor quality and should not be used in characterizing the mass. On a 3D shear wave elastogram (▶ Fig. 6.11h) no elevated Vs is noted.

## 6.11.3 Diagnosis

Focal columnar cell change and stromal fibrosis. There was no evidence of epithelial atypia or neoplasm.

## 6.11.4 Discussion

Epithelial hyperplasia is a condition in which there is an increase in the number of normal cells that line either the ducts (ductal hyperplasia) or the lobules (lobular hyperplasia) of the breast. This condition is also referred to as proliferative breast disease. Epithelial hyperplasia can be diagnosed by core needle biopsy or surgical biopsy.

When examined under a microscope, hyperplasia may be classified as follows:
1. Usual type, meaning there is an increase in the number of cells, but the cells look normal
2. Atypical, meaning there is an increase in the number of cells and the cells are not quite normal appearing

On average, about 70% of biopsy specimens do not contain any hyperplasia. About 26% have usual hyperplasia and only 4% have atypical hyperplasia.

In this case all of the SE techniques suggest this lesion is malignant. The shear wave imaging from one system does not color code a portion of the lesion. The other areas code soft (blue); however, the quality map is yellow (poor-quality shear waves) throughout the lesion. In general when the lesion is solid and the quality map is poor quality (yellow or red) the lesion, if not a simple cyst, has a high probability of being malignant.

In general benign solid lesions propagate shear waves well and usually have a high (green) quality map. Some cancers, for reasons not yet fully understood, do not generate shear waves that can be accurately measured. In some of these cases the lesion will not color code, whereas others may color code as soft inaccurately. The quality map can help determine which of these cancers codes incorrectly.

In this case, the area not color coded in the velocity map was rejected by the initial algorithm, but some areas with poor shear wave generation were color coded. The addition of the second algorithm (the quality map) rejects additional poor shear waves. Improved algorithms will allow for improved color coding so these lesions are not color coded as opposed to coding soft.[65] Some benign lesions, particularly sclerotic lesions, also have elastographic findings suggestive of a malignant lesion. Other lesions that may have false-positive elastography findings are fat necrosis and mastitis. These are discussed in Cases 23, 24, 25, 26, 29, and 30 in detail.

Presently there are no studies evaluating the elastographic findings in the spectrum of usual hyperplasia, atypical ductal hyperplasia, and DCIS. In our experience, both usual hyperplasia and atypical ductal hyperplasia have elastographic findings of benign lesions. DCIS is discussed in Case 7.1 and 7.2.

Based on the proposed elastography classification system (similar to the BI-RADS classification) presented in Chapter 5 we would consider this lesion to have a > 95% chance of malignancy (> 95% on SE; indeterminate on SWE due to poor-quality shear waves).

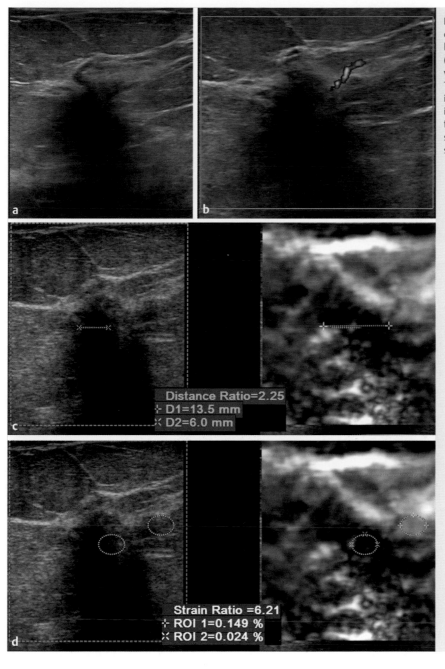

**Fig. 6.11** (a) B-mode imaging of the lesion noted on screening mammography demonstrates the lesion is irregular, hypoechoic with shadowing. (b) On power Doppler imaging there is a single vessel entering perpendicular to the lesion. (c) The lesion is stiffer than surrounding tissue and increased in size compared with the corresponding B-mode image, with an E/B ratio of 2.3. The findings are suspicious for a malignancy. (d) The strain ratio (lesion to fat ratio) of the lesion is 6.2 suggestive of a malignant lesion. (*Continued*)

# 6.12 Case 12: Sclerosing Lesion—Sclerosis Lobulitis

## 6.12.1 Clinical Presentation

The patient is a 36-year-old woman who had an abnormal area of enhancement on an MRI scan for further workup of a palpable mass in the right breast. The patient's recent mammogram was classified as BI-RAD 1 but was heterogeneously dense.

## 6.12.2 Ultrasound Findings

On B-mode imaging (▶ Fig. 6.12a) an isoechoic lesion with ill-defined borders is identified within glandular tissue. On color

Doppler (▶ Fig. 6.12b) there is no flow within the lesion. The lesion was classified as a BI-RADS category 3 lesion.

On strain imaging (▶ Fig. 6.12c) the lesion is stiffer than the adjacent glandular tissue. A fat lobule can be excluded based on this elastogram because the lesion is stiffer than other fat in the image as well as adjacent glandular tissue. If the lesion were a fat lobule it would have coded as soft as adjacent fat (white). The E/B ratio is difficult to calculate because the lesion's stiffness appears similar to that of the adjacent glandular tissue and cannot be accurately measured (▶ Fig. 6.12d). The strain ratio (lesion to fat ratio) is 3.35 (▶ Fig. 6.12e). On the 5-point color scale this lesion would be classified with a score of 3. On shear wave imaging (▶ Fig. 6.12f) the lesion has a Vs of 2.4 m/s (18 kPa).

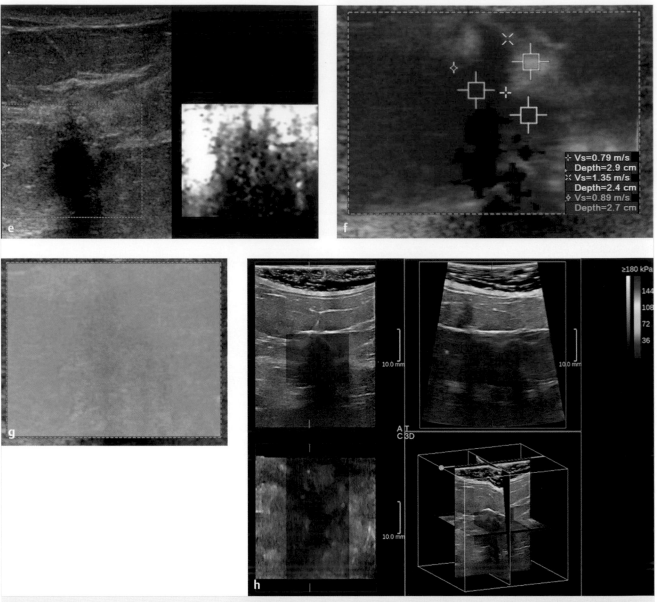

**Fig. 6.11** (*Continued*) (e) Using Virtual Touch Imaging (VTI, Siemens) (strain imaging using acoustic radiation force impulse [ARFI]) has similar findings to strain imaging using manual displacement (c). (f) On shear wave imaging a portion of the lesion does not color code, implying adequate shear waves were not generated. Other portions of the lesion have low Vs of 0.9 m/s (5 kPa). (g) The associated quality map codes yellow (poor quality) in the portions of the lesion that code blue in the velocity map (f). Thus the findings of low Vs should not be used in evaluation of the lesion. The quality map has greater sensitivity in evaluating the shear wave quality than the older algorithm that does not color code areas of poor shear waves. In this case, the area not color coded in the velocity map was rejected by the initial algorithm, but some areas with poor shear wave generation were color coded. The addition of the second algorithm (the quality map) rejects additional poor shear waves. (h) Three-dimensional shear wave elastography of the lesion. With this system the entire lesion has a low Vs of 2.6 m/s (20 kPa).

## 6.12.3 Diagnosis

Sclerosing lobulitis. The lesion was biopsied with a 12-gauge vacuum-assisted needle. The pathology was sclerosing lobulitis.

## 6.12.4 Discussion

Adenosis is an enlargement or excessive growth of lobular tissues (the outer end of the ducts). Sclerosing adenosis is a form of adenosis caused by distortion of the enlarged lobule by fi-

brous tissue. If a number of enlarged lobules are found near one another, the collection of lobules may be detected by palpation; otherwise, the condition is detected by mammography. Whether detected by palpation or by mammography, these lesions can be mistaken for cancer, so core needle biopsy is needed to determine whether cancer cells are present. In some instances, a surgical biopsy is required for a definitive diagnosis. Women with adenosis have about 1.5 to 2 times the risk of the general population for developing breast cancer.

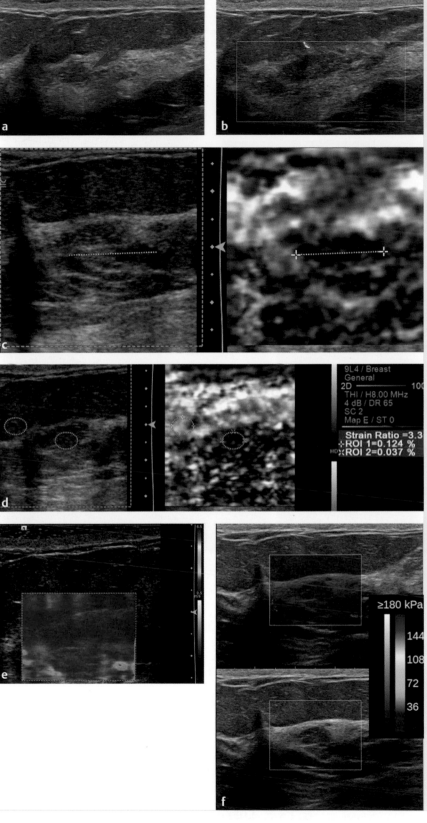

**Fig. 6.12** (a) On B-mode imaging there is a hypoechoic lesion (arrow) corresponding to the area of abnormality on the mammogram. The lesion is within an area of dense glandular tissue. (b) On color Doppler imaging there is minimal flow adjacent to the area of concern. (c) Strain imaging identifies a stiff area compared to adjacent fatty tissue. In this case the lesion is best identified on the elastogram. The lesion was measured on the elastogram (yellow dotted line) and the copy function used to locate the lesion on the B-mode image. Measuring the lesion on B-mode is problematic; therefore the E/B ratio cannot be accurately calculated. (d) The strain ratio (lesion to fat ratio) can be calculated measuring 3.3 suggestive of a benign lesion. (e) On shear wave imaging the lesion and surrounding area has a low Vs (blue) suggestive of a benign lesion. (f) Shear wave imaging on a different system also has similar benign findings.

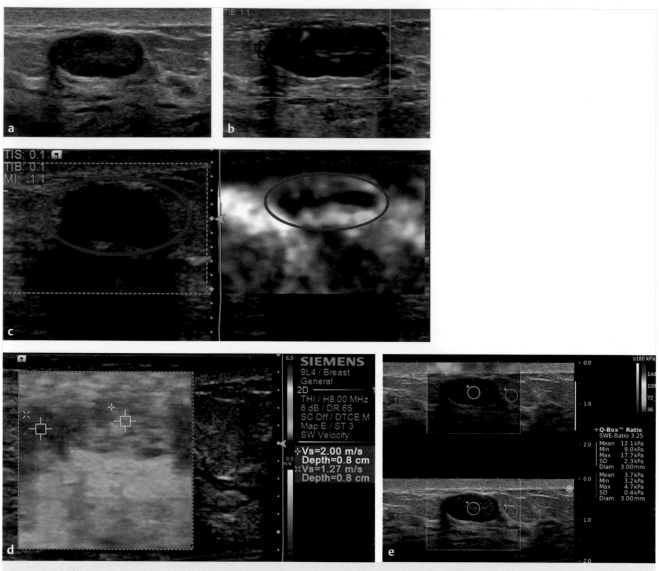

**Fig. 6.13** (a) The palpable mass is a 1.5 cm well circumscribed hypoechoic mass with refractive shadowing and through transmission. (b) On power Doppler imaging the lesion has moderate internal blood flow. (c) On strain elastography the lesion (circle) is mostly soft with stiffness similar to adjacent breast tissue. The lesion has a score of 2 on the 5-point color scale. The E/B ratio is less than 1, suggestive of a benign lesion. (d) On shear wave imaging the lesion has a Vs of 2 m/s (13 kPa) concordant with strain imaging of a benign lesion. (e) Shear wave imaging on a different system has similar benign findings with a Vs of 2 m/s (12.1 kPa).

In this case the lesion is stiffer than the adjacent breast tissue, but a closer look confirms that the stiff area on the strain elastogram also includes the adjacent glandular tissue. Therefore the lesion's stiffness is similar to that of glandular tissue, and an accurate E/B ratio cannot be caluclated, but it is probably benign. We can use the strain ratio (lesion to fat ratio) or the 5-point color scale, which in this case are both suggestive of a benign lesion. On both shear wave systems there is a low Vs suggestive of a benign lesion.

Based on the proposed elastography classification system (similar to the BI-RADS classification) presented in Chapter 5 we would consider this lesion to have an approximately 0% chance of malignancy.

# 6.13 Case 13: Fibroadenoma—Soft Fibroadenoma

## 6.13.1 Clinical Presentation

A 39-year-old woman presented with a palpable mass in the left breast. Mammography was not performed. Ultrasound was requested as the initial exam for workup.

## 6.13.2 Ultrasound Findings

B-mode imaging (▶ Fig. 6.13a) demonstrates a well-circumscribed 1.5 cm oval hypoechoic mass. There is moderate blood flow within the lesion on color Doppler imaging (▶ Fig. 6.13b). The lesion was classified as BI-RADS category 3.

On SE (▶ Fig. 6.13c) the lesion is stiffer than surrounding breast tissue and significantly smaller on the elastogram. On the 5-point color scale this lesion has a score of 3. On shear wave imaging (▶ Fig. 6.13d,e) the lesion has a Vs of 1.9 m/s (12 kPa) with the adjacent fat having a Vs of 0.7 m/s (3.7 kPa). Both the strain and shear wave findings are suggestive of a benign lesion.

### 6.13.3 Diagnosis

Fibroadenoma. The patient elected biopsy over a short-term follow-up. The lesion was biopsied using a 12-gauge vacuum-assisted core needle. The pathology was a fibroadenoma.

### 6.13.4 Discussion

Fibroadenomas are benign tumors made up of both glandular breast tissue and stromal (connective) tissue. They are most common in young women in their 20s and 30s, but they may be found in women of any age. The use of birth control pills before 20 is linked to an increased risk of fibroadenomas. Some fibroadenomas are too small to be palpated, but others can be several centimeters in length. They tend to be oval or round and have well defined distinct borders. They often feel like a marble within the breast. They can move under the skin and they are usually firm and not tender. Fibroadenomas can be solitary or multiple.

Fibroadenomas can be diagnosed by fine-needle aspiration (FNA) or core needle biopsy. Fibroadenomas may be simple, being composed of homogeneous tissue. But some fibroadenomas can contain other components (macrocysts, sclerosing adenosis, calcifications, or apocrine changes). These are called complex fibroadenomas. Women with fibroadenomas have been reported to have a slightly increased risk of breast cancer (about 1½ to 2 times the risk of women with no breast changes).

This case has the classical appearance of a fibroadenoma on ultrasound. The lesion is well circumscribed, is hypoechoic, and has refractive shadowing and through transmission. Lesions with this appearance are classified as BI-RADS category 3 lesions requiring short-term interval follow-up. Many women request biopsy to confirm the lesion is benign. If there are multiple bilateral well circumscribed cystic and solid lesions the lesions can be classified as BI-RADS 2, not requiring short-term interval follow-up. If there is a dominant lesion or a palpable lesion classification as BI-RADS category 2 should not be used. Elastography can be helpful to either upgrade or downgrade BI-RADS category 3 lesions. If the lesion has a benign appearance on SE and/or SWE the possibility of downgrading to BI-RADS category 2 has been suggested, but it is not yet suggested in the BI-RADS lexicon. Informing a patient that elastography is suggestive of a benign lesion may decrease the requests for biopsy and decrease the patient's concerns in waiting for a short-term interval follow-up.

The appearance of a fibroadenoma can be variable on elastography. A detailed study on the spectrum of fibroadenomas has not been published. In our experience the fibroadenomas can be very soft, as in this case, to very stiff, and in a small number of cases < 5% may have an E/B ratio and stiffness values suggestive of a malignant lesion. It is not known if the elastographic features can predict which fibroadenomas will continue to grow and have aggressive features.

Based on the proposed elastography classification system (similar to the BI-RADS classification) presented in Chapter 5 we would consider this lesion to have an approximately 0% chance of malignancy.

# 6.14 Case 14: Fibroadenoma— Intermediate Stiffness Fibroadenoma

## 6.14.1 Clinical Presentation

A 23-year-old woman presents with a new palpable mass in the right breast. Mammography was not performed. Ultrasound was requested as the initial imaging exam.

## 6.14.2 Ultrasound Findings

On B-mode imaging (▶ Fig. 6.14a) a 2.5 cm well circumscribed oval, wider than taller, heterogeneously hypoechoic mass was identified. The lesion has moderate blood flow on color Doppler imaging (▶ Fig. 6.14b). The lesion was classified as BI-RADS category 3.

The lesion has a similar stiffness to the adjacent breast tissue on strain imaging (▶ Fig. 6.14c). The lesion is classified with a score of 2 on the 5-point color scale. The lesion has an E/B ratio of 0.94 (▶ Fig. 6.14d) and a strain ratio (lesion to fat ratio) of 13.1 (▶ Fig. 6.14e). On VTI the lesion is stiffer than adjacent breast tissue with an E/B ratio of 0.9 (▶ Fig. 6.14f). On shear wave imaging the lesion has a Vs of 3.3 m/s (▶ Fig. 6.14g) on one system. On the other shear wave system (▶ Fig. 6.14h) the lesion has some areas with a Vs of 2.9 m/s (26 kPa) and a stiffer area with a Vs of 4.9 m/s (72 kPa). The adjacent fatty tissue has Vs of 2.4 m/s (18 kPa). On 3D SWE (▶ Fig. 6.14i) the lesion is shown to have heterogeneous stiffness with Vs ranging from 2.6 to 4.5 m/s (kPa values of 20–60).

## 6.14.3 Diagnosis

Fibroadenoma. The patient elected a biopsy instead of a short-term interval follow-up. The lesion was biopsied using a 12-gauge vacuum-assisted core needle. The pathology was a fibroadenoma.

## 6.14.4 Discussion

Fibroadenomas arise in the terminal duct lobular unit of the breast. They are the most common breast tumor in young women. They also occur in a small number of postmenopausal women. Their incidence declines with increasing age, and, in general, they appear before the age of 30. Fibroadenomas are partially hormone dependent and frequently regress after menopause.

Approximately 90% of fibroadenomas are < 3 cm in diameter. The vast majority of the remaining 10% that are 4 cm or larger occur mostly in women under 20 years of age. The tumor is round or ovoid, elastic, and nodular, and has a smooth surface.

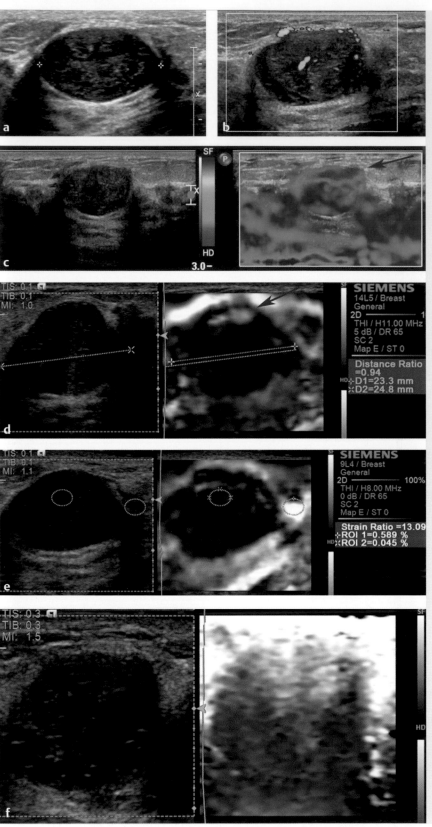

**Fig. 6.14** (a) The palpable mass is a 2.5 cm well circumscribed oval, wider than taller, heterogeneous hypoechoic mass. There is refractive shadowing and through transmission. (b) On power Doppler imaging the lesion has moderate internal blood flow. There are peripheral vessels that are parallel to the lesion surface. (c) On strain imaging using a color map with blue as hard demonstrates there is a soft area in the proximal portion of the lesion with the remainder of the lesion having a stiffness similar to the background tissues. The lesion has a score of 2 on the 5-point color scale. (d) The same lesion evaluated with strain elastography with a gray scale map. The lesion has the same soft area in the proximal portion of the lesion, and the remainder of the lesion is stiffer than surrounding tissue. The E/B ratio is 0.94 suggestive of a benign lesion. The borders of the lesion are better defined with the gray scale map as compared to the color map in (b). The yellow lines measure the lesion on B-mode and is copied to the elastogram. The green line measures the lesion on the elastogram. (e) The lesion has a strain ratio of 13.1 that is not concordant with the E/B ratio or the 5-point color scale. The fat measurement was taken in an area with shadowing and is softer than other fat in the image, suggesting it may be inaccurate. A repeat measurement using the "grayer" fat just proximal to this measurement has a strain value of 4 (not shown) now concordant with the E/B ratio and 5-point color scale. (f) On Virtual Touch imaging (VTI, Siemens) (strain imaging using acoustic radiation force impulse [ARFI]) the lesion appears as stiffer than surrounding tissue and slightly smaller, with an E/B ratio of 0.95. Note that the proximal portion of the lesion is softer similar to the strain images obtained with the manual displacement technique. (*Continued*)

The cut surface usually appears as homogeneous, firm, and gray–white or tan in color. The pericanalicular type (hard) has a whirly appearance with a complete capsule, whereas the intracanalicular type (soft) has an incomplete capsule.[75]

A growth rate of < 16% per month in women under 50 years of age, and a growth rate of < 13% per month in women over 50 years of age have been published as safe growth rates for continued nonoperative treatment and clinical observation.[76]

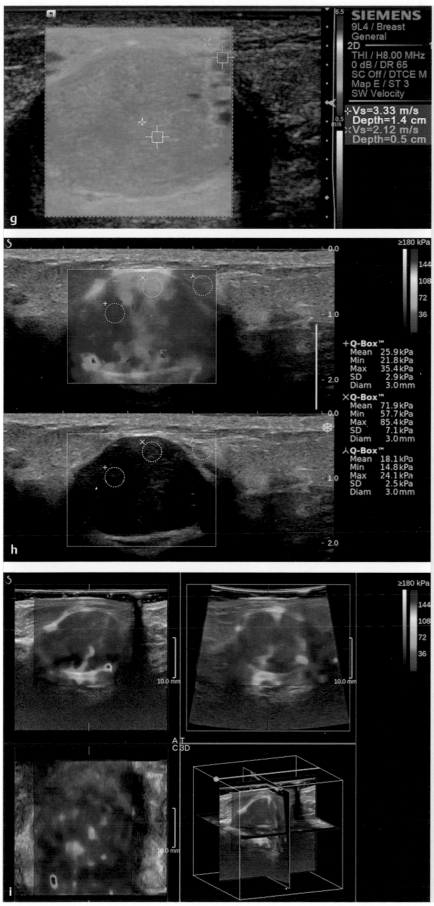

**Fig. 6.14** (*Continued*) (g) On shear wave imaging the lesion has a Vs of 3.3 m/s (32 kPa) consistent with the strain imaging findings of a benign lesion. (h) Three-dimensional (3D) SWE has similar findings as (g). (i) The same lesion using 3D shear wave elastography provides a better assessment of the stiffness throughout the entire lesion

The conventional ultrasound in this case is similar to that in Case 6.13. However, the elastographic features are very different. The fibroadenoma in Case 6.13 was very soft, whereas in this case the lesion is fairly stiff. In our experience there is a wide range of elastographic findings in fibroadenomas from very soft to very stiff. A small number (< 5%) of fibroadenomas in our experience are stiff enough to be suggestive of malignant lesions on SE and SWE. It is unknown if the elastographic features are predictive of the histology of the lesions, or if it can predict which fibroadenomas will be prone to grow rapidly.

The elastographic changes of a fibroadenoma can also change over time, and the elastographic features may reflect the hormonal changes (see Case 6.34, this chapter).

Based on the proposed elastography classification system (similar to the BI-RADS classification) presented in Chapter 5 we would consider this lesion to have a 2 to 95% chance of malignancy (~ 0% on SE; 2–95% on SWE).

## 6.15 Case 15: Fibroadenoma—Stiffer Fibroadenoma

### 6.15.1 Clinical Presentation

A 74-year-old presented woman with a remote history of invasive ductal carcinoma in the left breast. The patient is status postlumpectomy, chemotherapy, and radiation therapy. The patient now has a new mass in her left breast 3 cm inferior to her surgical scar. On a diagnostic mammogram there was the interval development of an 8 mm density. The mammogram was classified as BI-RADS category 0, and an ultrasound was requested for further workup.

### 6.15.2 Ultrasound Findings

On B-mode imaging (▶ Fig. 6.15a) a 5.5 mm well circumscribed oval hypoechoic lesion is identified. On color Doppler imaging (not shown) there was no blood flow within the lesion. The lesion was classified as a BI-RADS category 3 lesion.

On strain imaging the lesion has an E/B ratio of 1.3 (▶ Fig. 6.15b) and a lesion to fat ratio of 7.7 (▶ Fig. 6.15c). On the 5-point color scale this would be classified with a score of 4. On VTI imaging (▶ Fig. 6.15d) the lesion is stiffer than adjacent glandular tissue and appears larger than on B-mode. All the SE findings are suggestive of a malignant lesion. On shear wave imaging the lesion has a Vs of 1.6 m/s (9 kPa) on one system (▶ Fig. 6.15e) and a Vs of 1.9 m/s (11.4 kPa) (▶ Fig. 6.15f) on another. Both shear wave systems have findings suggestive of a benign lesion.

### 6.15.3 Diagnosis

Sclerosed fibroadenoma. Based on the strain elastography finding the lesion was upgraded to a BI-RADS 4A, and biopsy was recommended. The lesion was biopsied using a 12-gauge vacuum-assisted core biopsy needle. The pathology was a sclerosed fibroadenoma.

### 6.15.4 Discussion

Although fibroadenomas can be located anywhere in the breast, there may be a predilection toward the upper outer quadrant.

On mammography fibroadenomas have a spectrum of features from the well circumscribed discrete mass to the multilobulated mass. They may contain popcorn calcification. Calcification may also present as microcalcifications, which makes differentiation from malignancy very difficult. The lesions are especially prone to calcification in the postmenopausal woman, and the process is part of involution of the breast as a function of age.

On ultrasound fibroadenomas are typically seen as a well circumscribed, round to ovoid, or macrolobulated mass with generally uniform hypoechogenicity. Intralesional sonographically detectable calcification may be seen in ~ 10% of cases. Sometimes a *thin* echogenic rim or pseudocapsule may be seen sonographically.

On MRI scan fibroadenomas usually have the following findings:
1. **T1**—typically hypointense or isointense compared with adjacent breast tissue
2. **T2**—can be hypo- or hyperintense
3. **T1 C+(Gd)**—can be variable but a majority will show slow initial contrast enhancement and a persistent delayed phase (type I enhancement curve); nonenhancing internal septations may be seen

This case is the other part of the spectrum of elastographic findings of fibroadenomas compared with Case 13. This fibroadenoma has SE findings suggestive of a malignant lesion. The SWE findings are suggestive of a benign lesion. The discordant findings on SE and SWE should raise concerns about the lesion. The elastographic findings in this case cannot be used to downgrade the BI-RADS category score.

Based on the proposed elastography classification system (similar to the BI-RADS classification) presented in Chapter 5 we would consider this lesion to have a > 95% chance of malignancy (> 95% on SE and ~ 0% on SWE).

## 6.16 Case 16: Fibroadenoma—Stiffer Fibroadenoma

### 6.16.1 Clinical Presentation

A 28-year-old woman presented with a new palpable mass in the right breast. Ultrasound was requested as the initial imaging modality. Mammography was not performed.

### 6.16.2 Ultrasound Findings

On B-mode imaging (▶ Fig. 6.16a) a 2.2 cm well circumscribed hypoechoic lesion with some angular margins is identified. There is moderate blood flow within the lesion on color Doppler imaging (▶ Fig. 6.16b). The lesion was classified as BI-RADS category 4A due to the angular margins.

On SE the lesion is stiffer than adjacent breast tissue and has an E/B ratio of 0.63 (▶ Fig. 6.16c) and a lesion to fat ratio of 2.45 (▶ Fig. 6.16d). The lesion would have a score of 3 on the 5-point color scale. On shear wave imaging (▶ Fig. 6.16e) the lesion has a max Vs of 2.5 m/s (18 kPa). On 3D SWE (▶ Fig. 6.16f) the lesion did not color code, but the surrounding tissue all color codes with a low Vs. All SE and SWE findings are suggestive of a benign lesion.

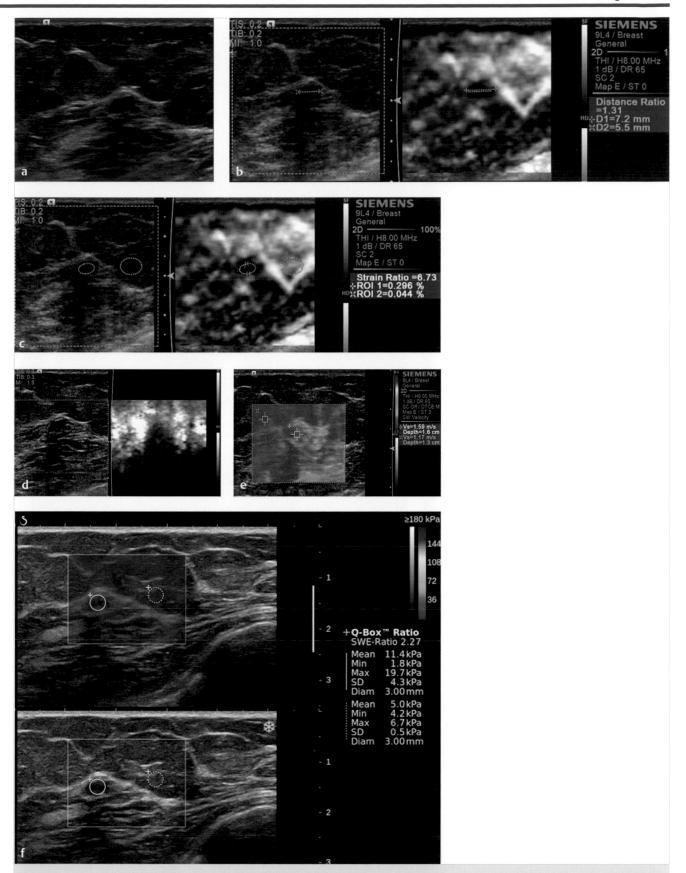

**Fig. 6.15** (a) The new density on the patient's mammogram was a 5.5 mm oval hypoechoic mass on B-mode ultrasound. No blood flow was identified in the lesion on color Doppler (not shown). (b) On strain imaging the lesion is stiffer than adjacent tissue and has an E/B ratio of 1.3, suggestive of a malignant lesion. The lesion has a score of 5 on the 5-point color scale. The lesion measures 5.5 mm on B-mode (yellow line) and 7.2 mm on SE (green line). (c) The lesion has a strain ratio (lesion to fat ratio) of 6.7 also suggestive of a malignant lesion. (d) On Virtual Touch Imaging (VTI, Siemens) (strain imaging using acoustic radiation force impulse [ARFI]) the lesion is stiffer than the surrounding tissue and has an EI/B ratio of > 1. (e) On shear wave imaging the lesion has a Vs of 1.6 m/s (8 kPa) suggestive of a benign lesion, not concordant with the strain results. (f) Similar benign finding are obtained with a different shear wave system (Vs of 1.9 m/s; 11 kPa).

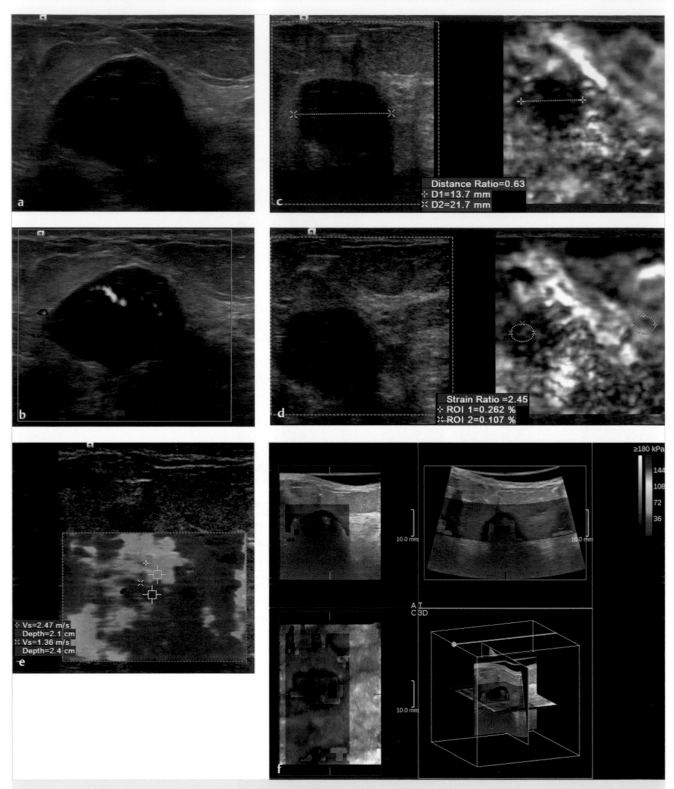

**Fig. 6.16** (a) The palpable mass is a slightly lobulated well circumscribed hypoechoic lesion on B-mode imaging. (b) There is internal blood flow noted on power Doppler imaging. (c) The lesion is stiffer than surrounding tissue with an E/B ratio of 0.6. The lesion has a score of 3 on the 5-point color scale, both suggestive of a benign lesion. The lesion measures 21.7 mm (yellow line left image) on B-mode and 13.7 mm (yellow line on right image) in SE. (d) On strain elastography the strain ratio (lesion to fat ratio) is 2.5, concordant with the other strain findings as suggestive of a benign lesion. (e) On shear wave imaging the lesion has a Vs of 2.5 m/s (19 kPa) suggestive of a benign lesion and concordant with the strain findings. (f) On three-dimensional (3D) shear wave imaging the lesion does not color code, and there is no increased Vs around the lesion. The lesion does not color code on the 3D shear wave images, most likely secondary to the lesion depth. Note that there is no color coding in the adjacent tissues at about the mid depth of the lesion.

### 6.16.3 Diagnosis

Fibroadenoma. The lesion was biopsied using a 12-gauge vacuum-assisted needle. The pathology was fibroadenoma.

### 6.16.4 Discussion

The conventional ultrasound findings in this fibroadenoma are slightly more suspicious, with the lesion being more round than oval and slightly lobulated. The SE findings and the SWE findings are concordant with a benign lesion. On the 3D strain images the lesion does not color code and therefore can be assessed as benign or malignant. The 2D SWE findings are suggestive of a benign lesion. The non–color coding on the 3D image can be secondary to the lesion being at a depth where the ARFI is attenuated and shear waves are not generated.

In this case the E/B ratio is 0.6, which is quite low. Although it has been suggested that an increasing E/B ratio in malignant lesions is suggestive of a higher tumor grade,[28] it is not known if a lower E/B ratio in benign lesions is more predictive of benignity. This case has conventional findings of a BI-RADS category 4A lesion. Downgrading one BI-RADS category based on elastographic findings would change the follow-up to a BI-RADS category 3. With the concordant findings of a benign lesion on SE and SWE and a very low E/B ratio consid-

eration of downgrading to a BI-RADS 2 lesion is an area of active research.

Based on the proposed elastography classification system (similar to the BI-RADS classification) presented in Chapter 5 we would consider this lesion to have an approximately 0% chance of malignancy.

## 6.17 Case 17: Fibroadenoma—False-Positive Fibroadenoma

### 6.17.1 Clinical Presentation

The patient is a 50-year-old female who has had a stable 1.6 cm lobular mass in her left breast, upper outer quadrant, which has been stable for 5 years on mammography. The patient feels the lump is increasing in size. Ultrasound is performed for further evaluation.

### 6.17.2 Ultrasound Findings

On B-mode ultrasound (▶ Fig. 6.17a) a 1.9 cm well circumscribed lobular hypoechoic mass is identified. The mass has increased in size since an ultrasound 3 years prior, when it measured 1.6 cm. The mass has moderate internal blood flow

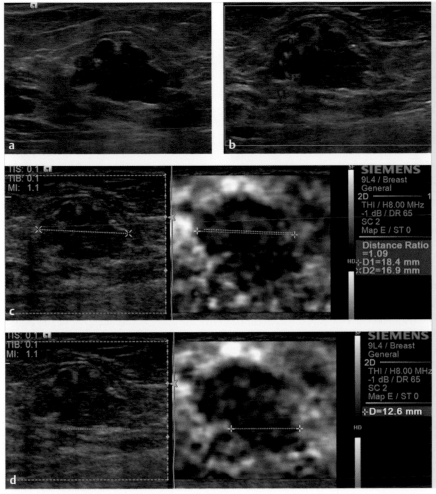

**Fig. 6.17** (a) The palpable mass in the left breast, which the patient believes is increasing in size, is a lobular well circumscribed hypoechoic mass with through transmission. (b) There is moderate blood flow in the lesion on power Doppler. (c) On strain imaging the lesion is stiffer than surrounding tissue. The lesion measures 16.9 mm (yellow line) on B-mode and 18.4 mm (green line) on SE with an E/B ratio of 1.1. The lesion has a score of 5 on the 4-point color scale, both suggestive of a malignant lesion. (d) Strain imaging in a different position demonstrates a stiff area (yellow line) in the posterior portion of the mass without a corresponding B-mode abnormality. (*Continued*)

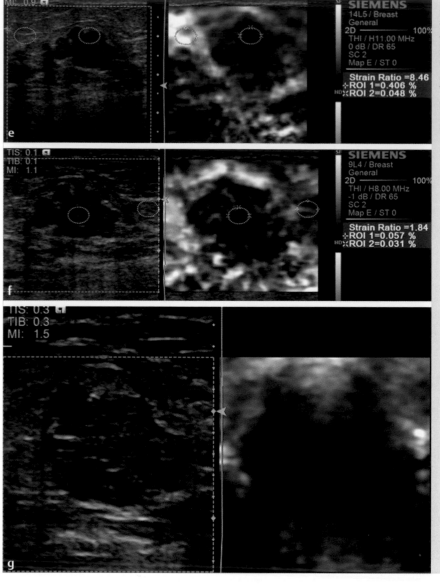

**Fig. 6.17** (*Continued*) (e) The strain ratio (lesion to fat ratio) is 8.5, consistent with the other strain findings suspicious for malignancy. (f) A repeat strain ratio using adjacent fat that is not as "soft" (white) is 1.8, now suggestive of a benign lesion. (g) The lesion is stiffer than adjacent tissue on Virtual Touch imaging (VTI, Siemens) (strain imaging with acoustic radiation force impulse [ARFI]) and appears larger than in the B-mode imaging. (*Continued*)

on color Doppler (▶ Fig. 6.17b). The lesion was classified as BI-RADS category 4B.

On strain imaging the lesion is stiffer than adjacent breast tissue and has an E/B ratio of 1.1 (▶ Fig. 6.17c). There is a stiffer area in the inferior portion of the lesion that appears as normal breast tissue on B-mode imaging (▶ Fig. 6.17d). The lesion to fat ratio is 8.5 (▶ Fig. 6.17e) on one image and 1.8 using a different location (▶ Fig. 6.17f) as the reference. On VTI (▶ Fig. 6.17g) the lesion is stiffer than surrounding breast tissue and appears larger than on the B-mode imaging, with an E/B ratio of 1.2. The lesion has a score of 5 on the 5-point color scale. The SE findings are more suggestive of a malignant lesion. On shear wave imaging the lesion has a Vs of 2.7 m/s (22 kPa) on one system (▶ Fig. 6.17h) and a Vs of 3.8 m/s (42 kPa) (▶ Fig. 6.17i) on another system, both suggestive of a benign lesion.

### 6.17.3 Diagnosis

Fibroadenoma. The lesion was biopsied under ultrasound guidance with a 12-gauge vacuum-assisted needle. The lesion

was a fibroadenoma. The patient elected to have the lesion removed surgically. The pathology at surgical resection was fibroadenoma.

### 6.17.4 Discussion

This case has conventional findings that are not classic for a fibroadenoma. On SE the findings are suggestive of a malignant lesion. In addition on strain there is the question of the lesion having a component on the posterior portion of the lesion that is not identified on B-mode imaging. On surgical resection of the lesion there was no evidence of malignancy. Unfortunately the pathology was not evaluated to determine the etiology of the area of stiffness not identified on B-mode imaging.

The SE and SWE findings are discordant in this case. The SE findings are suggestive of a malignant lesion, whereas the SWE findings are suggestive of a benign lesion. A reason for the discordant findings is not evident in this case. The lesion is well identified on both B-mode imaging and SE. The lesion is surrounded by fatty tissue; therefore the E/B ratio cannot be

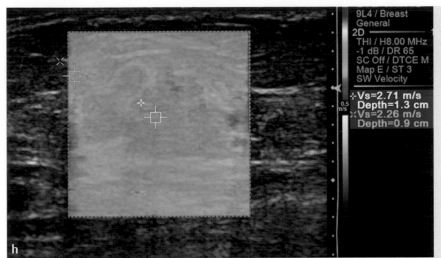

9L4 / Breast
General
2D
THI / H8.00 MHz
-1 dB / DR 65
SC Off / DTCE M
Map E / ST 3
SW Velocity

Vs=2.71 m/s
Depth=1.3 cm
Vs=2.26 m/s
Depth=0.9 cm

**Fig. 6.17** (*Continued*) (h) On shear wave imaging the lesion has a Vs of 2.7 m/s (21 kPa) consistent with a benign lesion and not concordant with the strain E/B ratio or the 5-point color scale. (i) Similar results are obtained with a different shear wave system.

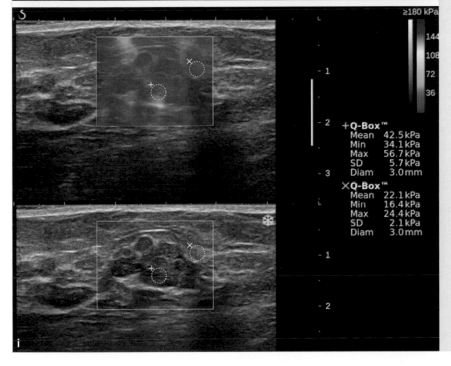

≥180 kPa

144

108

72

36

+Q-Box™
Mean 42.5 kPa
Min 34.1 kPa
Max 56.7 kPa
SD 5.7 kPa
Diam 3.0 mm
×Q-Box™
Mean 22.1 kPa
Min 16.4 kPa
Max 24.4 kPa
SD 2.1 kPa
Diam 3.0 mm

artificially elevated due to the lesion's blending in with glandular tissue on the elastogram. Also, if this were the case, the strain ratio (lesion to fat ratio) is 8.5, suggesting the lesion is much stiffer than normal glandular tissue, which usually has a strain ratio of 1.5 to 2.5. The quality map was green in this case, suggesting that the shear wave results are of high quality.

Because we cannot identify a reason why there are discordant findings on SE and SWE, the more suspicious findings should be used to determine the workup. In this case the elastographic findings should increase the suspicion for malignancy. Further investigation into why the elastographic findings are discordant as in this case, with the lesion appearing significantly stiffer on SE than on SWE, is needed. This constellation of elastographic findings is sometimes identified in malignant lesions; however, in the vast majority of these cases the quality map on SWE is of poor quality, confirming that the SWE data

are not reliable and more weight should be given to the SE findings (see Chapter 4.3.3).

Based on the proposed elastography classification system (similar to the BI-RADS classification) presented in Chapter 5 we would consider this lesion to have a 95% chance of malignancy (95% on SE and ~ 0% on SWE).

## 6.18 Case 18: Papillary Lesion– Hyalinized Intraductal Papilloma

### 6.18.1 Clinical Presentation

A 64-year-old woman presented with an enlarging left retroareolar mass on screening mammography. The mammogram was classified as BI-RADS category 0, and ultrasound was advised for further workup.

## 6.18.2 Ultrasound Findings

On B-mode imaging (▶ Fig. 6.18a) a 9 mm well circumscribed oval lesion with both cystic and solid components is identified. The lesion has significant peripheral blood flow on color Doppler imaging (▶ Fig. 6.18b). The lesion was classified as a BI-RADS category 4B lesion.

On strain imaging (▶ Fig. 6.18c) the cystic component has the bull's-eye artifact. The solid components appear stiffer than surrounding breast tissue. The solid component of the lesion has a lesion to fat ratio of 2.8 (▶ Fig. 6.18d). On the 5-point color scale this lesion would have a score of 2. On shear wave imaging the max Vs is 5 m/s (75 kPa), and no signal is identified in a portion of the cystic lesion (▶ Fig. 6.18e). The quality map of this shear wave elastogram (▶ Fig. 6.18f) has poor quality in the area of the cyst. On another shear wave system (▶ Fig. 6.18g) the max Vs is 4.2 m/s (52 kPa), and the cystic area does not color code, suggesting that it contains simple fluid.

## 6.18.3 Diagnosis

Hyalinized intraductal papilloma. The lesion was biopsied using a 12-gauge vacuum-assisted core biopsy under ultra-sound guidance. The pathology was a hyalinized intraductal papilloma.

## 6.18.4 Discussion

Papillomas of the breast can be divided into solitary papillomas, multiple papillomas, and juvenile papillomatosis. Solitary or central papillomas arise in the large retroareolar ducts. Pathologically, a papilloma is a masslike projection that consists of papillary fronds attached to the inner mammary duct wall by a fibrovascular core that is covered with ductal epithelial and myoepithelial cells. Ductal epithelial cells may undergo apocrine metaplasia, hyperplasia, or atypia.

Clinically, solitary papillomas commonly occur in perimenopausal women. Patients commonly present with spontaneous nipple discharge that may be bloody, serous, or clear. Women with solitary papillomas have a slightly increased risk of developing breast carcinoma (1.5–2 times greater).[77]

Central papillomas are usually solitary, but multiple central papillomas have been reported.[78] Central papillomas are typically small and are often mammographically occult. Sonography or ductography is usually necessary for visualization of the lesion. A solitary papilloma occasionally appears on mammography as a circumscribed retroareolar mass or as a

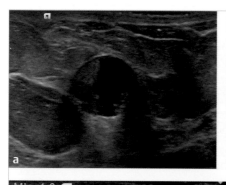
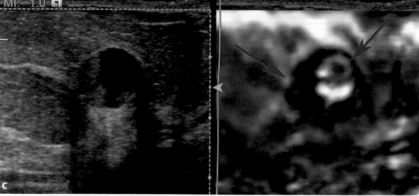
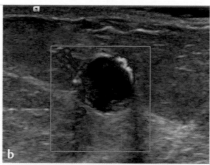
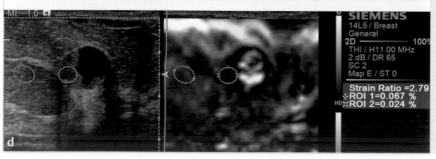

**Fig. 6.18** (a) The mass noted on mammography is a 9 mm well circumscribed, mixed solid and cystic lesion with through transmission on B-mode imaging. (b) There is significant blood flow in the periphery of the lesion on power Doppler imaging. (c) On strain elastography there is a bull's-eye artifact in the cystic portion of the lesion (arrow). The solid component is stiffer than surrounding breast tissue (dotted arrow). The lesion has an E/B ratio of 1. The lesion has a score of 2 on the 5-point color scale. (d) The solid component of the lesion has a strain ratio (lesion to fat ratio) of 2.8 on strain imaging, suggestive of a benign lesion. (*Continued*)

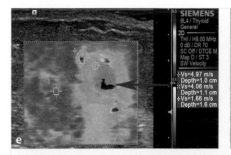

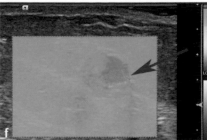

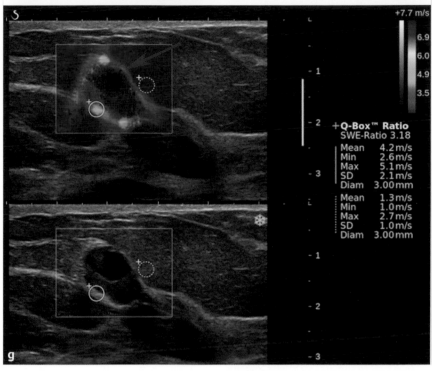

+Q-Box™ Ratio
SWE-Ratio 3.18

| | |
|---|---|
| Mean | 4.2 m/s |
| Min | 2.6 m/s |
| Max | 5.1 m/s |
| SD | 2.1 m/s |
| Diam | 3.00 mm |
| Mean | 1.3 m/s |
| Min | 1.0 m/s |
| Max | 2.7 m/s |
| SD | 1.0 m/s |
| Diam | 3.00 mm |

**Fig. 6.18** (*Continued*) (e) On shear wave imaging the central portion of the lesion is not color coded (arrow), consistent with the strain elastography findings of simple fluid. The other wall of the lesion and solid components has a Vs maximum of 5 m/s (75 kPa), suggestive of a malignant lesion and more suspicious than the strain findings. (f) The quality map confirms that the portion not color coded in the shear wave image (e) has poor-quality shear waves. In the areas with high Vs on the shear wave image the shear wave quality is good. (g) On a different shear wave system the cystic portion also does not color code (arrow), consistent with strain and the other shear wave system. The rim has areas of stiffness measuring up to 4.2 m/s (52 kPa), less suggestive of malignancy than the other shear wave system.

solitary dilated retroareolar duct. These lesions rarely calcify. On sonography, a papilloma is seen as an intraductal mass in a dilated duct, an intracystic mass, or a solid mass with a well-defined border.[77] Ductography may show an intraluminal filling defect or ductal dilatation due to partial or complete ductal obstruction. Recently, MRI has been reported to be a useful adjunct technique to detect intraductal papilloma of the breast.[79]

The characteristic ultrasound finding of a papilloma is a solid mural nodule within a dilated duct. Other features include an intracystic mass or a well circumscribed hypoechoic solid mass. Ductal dilation may be the only finding in a small papilloma. The vascular pedicle within the mural nodule can often be identified on color Doppler imaging. Ductography may show an intraluminal filling defect, ductal dilation, ductal wall irregularity, and distortion. Atypical papillomas may have imaging features similar to benign papillomas, and the diagnosis is usually based on histopathology.

Differentiating benign from malignant papillary lesions can be difficult. A nonparallel orientation, echogenic halo, posterior acoustic enhancement, and associated microcalcifications are reported to be more frequent in malignant lesions.[80]

A classification based on the relationship between the mass and the duct on sonography has been proposed; type I, intraluminal mass; type II, extraductal mass; type III, purely solid mass; type IV, mixed. Type I was subdivided into intraductal type, intracystic type, and solid type with an anechoic rim, depending on the degree of expansion and filling of the duct by the mass.[81]

This lesion has the appearance of a complex cystic lesion on conventional ultrasound. The SE demonstrates that the anechoic portion of the lesion is low-viscosity fluid because a bull's-eye artifact is present. The "solid" component of the mass is stiffer than surrounding tissue with an E/B ratio and strain ratio (lesion to fat ratio) suggestive of a benign lesion. Based on the SE finding the lesion can be a complicated cyst with adherent debris or high-viscosity fluid as the "solid" components or a benign complex cystic lesion. The SWE findings are not concordant with the SE findings because the "solid" component has elevated Vs.

Based on the proposed elastography classification system (similar to the BI-RADS classification) presented in Chapter 5 we would consider this lesion to have a 2–95% chance of malignancy (~ 0% on SE; 2–95% on SWE).

# 6.19 Case 19: Papillary Lesion—Intraductal Papilloma

## 6.19.1 Clinical Presentation

The patient is a 37-year-old woman who presents with a palpable right retroareolar mass and occasional white discharge. Mammography was not performed.

## 6.19.2 Ultrasound Findings

On B-mode imaging (▶ Fig. 6.19a) an isoechoic, well circumscribed, wider than taller lesion is identified. The lesion does not have internal blood flow on color Doppler imaging (▶ Fig. 6.19b). The lesion was classified as BI-RADS category 3 based on the conventional ultrasound findings.

On strain imaging (▶ Fig. 6.19c) the lesion is more conspicuous and stiffer than the surrounding breast tissue. The E/B ratio is 0.95. The lesion has a score of 3 on the 5-point color scale (▶ Fig. 6.19d). The strain ratio (lesion to fat ratio) is 3.8 (not shown). On shear wave imaging the lesion has a maximum Vs

of 3.5 m/s (38 kPa) on one system (▶ Fig. 6.19e) and a Vs of 2.1 m/s (14 kPa) on a different system (▶ Fig. 6.19f), both suggestive of a benign lesion.

## 6.19.3 Diagnosis

Intraductal papilloma. The lesion was biopsied with a 12-gauge vacuum-assisted needle under ultrasound guidance. The pathology was intraductal papilloma and mild stromal fibrosis.

## 6.19.4 Discussion

Classifying papillary lesions of the breast on core biopsy is challenging. Although traditionally all such lesions were surgically excised, at present, conservative management of benign lesions is being advocated; therefore, accurately classifying papillary lesions on core biopsy is all the more imperative. The change in diagnoses from core biopsy to surgical excision according to subspecialist training in breast pathology and interobserver agreement between specialized breast pathologists and nonbreast pathologists in classifying these lesions has been studied.[82]

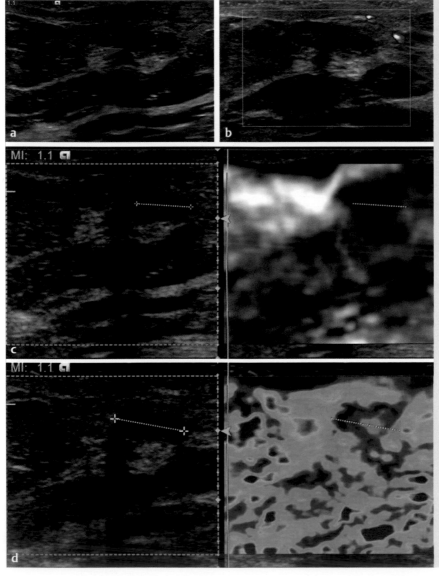

**Fig. 6.19** (a) At the site of the palpable abnormality B-mode imaging identifies an isoechoic, well circumscribed, wider than taller lesion. (b) On power Doppler imaging the lesion does not have blood flow. (c) On strain imaging the lesion (yellow line) is stiffer than surrounding tissue with an E/B ratio of 0.95. The lesion has increased conspicuity on strain imaging compared to B-mode imaging. The lesion has a score of 3 on the 5-point color scale. (d) The same image as in (c) using a color map (blue is stiff). Choice of the color map (colors or gray scale) is a personal preference. We prefer the gray scale map—we believe we can better define the lesion with a gray scale because there are not marked color changes in some areas with small changes in stiffness. The lesion is marked with the yellow line. (*Continued*)

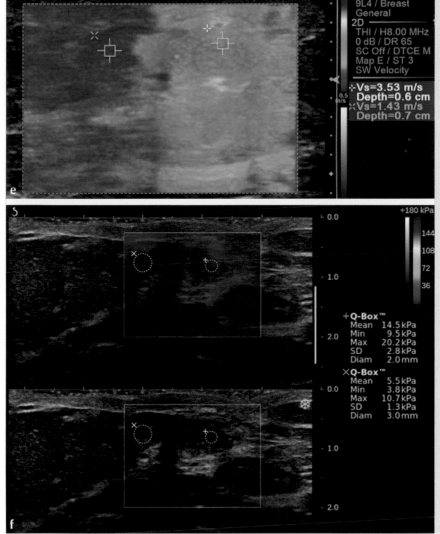

Fig. 6.19 (*Continued*) (e) On shear wave imaging the lesion has increased stiffness to surrounding breast tissue with a Vs of 3.5 m/s (38 kPa), suggestive of a benign lesion similar to the strain elastography findings. (f) Shear wave imaging on a different system also demonstrates the lesion has a Vs suggestive of a benign lesion.

This lesion does not contain a cystic component. The SE findings of an E/B ratio of 0.95, a score of 3 on the 5-point scale, and a strain ratio of 3.8 are all suggestive of a benign finding. The SWE finding of Vs of 3.5 m/s (38 kPa) are also suggestive of a benign lesion. The SE and SWE findings are concordant. In this case it is appropriate to consider downgrading the lesion to BI-RADS 2.

Based on the proposed elastography classification system (similar to the BI-RADS classification) presented in Chapter 5 we would consider this lesion to have an approximately 0% chance of malignancy.

# 6.20 Case 20: Papillary Lesion— Intraductal Papillomatosis

## 6.20.1 Clinical Presentation

The patient is a 64-year-old woman who was diagnosed at an outside facility with a 7 mm lobular mass in the right breast on ultrasound. The ultrasound was performed for increased density on a screening mammogram. The lesion was classified as BI-RADS 4A at the outside facility, and biopsy was recommended.

## 6.20.2 Ultrasound Findings

On B-mode imaging (▶ Fig. 6.20a) a 0.9 cm well circumscribed hypoechoic lesion with some angular margins is identified. There was a question of microcalcifications within the mass. On color Doppler imaging there is a small amount of internal blood flow (▶ Fig. 6.20b). The lesion was classified as BI-RADS category 4A.

On strain imaging (▶ Fig. 6.20c) the lesion is stiffer than adjacent breast tissue with an E/B ratio of 0.96. The lesion has a score of 3 on the 5-point color scale and a strain ratio (lesion to fat ratio) of 3. On shear wave imaging (▶ Fig. 6.20d) the Vs of the lesion is 3 m/s (27 kPa), with adjacent fatty tissue having a Vs of 1.3 m/s (6 kPa). On a different shear wave system (▶ Fig. 6.20e) the lesion had a Vs of 3.4 m/s (33 kPa), with the adjacent fatty tissue having a Vs of 1.5 m/s (8 kPa).

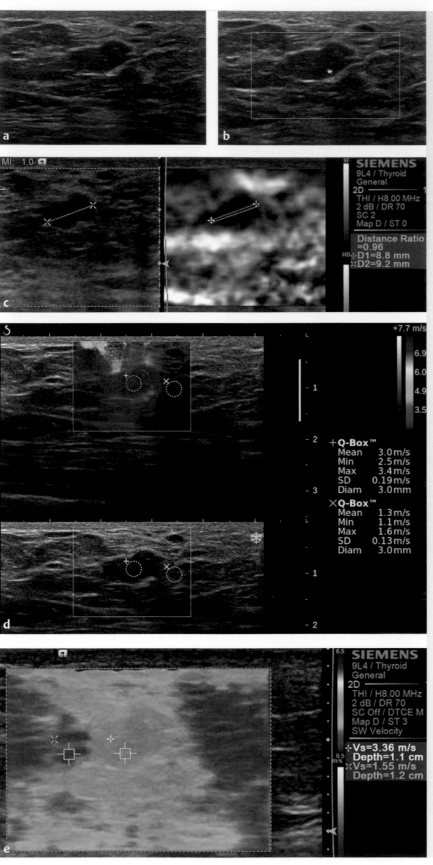

**Fig. 6.20** (a) On B-mode imaging the lesion is a 9 mm well circumscribed, isoechoic, irregular mass (arrows). (b) On color Doppler there is some flow within the lesion. (c) On strain imaging the lesion is stiffer than surrounding breast tissue. The lesion measures 9.2 mm on B-mode (yellow line) and 8.8 mm on elastography (green line) with an E/B ratio of 0.96. On the 5-point color scale the lesion has a score of 3. (d) On shear wave imaging the lesion has a Vs max of 3 m/s (27 kPa) compared with the background fatty tissue with a Vs max of 1.3 m/s (7 kPa). The shear wave findings are concordant with the strain findings of a benign lesion. (e) Shear wave imaging on a different system has similar results.

### 6.20.3 Diagnosis

Intraductal papillomatosis, apocrine metaplasia, proliferative fibrocystic changes with typical duct epithelial hyperplasia, and nodular stromal fibrosis. The lesion was biopsied using a 12-gauge vacuum-assisted needle under ultrasound guidance. The pathology was intraductal papillomatosis, apocrine metaplasia, proliferative fibrocystic changes with typical duct epithelial hyperplasia, and nodular stromal fibrosis.

### 6.20.4 Discussion

Multiple or peripheral papillomas arise in the terminal ductal lobular units. The basic histopathological features are similar to those of central papillomas, but ductal epithelial cells are more frequently associated with hyperplasia, atypia, DCIS, or invasive carcinoma, as well as with sclerosing adenosis or a radial scar. There is an increased risk of carcinoma in these patients that is related to the presence of proliferative epithelial change. Clinically, patients commonly present with palpable masses. Multiple papillomas are usually found bilaterally, and recurrence after surgical treatment is more common.[78] Mammographic findings of multiple papillomas are variable and include round, oval, or slightly lobulated well circumscribed or spiculated masses with or without calcifications, foci of microcalcifications, clusters of nodules, and asymmetric density. On sonography, multiple papillomas are seen as round, oval, or lobulated circumscribed solid masses or complex masses.[83]

This lesion has all benign characteristics on SE, an E/B ratio of 0.96, a score of 3 on the 5-point color scale, and a strain ratio (lesion to fat ratio) of 3. The SWE findings are also suggestive of a benign lesion with Vs of 3.4 m/s (33 kPa) or less. The SE and SWE findings are concordant. It is appropriate to consider downgrading this lesion from BI-RADS category 4A to BI-RADS category 3. Further studies are needed to determine if it is appropriate to downgrade the lesion to BI-RADS category 2.

Based on the proposed elastography classification system (similar to the BI-RADS classification) presented in Chapter 5 we would consider this lesion to have an approximately 0% chance of malignancy.

## 6.21 Case 21: Papillary Lesion—Intraductal Papilloma

### 6.21.1 Clinical Presentation

The patient is a 60-year-old woman referred for ultrasound evaluation of a new 1 cm lesion on screening mammography. The mammogram was classified as BI-RADS 0, and an ultrasound was advised for further workup.

### 6.21.2 Ultrasound Findings

On B-mode imaging (▶ Fig. 6.21a) a 1.3 cm hypoechoic well circumscribed lesion with some angular margins in the retro-

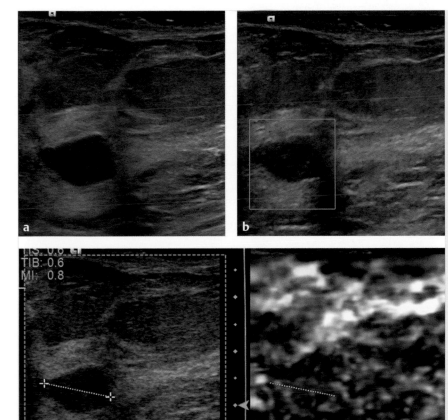

**Fig. 6.21** (a) The new mass identified on mammography is a 1 cm well circumscribed hypoechoic lesion with some lobulations. (b) On power Doppler imaging there is some internal blood flow noted. (c) On strain elastography the lesion has similar stiffness as the surrounding glandular tissue making it hard to calculate the E/B ratio (yellow lines). The E/B ratio is estimated at 0.9. The lesion has a score of 2 or 3 on the 5-point color scale. Because the lesion stiffness is similar to glandular tissue the lesion is most likely benign. (*Continued*)

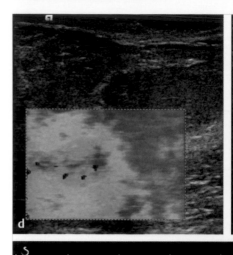

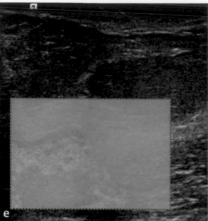

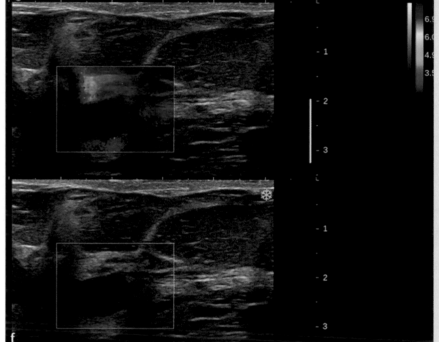

**Fig. 6.21** (*Continued*) (d) On shear wave imaging the lesion has a Vs of 3 m/s (27 kPa) concordant with the strain findings of a benign lesion. (e) The quality map has areas of yellow (poor quality) in the central portion of the lesion. The shear wave findings should be used with low confidence. (f) Shear wave imaging of the lesion on a different system has the lesion not color coded, consistent with poor-quality shear waves as noted in the other shear wave system (d,e).

areolar region of the right breast is identified. There is a small amount of blood flow in the lesion on color Doppler imaging (▶ Fig. 6.21b). The lesion was calcified as BI-RADS category 4A.

On SE (▶ Fig. 6.21c) the lesion is similar in stiffness to the surrounding glandular breast tissue. The E/B ratio is 0.9. The lesion has a score of 3 on the 5-point color scale. The strain ratio (lesion to fat ratio) is 2.4. On shear wave imaging (▶ Fig. 6.21d) the lesion has a Vs of 3 m/s (27 kPa); however, on the quality map (▶ Fig. 6.21e) the majority of the lesion is coded yellow, indicating the shear waves generated were not adequate for Vs estimation. On a different shear wave system (▶ Fig. 6.21f) the lesion is not color coded, consistent with the poor-quality map in ▶ Fig. 6.21e. The Vs (< 4.5 m/s; 60 kPa) is not elevated in the surrounding tissue.

### 6.21.3 Diagnosis

Intraductal papilloma. The lesion was biopsied with a 12-gauge vacuum-assisted needle. The pathology was intraductal papillo-

ma. The patient underwent a surgical excision of the lesion that confirmed the diagnosis.

### 6.21.4 Discussion

Papillary lesions can be broadly categorized as benign or malignant. Benign papillary lesions include a solitary intraductal papilloma, multiple intraductal papillomas, and atypical ductal hyperplasia within a papilloma. Malignant papillary lesions include DCIS arising in a papilloma, papillary DCIS, intracystic or encapsulated papillary carcinoma, solid papillary carcinoma, invasive papillary carcinoma arising in an intracystic papillary carcinoma, and invasive papillary carcinoma.[84]

Solitary papillomas arise from a large central duct, are more common in perimenopausal women, and present with nipple discharge. Multiple papillomas are usually peripheral lesions arising from the terminal duct lobular unit. These are less common, occur in a younger age group, and present as a palpable mass. Both can be associated with proliferative and high-risk lesions, such as radial scars, and with an increased risk of cancer.

Patients with a solitary papilloma without atypia have a twofold greater risk of cancer, whereas those with multiple papillomas have a threefold relative risk.[85,86]

The SE findings in this case are all suggestive of a benign etiology. The E/I ratio is 0.9, the strain ratio is 2.4, and the lesion has a score of 2 on the 5-point color scale. The SWE findings are indeterminate, with the lesion having a poor-quality map on one SWE system and not color coding on the other system. The findings of poor-quality map and non–color coding in SWE are often seen in malignant lesions. Therefore this author would consider the findings to be nonconcordant; as a result,downgrading the lesion from BI-RADS category 4A would be inappropriate.

Based on the proposed elastography classification system (similar to the BI-RADS classification) presented in Chapter 5 we would consider this lesion to have an approximately 0% chance of malignancy on SE, but it is indeterminate on SWE.

## 6.22 Case 22: Phyllodes Tumor

(Case courtesy of Professor Alexander Mundinger, Osnabrunk, Germany.)

### 6.22.1 Clinical Presentation

A 54-year-old woman presented with a palpable mass in the right breast. The patient had a mammogram that confirmed the presence of a large mass in the right breast. Ultrasound was performed for additional characterization of the lesion.

### 6.22.2 Ultrasound Findings

On B-mode imaging (► Fig. 6.22a, b) a 3.7 cm heterogeneous well circumscribed lobular mass is identified. Skin thickening of the breast was noted. On power Doppler (► Fig. 6.22c) no blood flow is identified within the lesion. The lesion was classified as a BI-RADS 4B lesion.

On shear wave imaging (► Fig. 6.22d, e) the lesion color codes blue with a Vs of 3.5 m/s (35 kPa). Strain imaging was not performed.

### 6.22.3 Diagnosis

Phyllodes tumor. The lesion was biopsied under ultrasound guidance with a pathology diagnosis of cystosarcoma phyllodes. The patient had the lesion surgically resected. It was very cellular and a size of 17 cm.

### 6.22.4 Discussion

Phyllodes tumor is a rare fibroepithelial neoplasm accounting for less than 1% of all breast tumors.[87] It is believed the tumor is underdiagnosed by pathologists and undertreated by surgeons.[88] Phyllodes tumors are rare breast tumors that, like fibroadenomas, contain two types of breast tissue: stromal (connective) tissue and glandular (lobular and ductal) tissue. They are most common in women in their 30 s and 40 s but can be found in women of any age. The patients usually present with a painless mass, which can grow quickly and stretch the skin.

These tumors are often difficult to distinguish from fibroadenomas on imaging tests and on small sample biopsies. The cytological features differentiating fibroadenomas from phyllodes tumors have been described.[89] Phyllodes tumors are classified as benign, malignant, or borderline. These tumors behave differently. Phyllodes tumors are usually treated by surgical removal. Recurrence is common if the lesion is not completely removed. They do not respond to hormone therapy and are less likely than most breast cancers to respond to radiation therapy or the chemotherapy drugs normally used for breast cancer. Less than 5% of phyllodes tumors metastasize. Those that metastasize are often treated like sarcomas.[90]

High-grade phyllodes tumors may contain sarcomatous elements such as chondrosarcoma, osteosarcoma, and leiomyosarcoma. The margins of these lesions may become less defined. Metastatic lesions may likewise exhibit sarcomatous elements, even when the primary lesion did not.[75] Prognosis is poor for lesions containing sarcomatous elements because they tend to follow the behavior of sarcomas.

On mammography, phyllodes tumors appear as lobulated, round, or oval masses. They are usually noncalcified and well

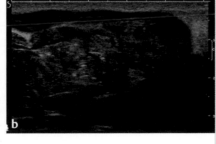

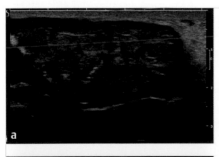

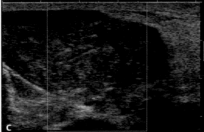

**Fig. 6.22** (a) B-mode imaging demonstrates a 3.7 cm lobular well circumscribed heterogeneous mass identified as the palpable mass. (b) B-mode image at a different location demonstrates the heterogeneity of the large lesion. (c) On power Doppler imaging no blood flow is identified within the lesion. (*Continued*)

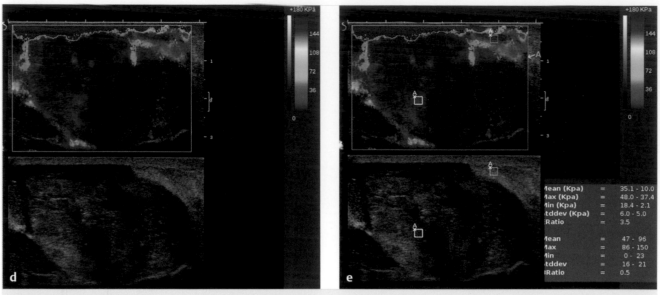

| Mean (Kpa) | = | 35.1 - 10.0 |
| Max (Kpa) | = | 48.0 - 37.4 |
| Min (Kpa) | = | 18.4 - 2.1 |
| Stddev (Kpa) | = | 6.0 - 5.0 |
| Ratio | = | 3.5 |
| | | |
| Mean | = | 47 - 96 |
| Max | = | 86 - 150 |
| Min | = | 0 - 23 |
| Stddev | = | 16 - 21 |
| Ratio | = | 0.5 |

**Fig. 6.22** (*Continued*) (d) On shear wave imaging the lesion has a low Vs of 3.4 m/s (35 kPa), suggestive of a benign lesion. (e) Shear wave imaging with demonstrating the placement of regions of interest (ROIs) to obtain measurements. The measurements include the *mean* value within the ROI, the *maximum* value within the ROI, the *minimum* within the ROI as well as the *standard deviation* of the measurements within the ROI. Most papers use the maximum value within the lesion to characterize the lesion. With the use of the color map the area with highest stiffness can be identified visually and an ROI placed at this location. Multiple ROIs can be used.

circumscribed. On sonography, phyllodes tumors are usually well defined, solid masses with heterogeneous internal echoes, without posterior acoustic attenuation.[91] Tumor size, irregular shape, internal nonenhanced septations, slitlike changes in enhanced images, and signal changes from T2-weighted to enhanced images on MRI have been reported to correlate significantly with the histologic grade.[92] No reports are present in the literature on the elastographic appearance of phyllodes tumors. In this case the tumor is soft with a Vs of 3.5 m/s (35 kPa). However, it is expected that some of these tumors, like fibroadenomas, would have stiffness values significantly higher within the range seen in malignant lesions. It is unknown if the stiffness value of the tumor would predict the behavior or pathology of the tumor.

Phyllodes tumors and fibroadenomas are the most common benign breast tumors. They arise from intralobular fibrous tissue as a unique lesion, and after a period of time they differentiate in two directions: to fibroadenoma and to phyllodes tumors. Fibroadenomas grow up to 2 to 3 cm and then stop growing, but phyllodes tumors grow continually, sometimes to 40 cm. Both these lesions have epithelial and stromal components. Clinically fibroadenomas are well circumscribed, hard, oval, movable lesions. They can be solitary, multiple, unilateral, and bilateral. They are hormone-dependent changes because they change their own consistency during menstrual cycle and gravidity. The most commonly used histologic classification consists of two types: pericanalicular and intracanalicular. Phyllodes tumors represent about 1% of all breast tumors. Starting as fibroadenomas in an intralobular stromal component they show continuous growth, and biologically they can be benign, borderline, or malignant.[93]

Based on the proposed elastography classification system (similar to the BI-RADS classification) presented in Chapter 5 we would consider this lesion to have an approximately 0% chance of malignancy.

## 6.23 Case 23: Mastitis—Mastitis with Abscess Formation

### 6.23.1 Clinical Presentation

A 68-year-old woman presented with a new palpable mass in the left breast. On diagnostic mammogram performed the same day a 3 cm irregular mass was identified. The mammogram was classified as BI-RADS category 0, and ultrasound was advised for further workup.

### 6.23.2 Ultrasound Findings

On B-mode imaging (► Fig. 6.23a) there is an irregular 4 cm complex-appearing mass corresponding to the palpable mass and mammographic abnormality. The mass has well defined borders and a hyperechoic rim. On color Doppler imaging (► Fig. 6.23b) the lesion has adjacent blood flow but no internal blood flow. The lesion was classified as BI-RADS category 4A.

On SE (► Fig. 6.23c) the mass is very soft with a thick stiff rim around the lesion. The lesion has a score of 2 on the 5-point color scale. The E/B ratio is > 1. The strain ratio (lesion to fat ratio) of the central area is 1.2 and 5 in the rim. On shear wave imaging (► Fig. 6.23d) the lesion has a similar appearance, with a soft center (kPa 15) and a stiff rim (with a maximum kPa value of 63). The appearance is similar on a different shear wave imaging system (► Fig. 6.23e).

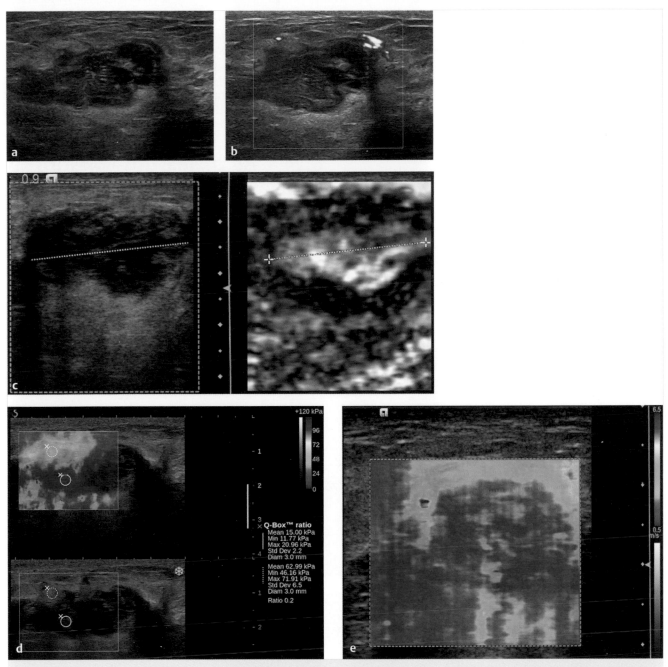

**Fig. 6.23** (a) B-mode image of the palpable mass demonstrates a 4 cm irregular, heterogeneous mass corresponding to the mammographic abnormality. (b) On power Doppler imaging there is peripheral blood flow but no internal blood flow. (c) On strain elastography the lesion has a very soft center with a thick stiff rim. (d) On shear wave imaging the hypoechoic lesion has a low Vs of 2.2 m/s (15 kPa). The stiff rim noted on strain elastography has a Vs of 4.5 m/s (62 kPa). (e) Shear wave imaging on another shear wave system has similar findings as (d), a soft central area with a stiff, thick rim.

## 6.23.3 Diagnosis

Mastitis with abscess formation. The lesion was biopsied using a 12-gauge vacuum-assisted needle. The pathology was chronic and acute mastitis with abscess formation.

## 6.23.4 Discussion

Mastitis is inflammation of the breast that may be either infectious or noninfectious in origin. Infectious mastitis is most commonly acute, occurs during lactation, and may progress to tissue necrosis and abscess formation. Patients with acute puerperal mastitis have localized edema and erythema of the breast with pain, tenderness, warmth, fever, and leukocytosis. A purulent nipple discharge may be present.[94]

Acute mastitis may also occur in nonlactating patients (nonpuerperal mastitis). These patients often have underlying duct ectasia or breast cysts. The inflammation in these patients may be chemical rather than infectious due to rupture of ectatic ducts or cysts. Secondary bacterial infection may supersede.[94]

Ultrasound findings include edema, skin thickening, and an ill-defined mass. Hypoechoic areas representing an abscess cavity can be seen. Color Doppler may demonstrate regional increased blood flow.

The elastographic findings in mastitis are very soft areas representing abscess cavities and stiff areas representing the inflammation and edema. Mastitis can have an elastographic appearance suggestive of a malignancy. Mastitis and fat necrosis are often false-positives for malignancy on elastography. It is rare that cancers have a very soft central area on elastography because liquefied necrosis is an uncommon finding in breast cancer. Mastitis should be a major consideration when elastography identifies a stiff lesion that appears larger on the elastogram and has a soft central area.

In this case the conventional imaging demonstrates an irregular mass with hypoechoic areas and some adjacent blood flow. The region around the mass is slightly hyperechoic. These findings are nonspecific and can be seen in malignant lesions as well as in mastitis. In the appropriate clinical setting of a lactating patient with other clinical signs of mastitis these findings are sufficient to assume a diagnosis of mastitis and treat the patient and follow up clinically. However, in the postmenopausal patient presented here, malignancy must be considered. The elastographic features in this case with a soft central area and thick stiff surrounding rim are more characteristic of mastitis

than a malignancy.[18] In this case aspiration of the soft central area to confirm pus is the appropriate next diagnostic step. Core biopsy is not required if pus is aspirated on FNA.

Based on the proposed elastography classification system (similar to the BI-RADS classification) presented in Chapter 5 we assign the lesion a > 95% chance of malignancy (> 95% on SE; 2 to 95% on SWE). However, we consider this soft center and stiff rim as a special case suggestive of mastitis.

# 6.24 Case 24: Mastitis—Mastitis with Abscess Formation

## 6.24.1 Clinical Presentation

A 43-year-old woman presents with a painful palpable breast mass. The patient had a mammogram at an outside facility that demonstrated a 2 cm left breast mass corresponding to the palpable abnormality. The mammogram was classified as BI-RADS category 0, and ultrasound was advised for further workup.

## 6.24.2 Ultrasound Findings

On B-mode imaging (▶ Fig. 6.24a) there is an irregular mass that has an ill-defined hyperechoic rim. On color Doppler imag-

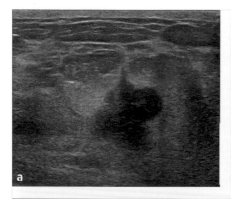
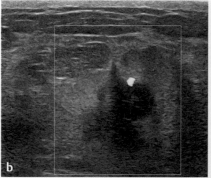
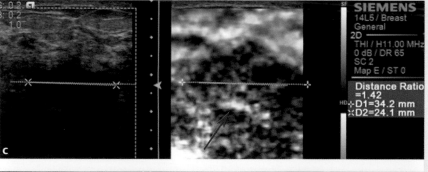
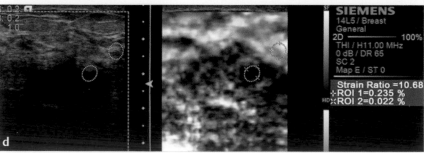

**Fig. 6.24** (a) On B-mode imaging there is an irregular 2.5 cm hypoechoic mass. There is a vague hyperechoic rim around the lesion. (b) On color Doppler imaging there is a small amount of peripheral blood flow. (c) On the B-mode image the lesion measures 24.1 mm (yellow line left images) and 34.2 mm (yellow line right images) on SE with an E/B ratio of 1.4, suggestive of a malignant lesion. There is a small softer area within the lesion (arrow). (d) The strain ratio of the periphery of the lesion is 10.7, suggestive of a malignant lesion. (*continued*) (e) The strain ratio of the softer central area is 2, which is significantly different than the rim of the lesion (d). (f) On shear wave imaging there are similar findings of a softer central area with a Vs of 0.8 m/s (8.5 kPa) and a stiff outer rim with a Vs of 4.5 m/s (60 kPa). (*Continued*)

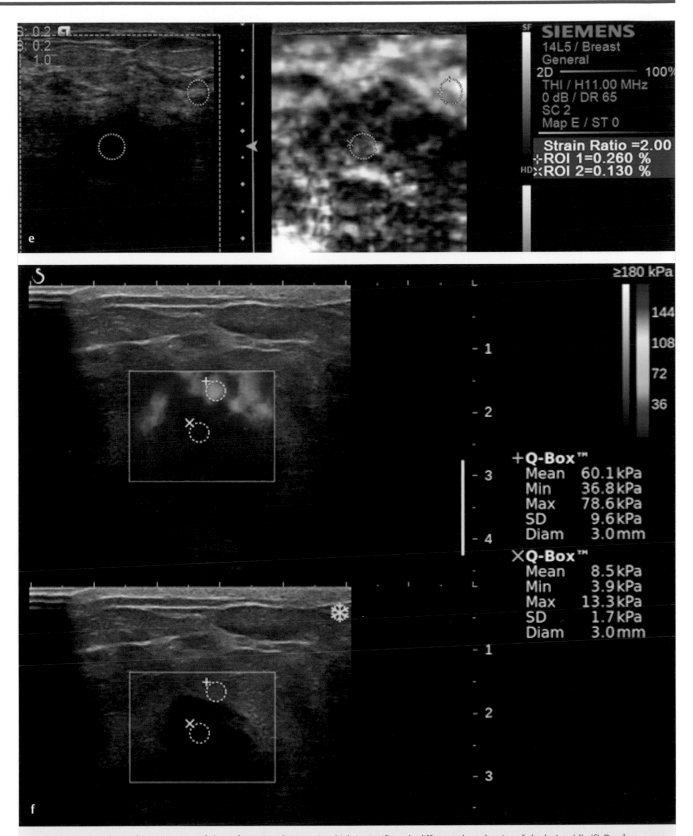

Fig. 6.24 (*Continued*) (e) The strain ratio of the softer central area is 2, which is significantly different than the rim of the lesion (d). (f) On shear wave imaging there are similar findings of a softer central area with a Vs of 0.8 m/s (8.5 kPa) and a stiff outer rim with a Vs of 4.5 m/s (60 kPa).

ing (► Fig. 6.24b) there is a small amount of adjacent blood flow. The lesion was classified as BI-RADS category 4C.

On SE (► Fig. 6.24c) the lesion is stiffer than surrounding tissue with an E/B ratio of 1.4 suggestive of a malignant lesion. There is a small softer area (white) within the lesion. To semi-quantify the stiffness of the two areas within the lesion the ratios of the areas to fat were calculated. The outer stiffer area has a lesion to fat ratio of 10.7 (► Fig. 6.24d), whereas the softer area has a lesion to fat ratio of 2 (► Fig. 6.24e). On shear wave imaging (► Fig. 6.24f) the lesion has a similar appearance with the outer stiffer area having a Vs of 4.5 m/s (60 kPa), whereas the center soft area has a Vs of 0.8 m/s (8.5 kPa).

### 6.24.3 Diagnosis

Mastitis with abscess formation. The soft portion of the lesion was aspirated using a 20-gauge needle under ultrasound, and 5 mL of frank pus were obtained. The patient was placed on antibiotics and the palpable mass resolved. The pathology of the lesion was moderate chronic active inflammation, focal fibrosis, and abscess formation.

### 6.24.4 Discussion

The pathophysiology and B-mode finding of mastitis are discussed in Case 6.23.

In this case an irregular hypoechoic mass with angular margins and a hyperechoic rim are demonstrated on B-mode imaging. There is peripheral blood flow noted on color Doppler. The appearance on conventional ultrasound is a BI-RADS category 4C lesion. When harmonic imaging is used there is significant shadowing from the lesion (B-mode image with elastogram, ► Fig. 6.24c). The lesion is larger on elastography than on B-mode imaging and has a central soft area (white), although not as prominent as seen in Case 6.23. The strain ratio (lesion to fat ratio) confirms that the rim is 10 times stiffer than fat, whereas the central area is only 2 times stiffer than fat. The findings are confirmed with shear wave imaging. Note that the stiffest areas of the lesion or surrounding tissue have stiffness values more suggestive of a malignancy than a benign lesion.

Based on the proposed elastography classification system (similar to the BI-RADS classification) presented in Chapter 5 we would assign this lesion a > 95% chance of malignancy. However, this pattern of a soft center and surrounding stiff rim is considered a special case, and mastitis should be considered.

## 6.25 Case 25: Mastitis—Mastitis without Abscess Formation

### 6.25.1 Clinical Presentation

A 45-year-old woman presented to her doctor with a palpable breast mass. An ultrasound obtained at an outside facility diagnosed a 3 mm simple cyst as the palpable abnormality (BI-RADS category 2). The referring doctor believed the mass was much larger, and the patient was sent for a second-look ultrasound with elastography.

### 6.25.2 Ultrasound Findings

Second-look B-mode ultrasound (► Fig. 6.25a) confirms the presence of the 3 mm cyst at the site of the palpable abnormality. The study was classified as BI-RADS category 3.

On SE (► Fig. 6.25b) there is a 1.5 cm stiff area in the area of the palpable mass that is not well seen on B-mode imaging. In this image with harmonics turned on there is shadowing without a definite mass. The area of shadowing corresponds to the stiff are on SE. An elastogram of the cyst (► Fig. 6.25c) demonstrates a bull's-eye artifact confirming the diagnosis of a benign cyst. On color Doppler (► Fig. 6.25d) there is generalized increased blood flow in the area. Because the lesion is identified only on SE, a biopsy was performed under SE guidance (► Fig. 6.25e). Shear wave imaging was not performed in this case.

### 6.25.3 Diagnosis

Mastitis without abscess formation. The specimen from the 12-gauge vacuum-assisted strain ultrasound-guided biopsy was mastitis without abscess formation on pathology.

### 6.25.4 Discussion

As illustrated by this case, some lesions that are not visualized on B-mode imaging can be identified with elastography. Mastitis without abscess formation may present with inflammation only, which may not be readily apparent on B-mode imaging. This inflammatory change is readily apparent on elastography because it significantly increases the stiffness value of the tissue. In cases where the elastogram demonstrates the lesion significantly better than B-mode imaging, elastography can be used in ultrasound-guided FNA or core biopsy of the lesion.

In this case a benign finding is present at the site of the clinically identified abnormality (palpable mass). However, the finding of a 3 mm cyst does not account for the clinical abnormality, and additional workup is required. Both strain and shear wave imaging were able to locate the "mass" felt on palpation and characterize the lesion and provide image guidance for biopsy of the lesion.

A probability of malignancy based on the proposed elastography classification system (similar to the BI-RADS classification) presented in Chapter 5 is not possible because an E/B ratio, strain ratio, and shear wave imaging were not able to be accurately calculated or not performed.

## 6.26 Case 26: Mastitis—Chronic Granulomatous Mastitis

(Case courtesy of Dr. Chandler Lulla, RIA Clinic, Mumbai, India.)

### 6.26.1 Clinical Presentation

A 34-year-old woman presents with recurring breast granulomatous mastitis and discharging sinuses.

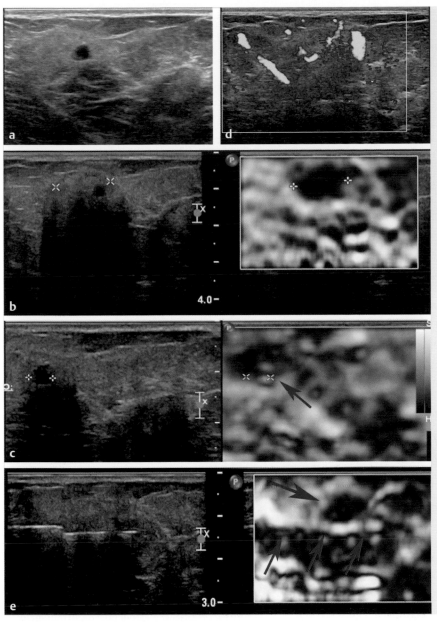

**Fig. 6.25** (a) B-mode imaging over the palpable abnormality in a 45-year-old woman. The 3 mm cyst is much smaller than the palpated mass. There is some subtle increased echogenicity around the cyst. (b) On strain elastography there is a larger stiff area adjacent to the cyst. With harmonic imaging on the B-mode image there is shadowing from the area of increased echogenicity. The size of the stiff lesion on strain elastography is similar to the size of the palpable abnormality. (c) A strain image in a slightly different location confirms the presence of a cyst with the bull's-eye artifact (arrow). (d) On power Doppler imaging there is significant diffuse increased blood flow in the area of the elastographic abnormality. (e) Because the lesion is seen well only on strain elastography, the area was biopsied under elastographic guidance. Solid arrows point to the needle positioned with the stylet deployed and the stiff abnormality (dotted arrow) within the trough of the needle.

## 6.26.2 Ultrasound Findings

B-mode imaging (▶ Fig. 6.26a) demonstrates a 2.2 cm ill-defined heterogeneous mass. On color Doppler imaging (▶ Fig. 6.26b) there is increased blood flow surrounding the lesion. The lesion was classified as BI-RADS category 4C.

On SE (▶ Fig. 6.26c) the lesion is stiffer than surrounding tissues and is larger than on B-mode imaging. On strain imaging (▶ Fig. 6.26d) using a color map with red as hard the lesion and surrounding tissue are stiffer than surrounding tissue.

## 6.26.3 Diagnosis

Chronic granulomatous mastitis (tuberculosis).

## 6.26.4 Discussion

Granulomatous inflammatory lesions of the breast can be a rare secondary complication of many conditions such as tuberculo-sis and other infections, sarcoidosis, and Wegener granulomatosis. Patients present with a palpable mass, nipple retraction, pain, inflammation of the overlying skin, nipple discharge, fistula, or enlarged lymph nodes. Peau d'orange skin changes rarely occur.

On B-mode ultrasound granulomatous mastitis is usually either a heterogeneous hypoechoic mass or an ill-defined hypoechoic mass. Multifocal abscess and enlarged lymph nodes can be seen. The imaging findings are often suspicious for malignancy.[95]

As opposed to the other cases of acute mastitis presented, this case of chronic mastitis has the additional finding of skin involvement. No soft areas suggestive of abscess formation are identified. The granulomatous process with chronic mastitis in general is stiffer than the inflammatory process seen in acute mastitis.

Based on the proposed elastography classification system (similar to the BI-RADS classification) presented in Chapter 5 this lesion would have a > 95% chance of malignancy.

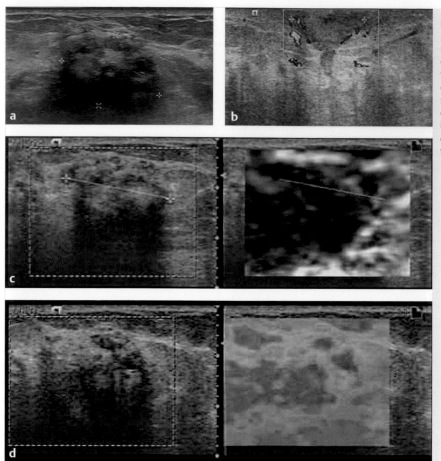

**Fig. 6.26** (a) On B-mode imaging there is a 2.2 cm ill-defined heterogeneous lesion. Corresponding to the area of chronic mastitis. (b) On color Doppler imaging there is increased blood flow surrounding the abnormality. (c) On strain elastography the area is stiff compared with the surrounding tissue. The lesion is larger on the elastogram than the B-mode image. (d) Strain imaging using a color map with red as stiff. Again demonstrating the lesion is stiffer than adjacent tissue.

# 6.27 Case 27: Surgical Scar— Benign Surgical Scar

## 6.27.1 Clinical Presentation

The patient is a 71-year-old woman with a history of invasive ductal cancer with lumpectomy 1 year prior. A 3 × 2 cm mass is present at the site of surgery. No old post-lumpectomy films are available for comparison. The patient believes the scar has been changing recently. The mammogram was classified as a BI-RADS category 0, and an ultrasound was advised for further workup.

## 6.27.2 Ultrasound Findings

The B-mode image (▸ Fig. 6.27a) at the site of the abnormality demonstrates a 2.9 × 3 cm markedly hypoechoic irregular mass with marked shadowing consistent with a surgical scar. This is at the site of the patient's prior lumpectomy. On power Doppler (▸ Fig. 6.27b) there is some blood flow in the proximal portion of the surgical scar. The lesion was classified as BI-RADS category 3.

On the strain elastogram (▸ Fig. 6.27c) the scar is of mixed stiffness but appears stiffer than the surrounding fatty tissue. There is no increased stiffness at the site of the increase vascularity on color Doppler. Note the artifact in the mid to posterior portion of the scar. This artifact is caused by the lack of B-mode signal due to the marked shadowing. The E/B mode ratio is 1.4; however, the right side (on image) of the elastogram may not correspond to the true lesion because the conspicuity on the elastogram is poor. With the use of VTI (strain imaging with AR-FI) at a slightly different location the lesion appears smaller on the elastogram (▸ Fig. 6.27d). The artifact from B-mode shadowing is again noted. Note that the artifact as a different appearance (more black) than the artifact on the strain imaging using the manual displacement technique. This is due to differences in the algorithm between the manual displacement and VTI techniques. An area of increased stiffness was noted during evaluation of a different location of the scar (▸ Fig. 6.27e). Note that in this image the scar is soft but the slightly hyperechoic area adjacent to the scar is stiff. The surrounding fatty tissue is very soft (white). On shear wave imaging (▸ Fig. 6.27f) a portion of the proximal scar is soft (blue) with a Vs of 1.8 m/s (10 kPa), whereas the area of increased stiffness on strain has a Vs of 2.4 m/s (17 kPa). The majority of the scar is not color coded because shear waves are not detected within the area of shadowing. This may be because the monitoring B-mode signals are too weak to evaluate the displacement caused by the shear wave, or a shear wave is not generated. On 3D shear wave imaging (▸ Fig. 6.27g) the portions of the lesion that have adequate shear waves within the lesion are coded soft (1.8 m/s), whereas the central portion of the scar is not color coded.

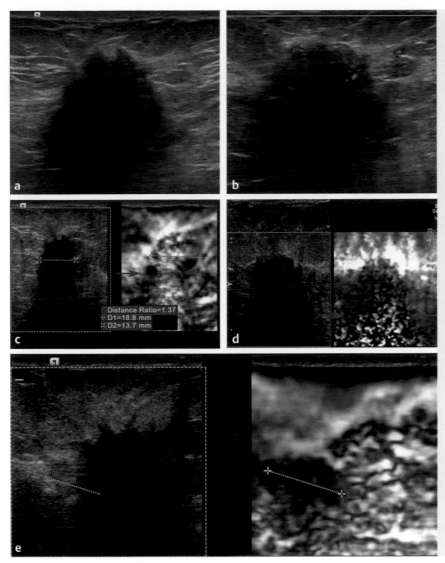

**Fig. 6.27** (a) B-mode image of the palpable mass at the site of prior lumpectomy measuring 2.9 × 3 cm markedly hypoechoic irregular mass with marked shadowing. (b) On power Doppler imaging there is blood flow present in the proximal portion of the lesion felt to be the patient surgical scar. (c) On strain elastogram the scar (yellow line) is of mixed stiffness and appears stiffer than the surrounding fatty tissue. There is no increased stiffness in the area of increased blood flow on power Doppler imaging. Note the artifact (arrows) in the mid and posterior portion of the scar. This artifact is caused by the lack of B-mode signal due to the marked shadowing. The E/B ratio is 1.4. (d) On Virtual Touch imaging (VTI, Siemens) (strain imaging using acoustic radiation force impulse [ARFI]) at a slightly different location demonstrates the elastogram lesion to be smaller than the B-mode image. Note the artifact from shadowing (arrows), which has a different appearance than on strain imaging using manual displacement. (e) A strain image using manual displacement method demonstrates a very stiff area (yellow line) adjacent to the surgical scar. On the corresponding B-mode image the area is hyperechoic. (*Continued*)

## 6.27.3 Diagnosis

Dense fibrocollagenous scar with remote focal hemorrhage, negative for malignancy. Vacuum-assisted ultrasound-guided biopsies were taken of the area with increased vascularity (proximal portion of lesion) as well as the area of stiffness next to the scar. Pathology confirmed surgical scar. Both specimens showed no evidence of malignancy.

## 6.27.4 Discussion

This case is typical of surgical scars. The surgical scar is relatively soft with shear wave velocities of 1.8 to 2.9 m/s (10–25 kPa). This result is unexpected because the lesions are often perceived as very stiff on manual palpation. Surgical scars often have intense shadowing, which leads to artifacts on strain imaging and non–color coding on shear wave imaging. It is important to evaluate the surrounding tissue for areas of relative stiffness. Areas of increased stiffness are of concern for residual or recurrent tumor. On shear wave imaging these areas will have Vs suggestive of a malignancy. If residual tumor or recurrence occurs within the area of dense shadowing it will not be identified on either SE or SWE. However, most recurrences occur at the margins of the scar and should be able to be identified with elastography. Minimal published results are available for surgical scars.

In this case the proximal area of increased blood flow is concerning for recurrence, although elastography demonstrated these areas as soft on both strain and shear wave imaging, correctly predicting a benign pathology. The area of relative stiffness adjacent to the scar is identified on both strain and shear wave imaging. On strain the area is stiffer than the scar and adjacent tissues, but we can't assess if it is stiff enough to be suggestive of a malignancy. However, on shear wave imaging a quantitative measure suggestive of a benign pathology is obtained that correlates with the biopsy pathology. The area of increased stiffness was denser breast tissue that is stiffer than the adjacent fatty tissue and in this case stiffer than the scar tissue. Thus the area is the stiffest tissue in the strain imaging FOV and is therefore colored blacker. However, with the quantitative measurement on shear wave imaging the tissue is soft enough to be suggestive of benign tissue.

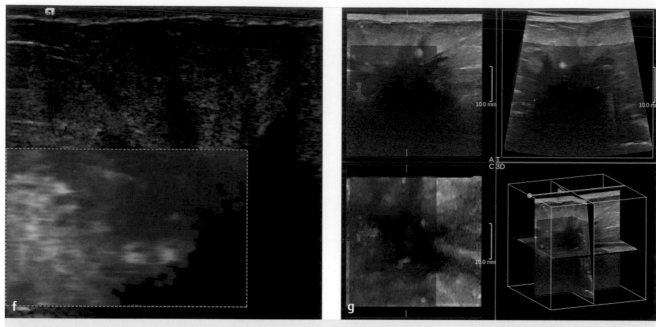

Fig. 6.27 (*Continued*) (f) On shear wave imaging the field of view (FOV) box cannot cover the entire surgical scar. The FOV box can be placed at different locations to evaluate the entire scar. It is helpful to always include some normal breast tissue in the FOV for reference. The portions of the lesion that color code are soft with low Vs values. Other areas do not code secondary to the marked shadowing. B-mode tracking pulses in the areas of marked shadowing cannot identify the tissue movement of the shear wave due to the lack of signal. (g) Three-dimensional shear wave image of the scar allows for visualization of the shear wave results through the whole lesion.

Because it is important to evaluate all the tissue surrounding the surgical scar the use of 3D elastography is helpful in confirming that all surrounding tissue is evaluated. Unfortunately, in most surgical scars the intense shadowing will not allow accurate evaluation of tissues within or distal to the shadowing.

Based on the proposed elastography classification system (similar to the BI-RADS classification) presented in Chapter 5 this lesion would have a > 95% chance of malignancy. (> 95% on SE and ~ 0 on SWE).

# 6.28 Case 28: Surgical Scar— Surgical Scar with Recurrence

## 6.28.1 Clinical Presentation

A 52-year-old woman with a history of invasive ductal cancer presents for routine yearly screening mammography. The patient is status postsurgical resection 5 years prior and has had chemotherapy and radiation. The patient believes the surgical scar is changing. The mammogram was interpreted as BI-RADS category 3.

## 6.28.2 Ultrasound Findings

On B-mode image (► Fig. 6.28a) at the site where the patient believes the scar is changing the surgical scar is identified as an irregular hypoechoic mass. Adjacent to the scar is a 2 cm irregular hypoechoic mass without shadowing. A better evaluation of the smaller lesion is presented in ► Fig. 6.28b. On power Doppler (► Fig. 6.28b) the scar does not have visualized blood flow;

however, the smaller lesion has significant internal blood flow. The ultrasound was classified as BI-RADS category 4B.

On SE (► Fig. 6.28c,d) the larger surgical scar is relatively soft, whereas the adjacent vascular nodule is very stiff and is larger on the elastogram, with an E/B mode ratio of 1.2 highly suggestive of recurrent neoplasm. SWE is not available for this case.

## 6.28.3 Diagnosis

Invasive ductal carcinoma, surgical scar. Patient underwent a vacuum-assisted biopsy with a 12-gauge needle of the smaller stiff nodule and the adjacent larger lesion. The larger lesion was a benign surgical scar, whereas the adjacent smaller lesion was invasive ductal cancer.

## 6.28.4 Discussion

Surgical scars are relatively soft opposed to the finding on clinical palpation where they "feel" very stiff. However, residual or recurrent tumors are very stiff and can be identified attached to or adjacent to the surgical scar by their relative stiffness. When evaluating a surgical scar imaging of the entire surgical scar and surrounding tissue should be performed. In this case the patient was able to locate the recurrence by the change in the surgical scar allowing for targeting of the elastographic evaluation. Because most scars have significant shadowing recurrences within the areas of shadowing, including distal to the scar, cannot be evaluated with elastography. Because no studies have been published the accuracy of elastography on detection of recurrence is not available.

Shear wave imaging is not available for this case. For areas of residual or recurrent tumor Vs values of greater than 4.5 m/s

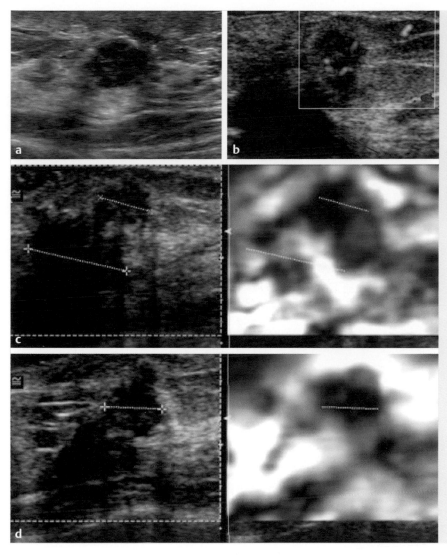

**Fig. 6.28** (a) B-mode image of a 52-year-old woman at the site of a lumpectomy scar demonstrates a 2 cm irregular hypoechoic mass with some through transmission adjacent to the surgical scar (not included in image). (b) Power Doppler image of the nodule demonstrates a significant amount of internal blood flow. The relationship of the nodule to the patient's surgical scar (arrows) is demonstrated in this image. (c) On strain imaging the nodule (upper yellow line) is very stiff with an E/B ratio of 1.2, suggestive of a recurrence or new malignancy. The surgical scar (lower yellow line) is soft on elastography. (d) Strain imaging in another location confirms the stiffness of the nodule (dotted line) adjacent to the soft surgical scar.

(60 kPa) would be expected. The use of 3D shear wave is helpful to screen the scar and surrounding tissue for areas of increased stiffness suspicious for recurrent tumor.

Based on the proposed elastography classification system (similar to the BI-RADS classification) presented in Chapter 5 the lesion would have a > 95% chance of malignancy.

## 6.29 Case 29: Fat Necrosis

### 6.29.1 Clinical Presentation

The patient is a 58-year-old woman with a recent (3 months) lumpectomy for invasive ductal cancer in her left breast. The patient believes the surgical scar is increasing in size. On mammography a surgical scar is noted, but no previous postoperative films are available for comparison. The mammogram was classified as BI-RADS category 0, and an ultrasound was advised for further workup.

### 6.29.2 Ultrasound Findings

On B-mode image (▶ Fig. 6.29a) there is a heterogeneous lesion that is mostly hyperechoic with one adjacent hypo-echoic area. The lesion borders are indistinct. There is some internal blood flow noted on color Doppler imaging (▶ Fig. 6.29b). The lesion was classified as BI-RADS category 4B.

On SE (▶ Fig. 6.29c) the lesion is stiffer than surrounding tissue, with an E/B ratio of 0.9. However, it is difficult to determine the exact size of the lesion on B-mode imaging due to indistinct borders. The measurement was made based on the refractive shadowing artifacts on the B-mode image. Strain imaging on a different system using a color scale with red as soft and blue as hard (▶ Fig. 6.29d) has similar findings. The lesion has a score of 2 on the 5-point color scale. The strain ratio (lesion to fat ratio) was 1.2 (▶ Fig. 6.29e); that is, the lesion is 1.2 times stiffer than fat. The SE findings are concordant, suggestive of a benign lesion.

On shear wave imaging (▶ Fig. 6.29f) the lesion has a Vs of 7.6 m/s (175 kPa) compared to a Vs of adjacent normal tissue of 1.7 m/s (9 kPa). On a different shear wave system (▶ Fig. 6.29g) the lesion again has a central area of higher stiffness of Vs of 6.6 m/s (128 kPa), with the remainder of the lesion having a stiffness of Vs 4.8 m/s (70 kPa). The SWE findings on both machines are suggestive of a malignancy.

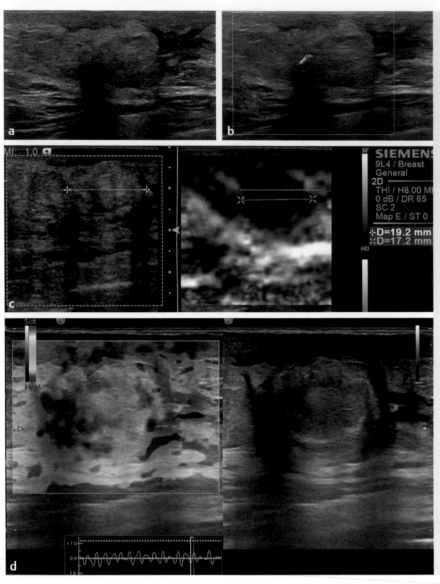

Fig. 6.29 (a) The B-mode image of a 58-year-old with a recent lumpectomy for invasive ductal carcinoma (IDC) demonstrates a heterogeneous lesion that is mostly hyperechoic with an adjacent hypoechoic area. (b) There is some internal blood flow within the lesion on color Doppler evaluation. (c) On strain elastography the lesion is stiffer than surrounding tissue. The lesion measures 19.2 mm (yellow line) on B-mode and 17.2 mm on SE (green line ) with an E/B ratio of 0.9, suggestive of a benign lesion. The lesion (or least a portion of the lesion) is more conspicuous on the elastogram. (d) The same lesion in (c) using a color map with blue as stiff. On this system, which requires a mild displacement technique, a scale is provided that allows monitoring of the frequency and amount of tissue displacement while acquiring the elastogram. (Continued)

### 6.29.3 Diagnosis

Organizing fat necrosis. A vacuum-assisted 12-gauge core biopsy of the lesion was performed. The pathology was focal reactive fibrosis and organizing fat necrosis.

### 6.29.4 Discussion

Fat necrosis can be seen after surgery, radiation therapy, or trauma. Pathologically, hemorrhage within fat evolves into cystic degeneration that can be associated with calcifications and eventually continues toward fibrosis and scar formation. Patients with fat necrosis are usually asymptomatic but can present with a palpable mass that can be tender. These lesions can often be diagnosed by classic mammographic classic appearance of oil cysts and dystrophic calcifications.

On sonography the appearance of fat necrosis varies according to the chronicity of the process. The appearance can range from a solid mass, complex mass with mural nodules or echogenic bands, to an isoechoic or anechoic mass with or without shadowing or posterior acoustic enhancement. Increased echo-

genicity of the subcutaneous fat and hyperechoic lesion almost always indicates a benign finding. However, varying degrees of fibrosis may give the appearance of a malignancy.[96]

Fat necrosis is one lesion that can be false-positive on both SE and SWE.[18] A detailed study of fat necrosis appearance on elastography has not been performed. The appearance on elastography is variable with some cases being very soft and others being very stiff as in this case. The elastic properties of fat necrosis may vary depending on the chronicity of the lesion. When there is acute inflammation associated with the fat necrosis, the stiffness should increase similar to that seen in mastitis.

In this case the strain findings (E/B ratio and strain ratio) are suggestive of a benign lesion. On the 5-point color scale the lesion would be classified with a score of 2, given there are both soft and stiff regions in the lesion, although the stiff components dominate. On both shear wave systems the lesion codes as being very stiff, well within the malignant range. The quality measure of the shear wave image was good (green). Whenever SE and SWE give discordant results an explanation based on principals of those techniques should be sought. If one cannot

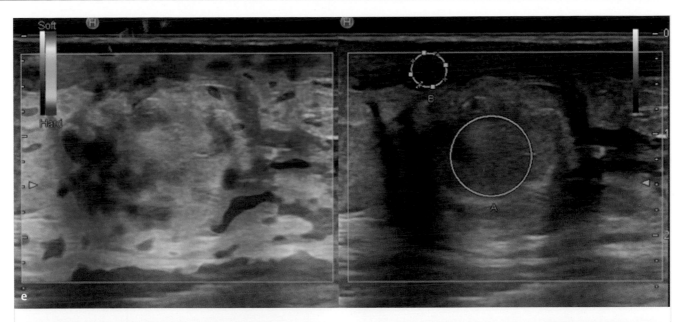

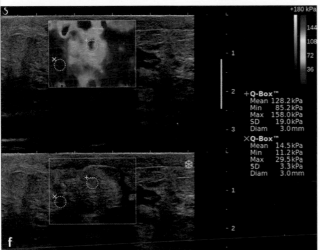

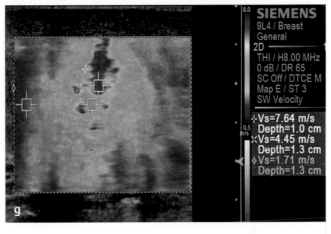

Fig. 6.29 (Continued) (e) The strain ratio (lesion to fat ratio) is calculated at 1.2, suggestive of a benign lesion. (f) On shear wave imaging the lesion has a high Vs of 7.6 m/s (175 kPa), suggestive of a malignant lesion. (g) Shear wave imaging on a different system has similar results to that in (f).

be identified, the more suspicious findings should be used in characterizing the lesion. Both fat necrosis and mastitis can give false-positive elastography results, and if other imaging modalities or the clinical presentation are diagnostic of one of those lesions the elastography results should not overrule that diagnosis.

Based on the proposed elastography classification system (similar to the BI-RADS classification) presented in Chapter 5 the lesion would have a > 95% chance of malignancy (~ 0% on SE and > 95% on SWE).

# 6.30 Case 30: Fat Necrosis—False-Positive Fat Necrosis

## 6.30.1 Clinical Presentation

A 68-year-old woman with a history of lumpectomy for an invasive ductal carcinoma presents with a change in the surgical scar. The mammogram demonstrates dystrophic calcification suggestive of fat necrosis. The mammogram was classified as BI-RADS category 3.

## 6.30.2 Ultrasound Findings

On B-mode imaging (▶ Fig. 6.30a) the lesion is a complex heterogeneous dumbbell-shaped lesion with shadowing. On color Doppler imaging (▶ Fig. 6.30b) there is some peripheral blood flow but no adjacent internal blood flow. The lesion was classified as BI-RADS category 4A.

The strain elastogram (▶ Fig. 6.30c) taken in a different plane demonstrates the lesion to have an E/B ratio of 1.8, suggestive of a malignant lesion. Note that there is marked shadowing on the B-mode image. There is artifact in the elastogram (circle in ▶ Fig. 6.30d) caused by a lack of returning ultrasound signal for the algorithm to determine changes due to the compression/decompression cycle (de-correlation). Shear wave imaging is not available in this case.

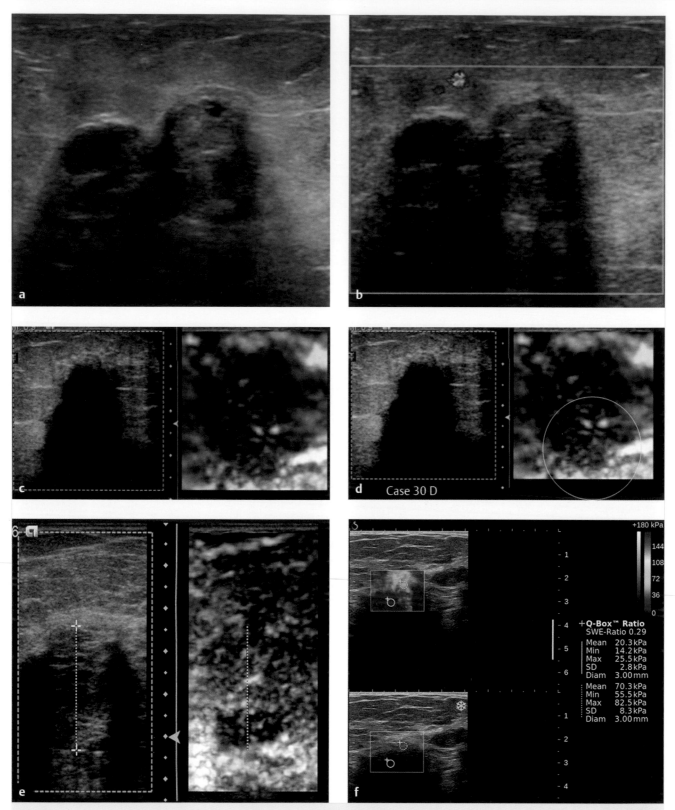

**Fig. 6.30** (a) B-mode image demonstrates a complex heterogeneous lesion with shadowing. (b) There is some color Doppler flow noted adjacent to the lesion, but no flow within the lesion. (c) On strain elastography the lesion is stiffer than the adjacent breast tissue, and the lesion has an E/B mode ratio of 1.8, suggestive of a malignant lesion. (d) Note the artifact (circle) caused by the shadowing from the mass. If the B-mode signal is minimal due to shadowing this artifact is produced. (e) In a different patient with fat necrosis, the strain elastogram demonstrates that the fat necrosis (yellow lines) is mostly very soft. This shows the varied appearance of fat necrosis as compared to the first patient, where the fat necrosis is very stiff. (f) In the same patient as in (e), the shear wave elastogram also codes the area of fat necrosis as soft with a Vs of 2.6 m/s (20 kPa).

### 6.30.3 Diagnosis

Fat necrosis. The lesion was biopsied with a 12-gauge vacuum-assisted core needle. Pathology was organizing fat necrosis with dystrophic calcifications and no evidence of malignancy.

### 6.30.4 Discussion

The pathophysiology and B-mode findings of fat necrosis are discussed in Case 6.29. In this case the lesion has an E/B mode ratio suggestive of a malignant lesion. The dense shadowing in this case causes a de-correlation artifact. The algorithm evaluates the frame-to-frame changes in tissue signal during the compression/decompression cycle. If no returning ultrasound signal occurs when there is marked shadowing, the algorithm can not calculate a stiffness value in this area, and a mixed pattern of black and white blotches code this area.

In this case the mammographic findings were highly suggestive of fat necrosis. Because fat necrosis is often false-positive on both stain and shear wave imaging, the elastography results in this case should not increase the BI-RADS score given on mammography.

Fat necrosis can have a varied appearance on elastography. The difference in appearances may be related to the chronicity of the condition. In a different patient with fat necrosis, the strain elastogram (▶ Fig. 6.30e,f) codes the lesion as very soft with an appearance similar to a hematoma. On shear wave imaging this lesion has a stiffness of Vs of 2.6 m/s (20 kPa). The two cases presented here demonstrate the two extremes that can be seen in fat necrosis with shear wave imaging.

Based on the proposed elastography classification system (similar to the BI-RADS classification) presented in Chapter 5 the lesion would have a > 95% chance of malignancy.

## 6.31 Case 31: Hematoma

### 6.31.1 Clinical Presentation

A 69-year-old woman presents with a new palpable right breast mass. Previous mammograms were negative (BI-RADS category 1). No history of trauma.

### 6.31.2 Ultrasound Findings

A well-circumscribed hypoechoic mass with through transmission and some internal echoes is identified on B-mode image (▶ Fig. 6.31a) corresponding to the palpable mass. The lesion is taller than wider. On color Doppler evaluation of the mass (▶ Fig. 6.31b) there are some peripheral vessels but no internal blood flow. The lesion was classified as BI-RADS category 4A.

On strain elastography (▶ Fig. 6.31c,d) the lesion has a fine stiff rim and is soft centrally. The lesion is smaller on the elastogram (E/B ratio of 0.9). A bull's-eye artifact is not identified. On VTi (strain imaging with ARFI) (▶ Fig. 6.31e) the lesion has a similar appearance to strain elastography with a soft (white) center and a stiffer rim.

On shear wave imaging the central area of the lesion is coded very soft or is not coded in this case (▶ Fig. 6.31f). There is an area of increased stiffness surrounding the central softer area with the Vs of 2.8 m/s (24 kPa) within the range of benign lesions. On SWE the lesion has poor shear wave generation centrally in the area that is not color coded on the quality map (▶ Fig. 6.31g). Elsewhere the lesion is soft with Vs values of less than 2.8 m/s. On another shear wave system the majority of the lesion is not color coded with slight increase in stiffness with Vs of 4.1 m/s (50 kPa) adjacent to the lesion (▶ Fig. 6.31h).

### 6.31.3 Diagnosis

Hematoma. The lesion was aspirated with a 20-gauge needle and resolved after aspiration. The aspirated material was old-appearing blood. On pathology the aspirated material was old blood without evidence of malignancy.

### 6.31.4 Discussion

Hematomas are typical after surgery, image-guided biopsy, or trauma, but they can occur spontaneously, particularly if the patient is on anticoagulant therapy. The age of the blood products determines the imaging appearance of the lesion. A hyperacute hematoma may appear as a simple cyst on B-mode imaging, which rapidly becomes a complicated cyst. Eventually all hematomas will have the appearance of a complicated cyst with internal debris and a thick echogenic wall. They are avascular, and any vascularity in the lesion should raise the question of an associated lesion and a malignancy should be excluded. Mural nodularity and septa are common.[96]

In general the bull's-eye artifact or BGR appearance is not seen with hematomas. Even when the hematoma is anecholc there is enough viscosity in the lesion to prevent the occurrence of these strain artifacts. If the hematoma is chronic and the fluid within the lesion is mostly serous with or without some free-floating debris the lesion may have the cyst artifact appearance. As in this case the usual appearance on SE is a soft (white) lesion with a stiff (black) fine wall.

On shear wave imaging the hematoma will usually allow for generation of shear waves regardless of chronicity. The lesion will usually color code as soft (blue). As seen in ▶ Fig. 6.31f in the areas that are not color coded the quality measure is poor. The poor generation of shear waves may be due to multiple interfaces within the hematoma, allowing for reflection of the shear waves leading to decreased signal to noise and rejection of color coding of the area.

If there is a stiff area within or adjacent to the soft hematoma, the possibility of a second lesion should be considered. In this situation a malignancy should be excluded.

Based on the proposed elastography classification system (similar to the BI-RADS classification) presented in Chapter 5 the lesion would have an approximately 0% chance of malignancy.

## 6.32 Case 32: Hematoma—False-Positive on E/B Ratio

### 6.32.1 Clinical Presentation

The patient is a 77-year-old woman with a thickening in her right breast. A diagnostic mammogram identifies a 6 cm right

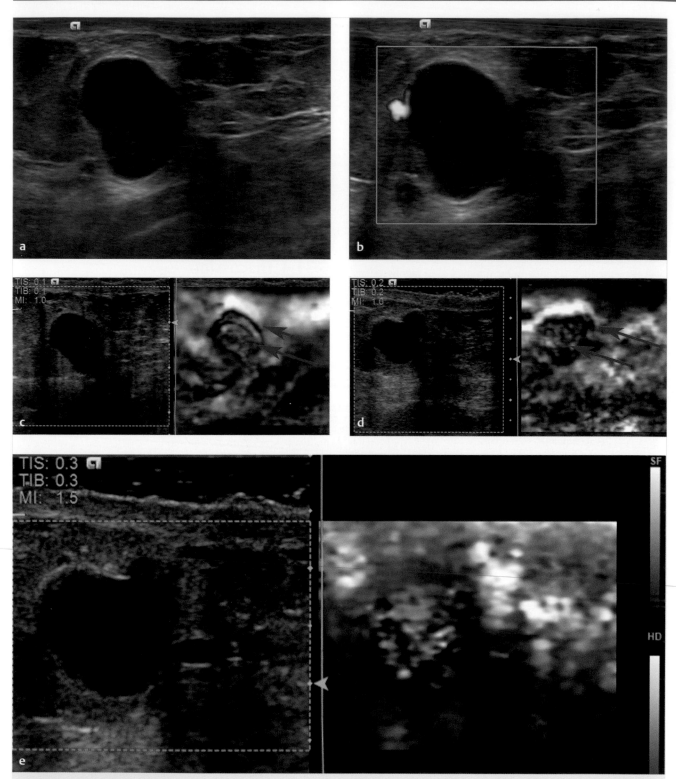

**Fig. 6.31** (a) On B-mode imaging the palpable mass is a well circumscribed, taller than wider, complex cystic lesion. There is through transmission. The echoes in the posterior portion of the lesion do not change on repositioning of the patient. The E/B ratio is 0.9, suggestive of a benign lesion. (b) On power Doppler imaging there is some peripheral blood flow but no internal blood flow. (c) Strain elastography demonstrates a soft (white) lesion (solid arrow) with a thin surrounding black rim (dotted arrow). A bull's-eye artifact is not identified. (d) Strain elastography at a different position again confirms the lesion is soft (white) with a rim of stiffness. No bull's-eye artifact is identified. (e) Using Virtual Touch Imaging (VTI, Siemens) (strain imaging using acoustic radiation force impulse [ARFI]) we get similar findings to strain imaging with manual displacement, a soft (white) center with a circumferential stiff rim. (*Continued*)

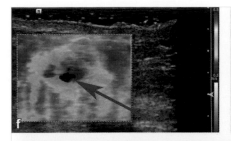

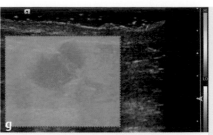

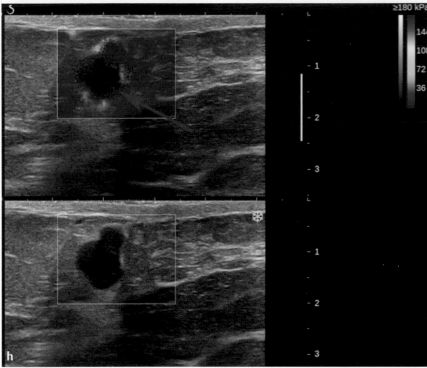

Fig. 6.31 (*Continued*) (f) On shear wave imaging a portion of the center of the lesion does not color code (arrow). Otherwise the center codes with low Vs of 1.2 m/s (7 kPa) with the rim of higher Vs of 2.8 m/s (24 kPa). (g) The quality map confirms that there are poor-quality shear waves generated in the central portion of the mass. This is most likely representative of simple fluid given the B-mode findings. (h) Shear wave imaging on a different system does not code a larger area of the central portion of the lesion (arrow). The stiffer rim is noted with teal color coding.

breast mass corresponding to the thickening new from her prior mammogram 3 years prior. The mammogram was classified as BI-RADS category 0, and an ultrasound was advised for further workup.

## 6.32.2 Ultrasound Findings

On B-mode imaging (▶ Fig. 6.32a) there is a well circumscribed 7 cm hypoechoic lesion with through transmission. Refractive shadowing is noted at the periphery of the lesion. Color Doppler imaging (▶ Fig. 6.32b) demonstrates a small amount of adjacent blood flow but no internal or peripheral blood flow. The lesion was classified as BI-RADS category 3.

On strain elastography (▶ Fig. 6.32c) there is a thin stiff (black) rim with a softer (white) center. The lesion to fat ratio is 1.07, suggestive of a benign lesion (▶ Fig. 6.32d). The E/B ratio is 1.11 (▶ Fig. 6.32e). On shear wave imaging (▶ Fig. 6.32f) the lesion is soft with a Vs of 3.2 m/s (30 kPa).

## 6.32.3 Diagnosis

Hematoma. The lesion was aspirated with a 20-gauge needle. The fluid was visually old blood that was confirmed on pathology. There was no evidence for malignancy.

## 6.32.4 Discussion

This case is similar to Case 6.31, except that regions of the lesion wall are not well defined. On strain imaging the lesion has the classic appearance of a hematoma with a soft center (white) with a fine stiff (black) rim seen only on anterior and lateral margins in this case. The lack of the stiff rim in the other areas may be secondary to the lesion being more acute and a well formed wall has not occurred. The bull's-eye or BGR patterns do not occur because the contents are too viscous to allow the conditions needed to have the artifact. The lesion to fat ratio is 1.07, demonstrating that the lesion is minimally stiffer than fat and benign. In this case the E/B ratio is 1.1, suggestive of a malignant lesion. However, the markedly soft appearance of the lesion should suggest this is a false-positive finding. The false-positive finding in this case may be due to the wall of the lesion not being well defined. On the 5-point color scale this lesion would be classified as a 1 (benign). When a lesion has a score of 1 or 2 on the 5-point color scale the E/B ratio can be difficult to measure, and the lesion should be considered benign.

This lesion is too large for the FOV available for shear wave imaging. In this situation shear wave imaging can be performed in a selected region. The FOV should be placed to include some surrounding tissue to evaluate for a stiff ring around the lesion. Repeat measurements with the FOV moved to all areas of the

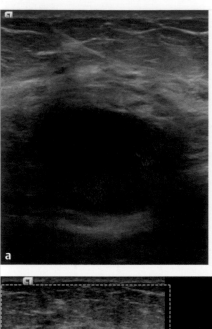
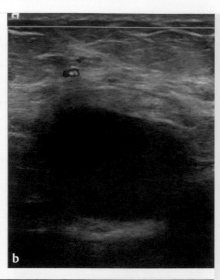
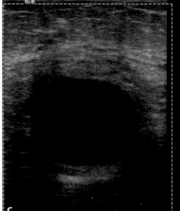
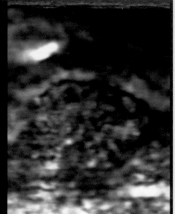

**Fig. 6.32** (a) At the site of the mammographic abnormality there is a well circumscribed 7 cm hypoechoic mass with through transmission. (b) On power Doppler imaging there is some blood flow in adjacent tissue but no peripheral or internal blood flow. (c) On strain elastography the central portion of the mass is soft (white) with a stiff rim around the lesion. A bull's-eye artifact is not identified. (*Continued*)

lesion should be performed to exclude a stiffer area within or adjacent to the lesion.

Shear wave imaging is limited by depth because the ARFI push pulse is attenuated as it transverses through tissue. In general shear wave imaging in the breast is limited to 4 to 5 cm depth. In this case a shear wave measurement at the posterior border of the lesion could not be obtained. As a general rule SE is not limited in depth for breast elastography because one can adjust the amount of compression/release to be appropriate for the depth of the lesion. This may lead to a poor elastogram in other areas. For example, on systems that use the minimal motion technique the patient can be asked to breathe more deeply to increase the compression/release motion if it is not sufficient for an optimal strain elastogram.

Based on the proposed elastography classification system (similar to the BI-RADS classification) presented in Chapter 5 this lesion would have an ~ 0% chance of malignancy.

## 6.33 Case 33: Pregnancy Changes —Pregnancy-Related Changes

### 6.33.1 Clinical Presentation

A 29-year-old patient, 32 weeks pregnant, presents with an enlarging palpable mass in the left breast over a month. Mammography was not performed.

### 6.33.2 Ultrasound Findings

Over the palpable mass a heterogeneous hypoechoic mass is identified with relatively well defined borders (▶ Fig. 6.33a). There is increased blood flow in both the lesion and the surrounding tissues on color Doppler (▶ Fig. 6.33b). The lesion was classified as BI-RADS category 3.

On SE (▶ Fig. 6.33c) the lesion blends in with surrounding tissues or may be slightly stiffer in some areas. The stiffness of the lesion is therefore similar to adjacent benign tissue. The lesion has a score of 2 on the 5-point color scale. On SWE (▶ Fig. 6.33d) the lesion is soft with a Vs of 1.9 m/s (12 kPa), whereas background tissue has a Vs of 2.1 m/s (14 kPa).

### 6.33.3 Diagnosis

Pregnancy-related changes. Because both the SE and SWE features were benign, biopsy was not performed. The mass resolved completely after delivery. The mass was felt to represent pregnancy changes.

### 6.33.4 Discussion

During pregnancy the ductal-lobular-alveolar system undergoes considerable hypertrophy, and prominent lobules are formed under hormonal stimulation. Ultrasound of the breast

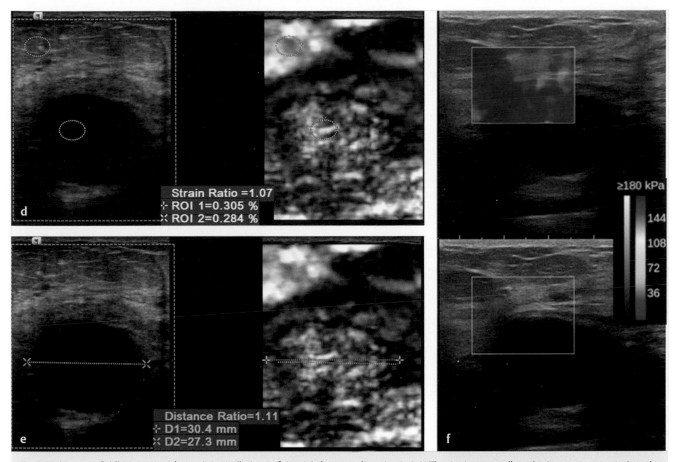

**Fig. 6.32** (*Continued*) (d) Measuring the strain ratio (lesion to fat ratio) the central portion is 1.1. The rim is too small to obtain an accurate strain ratio. (e) The lesion measures 27.3 mm on B-mode (yellow line) and 30.4 mm on SE (green line). The E/B ratio is 1.1, suggestive of a malignant lesion, in contradiction to the overall appearance, which is soft. This lesion would have a score of 1 or 2 on the 5-point color scale. (f) Due to the large size of the lesion shear wave imaging has to be performed in segments. In this representative sample the lesion as well and the rim have a low Vs of 3.2 m/s (30 kPa).

during pregnancy is characterized by diffuse, inhomogeneous, hypoechogenicity due to lobular hyperplasia and duct dilation. Palpable masses that occur during pregnancy include breast cancer, mastitis with or without abscess formation, lactating adenoma, galactocele, lobular hyperplasia, and fibroadenoma.[97]

Ultrasound is the first choice for examination of pregnancy-related breast lesions. Mammography is limited during pregnancy secondary to increased breast density and tenderness, limiting compression. Any suspicious lesions found on ultrasound are usually recommended for ultrasound-guided biopsy. In a study with a small number of patients, all lesions classified as BI-RADS 2 or BI-RADS 3 were found to be benign on biopsy.[97] Galactoceles can have a varying appearance from that of a simple anechoic cyst, a lobulated, fat-fluid level mass, or masses with internal heterogeneous echoes. In these lesions the Bull's-eye artifact is helpful in characterizing the lesion as a benign cystic lesion. However, if the viscosity of the fluid within the galactocele is high a bull's-eye artifact may not be identified, and lesions will code as soft on both strain and shear wave imaging. Well circumscribed solid lesions that can be detected during pregnancy include lactating adenomas and fibroadenomas. Elastography can help characterize these lesions for appropriate follow-up. An elastogram suggestive of a benign etiology can increase confidence of watching the lesion, whereas an elastogram suggestive of a malignancy increases suspicion leading to a biopsy.

Mastitis with or without abscess can have a varied appearance on B-mode imaging. Increased vascularity is usually present but can also be seen with malignant lesions. On elastography the inflamed breast from mastitis is stiff and can lead to a false-negative diagnosis. The area of increased stiffness is usually larger than the B-mode findings. If an abscess is present this codes very soft on both SE and SWE. A soft necrotic center is rare in breast cancer. The appearance of a very soft central area with a very stiff thick rim should raise the suspicion of mastitis with abscess.

Breast cancers in pregnancy will have elastographic features similar to those in the nonpregnant patient, which are described in detail in Chapter 7. Abnormal SE or SWE features should increase suspicion of a malignancy even if the B-mode characteristics are less suspicious.

In this case the lesion cannot be measured accurately in the strain elastogram so that an accurate E/B ratio cannot be obtained for lesion characterization. The use of the 5-point color scale can be used if the FOV is selected to include fat and pectoralis muscle to accurately set the relative color scale used in strain imaging. The strain ratio (lesion to fat ratio) can also be used to help characterize the lesion. In these situations where the B-mode properties of the lesion are very dissimilar from adjacent normal tissue (hypoechoic to background tissue) and the elastic properties are similar (lesion is not clearly identified on

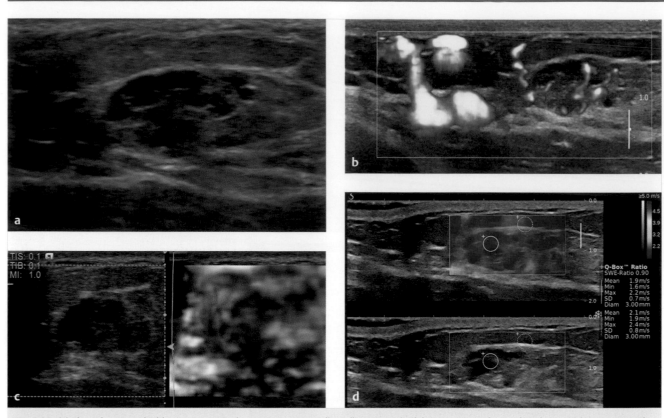

**Fig. 6.33** (a) The enlarging palpable mass on B-mode imaging is a partially well circumscribed, heterogeneous hypoechoic lesion with septations. The posterior portion of the lesion is less well defined. (b) On power Doppler imaging there is marked increased blood flow within the lesion as well as in the surrounding tissue. (c) On strain elastography the lesion is of slightly higher stiffness than surrounding tissue. The borders of the lesion are not well defined. An accurate E/B ratio can therefore not be obtained. (d) On shear wave imaging the lesion has a similar low Vs of 1.9 to 2.1 m/s (11–14 kPa), suggestive of a benign lesion.

elastography) shear wave imaging is helpful in increasing confidence that the lesion is benign.

In this case, the abnormality that resolved after delivery most likely represented lobular changes of pregnancy (although this was not biopsied). These changes are usually hypoechoic and have an irregular appearance and may be characterized as BI-RADS 3 or BI-RADS 4A. The addition of elastography can be helpful in determining if the lesion can be watched (downgrade of BI-RADS score) when the elastogram is suggestive of a benign lesion or if a biopsy is required when the elastogram is suggestive of a malignancy (upgrade of BI-RADS score). The elastographic findings of a benign lesion on both strain and shear wave imaging in this case increased confidence to monitor the lesion and not perform a biopsy.

Based on the proposed elastography classification system (similar to the BI-RADS classification) presented in Chapter 5 the lesion would have an approximately 0% chance of malignancy.

## 6.34 Case 34: Pregnancy Changes —Lactating Fibroadenoma

### 6.34.1 Clinical Presentation

A 25-year-old patient who is 20 weeks present presents with a palpable mass in the left breast. The mass has been increasing in size during the pregnancy. Ultrasound was requested as the initial imaging modality.

### 6.34.2 Ultrasound Findings

On B-mode imaging (► Fig. 6.34a) an 8.6 cm well circumscribed, slightly hypoechoic, wider than taller lesion is identified. On color Doppler (► Fig. 6.34b) there is a large peripheral vessel and internal blood flow noted. The lesion was classified as BI-RADS category 3.

SE (► Fig. 6.34c) was performed at the periphery of the lesion secondary to the large size of the lesion. The lesion is stiffer than adjacent glandular tissue and appears to be smaller on the elastogram than on the B-mode image. The strain ratio (lesion to fat ratio) was 4. On shear wave imaging (► Fig. 6.34d) the lesion has a Vs of 2.2 m/s (15 kPa).

The patient returned 1 year later (7 months postpartum) for follow-up. At that time the lesion had decreased to 5.6 cm in maximum length on B-mode imaging (► Fig. 6.34e). The lesion now had areas that were hyperechoic (► Fig. 6.34f) and a macrocalcification (► Fig. 6.34h). On strain imaging (► Fig. 6.34g) the lesion is now softer than the surrounding breast tissue. Strain imaging in a different location (► Fig. 6.34h) demonstrates the lesion to fat ratio is 2.4. The macrocalcification is noted at this level and codes extremely stiff on the elastogram. SWE (► Fig. 6.34i) at the site of the macrocalcification demonstrates the macrocalcification is extremely stiff with Vs of

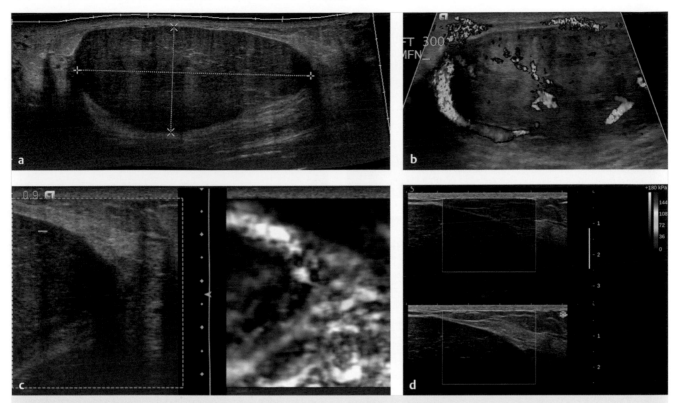

**Fig. 6.34** (a) The large palpable mass is found to be an 8.6 cm well circumscribed relatively homogeneous mass on panoramic B-mode imaging. (b) On color Doppler imaging there is some internal blood flow and a large vessel parallel to the lesion surface. (c) Due to the large size of the lesion obtaining strain elastography can be problematic. In order to have adequate color scale dynamic range, a portion of the lesion and portions of the surrounding breast tissue are required. If a strain elastogram is performed with only the lesion in the field of view (FOV), no useful information is obtained. In this case all the tissues within the FOV will be similar, and the determination of the relative stiffness of the lesion cannot be assessed. In this case the E/B ratio cannot be calculated. Assignment of a score on the 5-point color scale is difficult, but because the mass appears smaller on the elastogram a score of 3 would be assigned. However, the mass is stiffer than the adjacent breast tissue. A strain ratio (lesion to fat ratio) can be obtained and is 4. (d) As in strain imaging the lesion is too large for adequate evaluation with one shear wave imaging FOV. The FOV has to be placed serially over different portions of the mass. In shear wave imaging the inclusion of adjacent breast tissue is not as critical as in strain imaging because a quantitative measurement is obtained. (*Continued*)

9.7 m/s (> 180 kPa). Distal to the calcification no color coding occurs because the ARFI push pulse is attenuated by the calcification and/or the intense shadowing does not allow for the B-mode tracking pulses to monitor the tissue displacement of the shear wave. Another location in the lesion (▶ Fig. 6.34j) has Vs of 1.6 m/s (9 kPa). Shear wave imaging on a different system at a different location demonstrates Vs of 1.5 m/s (7 kPa).

### 6.34.3 Diagnosis

Lactating fibroadenoma. The lesion was biopsied using a 12-gauge vacuum-assisted core needle under ultrasound guidance at time of initial presentation. The pathology was a lactating fibroadenoma.

### 6.34.4 Discussion

Lactating fibroadenoma is a benign condition representing the most prevalent breast lesion in pregnant women and during puerperium, usually appearing during the third trimester of gestation and regressing spontaneously after delivery. Lactating fibroadenomas are benign stromal alterations and felt to be tubular adenomas with lactational changes.[98] Necrosis and

hemorrhage are not prominent features, occurring in only 5% of cases. Lactating fibroadenomas are not thought to carry an increased risk of breast carcinoma.[98]

The physiological changes occurring in the breast during pregnancy and lactation make the detection and management of breast abnormalities challenging. Routine ultrasound or mammography screening in asymptomatic pregnant women is not indicated. However, ultrasound should be performed for a pregnant or lactating patient with a palpable mass, presence of bloody nipple discharge, persistent axillary adenopathy, suspicious abscess or inflammatory disease, and pagetoid alterations of the nipple. Ultrasound can identify simple or complicated cysts, galactoceles, lymph nodes, as well as solid masses in the breast.

Our patient presented with a large palpable mass. The ultrasound findings of a well circumscribed mass with internal blood flow can be identified in both benign and malignant lesions. The appearance of a lactating adenoma can be identical to a fibroadenoma. The major clinical problem of a mass identified in a pregnant or lactating woman is characterizing the mass as benign or malignant. There are limited studies on the use of elastography to characterize lesions in pregnancy as benign or malignant, but there is no reason to expect elasto-

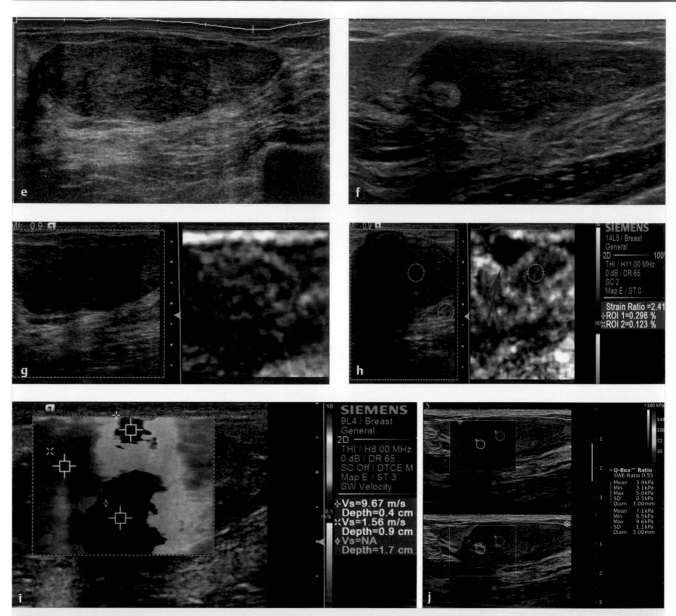

**Fig. 6.34** (*Continued*) (e) The patient returned for follow-up after delivery. The mass has decreased in size to 5.6 cm and become more heterogeneous. (f) An additional B-mode image demonstrating the heterogeneity of the lesion. (g) On strain elastography the mass is now softer than adjacent tissue, significantly different than in the initial presentation. (h) The strain ratio (lesion to fat ratio) is now 2.4 measuring the stiffest portion of the mass. Note that a very stiff area is present on the elastogram (arrow) that corresponds to a macrocalcification and should not be used to calculate the strain ratio. (i) On shear wave imaging the calcification codes very stiff with aVs of 9.7 m/s (> 180 kPa) as one would expect. Distal to the calcification no color coding is present due to the marked shadowing. The lesion has a Vs of 1.6 m/s (9 kPa). (j) Shear wave imaging on a different system at a different location again demonstrates the lesion has a Vs of < 1.5 m/s (3.9–7.1 kPa).

graphic findings would change during pregnancy. There have been too few studies of elastography performed during pregnancy to change the workup of these lesions. However, elastographic changes suggestive of a malignancy should warrant an image-guided biopsy of the lesion.

In this case the follow-up study after delivery demonstrates the lesion has decreased significantly in size and become more heterogeneous, contains macrocalcifications, and has become softer on elastographic studies. To our knowledge there is no other literature on the involutional changes of a lactating fibroadenoma in the literature.

Based on the proposed elastography classification system (similar to the BI-RADS classification) presented in Chapter 5 the lesion would have an approximately 0% chance of malignancy.

# 6.35 Case 35: Gynecomastia

## 6.35.1 Clinical Presentation

The patient is a 90-year-old man presenting with a painful palpable mass in this right breast.

## 6.35.2 Ultrasound Findings

On B-mode imaging a 2.3 × 0.7 cm hypoechoic, irregular mass is identified corresponding to the palpable abnormality (▶ Fig. 6.35a). There was moderate blood flow in the lesion on color Doppler (▶ Fig. 6.35b). The lesion was classified as BI-RADS category 3.

Elastography (▶ Fig. 6.35c,d) shows the lesion to be of similar stiffness to background tissue. The use of the copy, mirror, or shadow function is helpful in confirming the location of the lesion on the elastogram in this case. Although the E/B ratio cannot accurately be determined the stiffness of the lesion is similar to background benign tissue and therefore also has a high probability of being benign. If the lesion were a

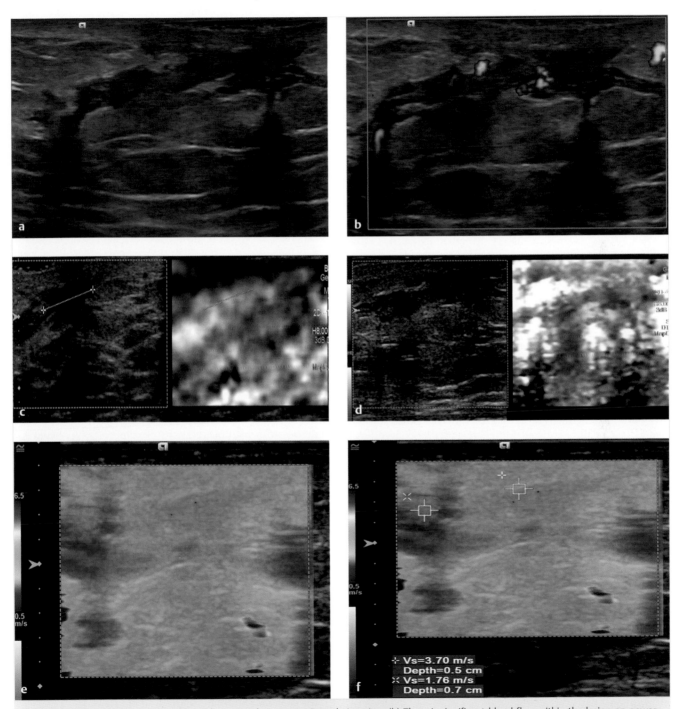

**Fig. 6.35** (a) The palpable mass is a hypoechoic irregular mass on B-mode imaging. (b) There is significant blood flow within the lesion on power Doppler imaging. (c) The lesion (yellow line) has similar stiffness to the surrounding breast tissue on strain elastography. (d) On Virtual Touch imaging (VTi, Siemens) (strain imaging using acoustic radiation force impulse [ARFI]) the lesion is slightly stiffer than the surrounding breast tissue. (e) On shear wave imaging the mass has a slightly higher Vs of 3.7 m/s (40 kPa) than the surrounding tissue, which has a Vs of 1.8 m/s (10 kPa). (f) On shear wave imaging the mass has a slightly higher Vs of 3.7 m/s (40 kPa) than the surrounding tissue, which has a Vs of 1.8 m/s (10 kPa).

malignancy it would display significantly stiffer (black) than the background tissue. The lesion would have a score of 2 on the 5-point color scale. The strain ratio (lesion to fat ratio) was not calculated in this case. On SWE (▶ Fig. 6.35e,f) the lesion has a Vs of 3.7 m/s (40 kPa), which is faster than the Vs of background tissue of 1.8 m/s but still in the range of normal breast tissue.

### 6.35.3 Diagnosis

Gynecomastia. The lesion was biopsied with a 12-gauge vacuum-assisted core biopsy. The pathology was gynecomastia.

### 6.35.4 Discussion

Gynecomastia is one of the most common diseases of the male breast. It is a benign proliferation (hypertrophy) of the ductal and glandular elements in the male breast.[99] The diagnosis of gynecomastia can usually be made based on clinical findings. However, when the clinical suspicion of gynecomastia is less certain imaging is often performed. The imaging findings of gynecomastia have been categorized into four patterns: (1) nodular—discrete round or oval hypoechoic area in the retroareolar region, (2) poorly defined—vague hypoechoic area in the retroareolar region, (3) flame shaped—irregular hypoechoic area with extensions into the surrounding tissue, and (4) increased anteroposterior depth at the nipple, defined as > 1 cm depth of breast parenchyma at the nipple (which may be isoechoic, hypoechoic, or hyperechoic).[99]

Carcinoma of the male breast is unusual with a frequency equaling only about 0.9% of the occurrence of female breast cancer and 0.2% of all malignancies in men.[100] Causes of gynecomastia include hormones, increased serum estrogen, decreased testosterone production, androgen receptor defects, chronic kidney disease, chronic liver disease, human immunodeficiency virus treatment, and chronic illness.[101] The peak incidence is in the fifth and sixth decades. Gynecomastia is not always readily differentiated from carcinoma by conventional imaging.[99] An eccentric location of the lesion should raise suspicion because this is more pronounced in carcinoma. A B-mode appearance of an irregular mass with microlobulated margins should raise the concern of a malignancy. Evaluation of the axilla can be helpful as axillary nodal involvement of cancer is seen in 47% of patients with a malignant lesion.[102] The pattern of calcifications if present is generally not as diagnostic in men as in women because the calcifications in male breast cancer often appear benign.[103]

No studies have been published on the accuracy of elastography in the diagnosis of gynecomastia versus male breast carcinoma. In our experience gynecomastia has a similar appearance to benign glandular tissue in the female patient. On SE the lesion has a similar stiffness to surrounding tissue as seen in ▶ Fig. 6.35c, d. On SWE gynecomastia has a Vs value similar to glandular breast tissue in the female patient. The findings in male breast carcinoma are felt to be similar to those in the female patient; however, a large study has not been reported to confirm that the same cutoff values for both SE and SWE will be similar to those of the female patient.

Based on the proposed elastography classification system (similar to the BI-RADS classification) presented in Chapter 5 this lesion would have an ~ 0% probability of malignancy.

## 6.36 Case 36: Lipoma

### 6.36.1 Clinical Presentation

A 49-year-old woman presents with a palpable mass in her right breast. On mammography the area of the palpable mass is only fat density. The mammogram was classified as BI-RADS category 2. The referring doctor ordered a diagnostic ultrasound for further evaluation.

### 6.36.2 Ultrasound Findings

On B-mode imaging (▶ Fig. 6.36a) a well circumscribed 1.5 cm lesion is identified. The lesion has slightly increased echogenicity over surrounding fat and some through transmission. No blood flow is noted in the lesion on color Doppler imaging (▶ Fig. 6.36b). The lesion was classified as BI-RADS category 2.

On SE (▶ Fig. 6.36c) the lesion is coded very soft (white). When a lesion codes similar to fat stiffness on SE, calculation of the E/B ratio is not required. The lesion would have a score of 1 on the 5-point color scale. The strain ratio (lesion to fat ratio) was not calculated in this case but would have been expected to be approximately 1. On shear wave imaging (▶ Fig. 6.36d) the lesion has a Vs of < 9 m/s (2.4 kPa), whereas that of adjacent fatty breast tissue has a Vs of < 9 m/s (2.7 kPa).

### 6.36.3 Diagnosis

Lipoma. The lesion had fat density on mammography, conventional ultrasound imaging consistent with a lipoma, and elastography features of a lipoma so the lesion was classified as BI-RADS 2 and felt to be a benign lipoma.

### 6.36.4 Discussion

Lipomas are benign overgrowths of adipose tissue. Many patients with breast lipomas have lipomas elsewhere in the body. Most lipomas arise within the subcutaneous fat layer but can occur in any location containing fat. Lipomas usually present as nontender, soft, mobile, palpable masses. If the lesion is tender fat necrosis should be considered.

Lipomas are well defined lesions with a thin capsule. The fat within lipomas is indistinguishable grossly from normal fat lobules that occur in the breast. Lipomas typically have one of three sonographic appearances: (1) completely isoechoic to normal fat lobules, (2) mildly hyperechoic to fat lobules, and (3) isoechoic to fat lobules but having numerous thin, internal echogenic septa that course parallel to the skin line. The diagnosis of lipoma has been suggested by confirming the softness of the lesion using palpation. The compressibility can be demonstrated by deforming the lipoma in the anteroposterior dimension with the ultrasound transducer. Lipomas can usually compress about 30%.[94]

The key to diagnosis of a lipoma is its softness. This can be assessed by clinical palpation or by compression with the ultrasound transducer. Elastography can provide a more quantitative method of characterizing a lesion as a lipoma. Although SE is qualitative it can be used to confirm that a lesion is fat containing because fat is always the softest tissue in the breast. On

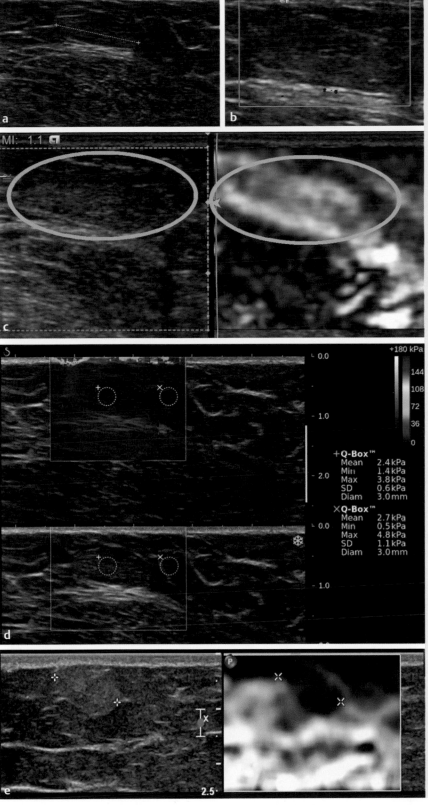

**Fig. 6.36** (a) On B-mode imaging the palpable mass corresponds to an isoechoic well circumscribed mass (white line). (b) On color Doppler imaging no blood flow is identified within the lesion. (c) On the strain elastogram the lesion (circle) is very soft (white) and softer than the underlying glandular tissue. (d) On shear wave imaging the lesion has a Vs of < 1 m/s (2.4 kPa), consistent with fatty tissue similar to the adjacent fatty tissue with a Vs of < 1 m/s (2.7 kPa). (e) In a different patient with a lipoma, the lipoma appears stiffer than the adjacent breast tissue. Note that only fatty tissue is included in the field of view. Therefore the relative stiffness of the lipoma is greater than the adjacent fatty tissue, but it is still soft because the dynamic range of the color scale is set very low at the soft end of stiffness. The dynamic range of the color scale is set so that the lipoma is the stiffest tissue, and the fatty breast tissue is the softest tissue. If we would have included glandular tissue or the pectoralis muscle the lipoma would code significantly whiter.

strain imaging a lipoma will always code as the softest tissue and be similar to adjacent fat lobules. However, it is important to remember that accurate color coding requires a variety of tissue types in the FOV. If an elastogram is obtained with only the lipoma and adjacent fat in the FOV the lipoma may code "stiffer" than the surrounding fat because the dynamic range of color coding is set to display differences between very soft tissues (i.e., all the tissues in the FOV are very soft).

On shear wave imaging the lesion will code very soft with Vs values similar to the adjacent fat. In general fat has a Vs of approximately 1 to 1.4 m/s (3–8 kPa). This method is quantitative and therefore can confirm that the lesion is fatty and benign. Care must be taken not to apply precompression when performing elastography because this can significantly increase the Vs of fat.[19]

Occasionally lipomas may contain small amounts of lobular or glandular tissue (adenolipomas), proliferating capillaries (angiolipomas), or a spindle cell type. If the nonadipose tissue is macroscopic in these variants, it may lead to stiffer areas within the soft lipoma.

Remember that for appropriate color coding the FOV must contain tissues of varying stiffness. In a different patient with a lipoma, the lipoma appears stiffer than the adjacent breast tissue (▶ Fig. 6.36e). Note that only fatty tissue is included in the FOV. Therefore the relative stiffness of the lipoma is greater than the adjacent fatty tissue, but it is still soft because the dynamic range of the color scale is set very low at the soft end of stiffness. The dynamic range of the color scale is set so that the lipoma is the stiffest tissue and the fatty breast tissue is the softest tissue. If we would have included glandular tissue or the pectoralis muscle the lipoma would code significantly whiter.

Based on the proposed elastography classification system (similar to the BI-RADS classification) presented in Chapter 5 this lesion has a 0% probability of malignancy.

## 6.37 Case 37: Epidermal Inclusion Cyst/Sebaceous Cyst

### 6.37.1 Clinical Presentation

The patient is a 56-year-old woman who presents with a new palpable lump in the left breast at 8 o'clock. The patient has a history of right mastectomy for invasive ductal cancer. On mammography no abnormality is identified; however, the breast is extremely dense. The mammogram was classified as BI-RADS category 0, and an ultrasound was advised for further workup.

### 6.37.2 Ultrasound Findings

On B-mode imaging (▶ Fig. 6.37a) a well circumscribed 1.2 cm lesion is identified at the site of the palpable abnormality. The

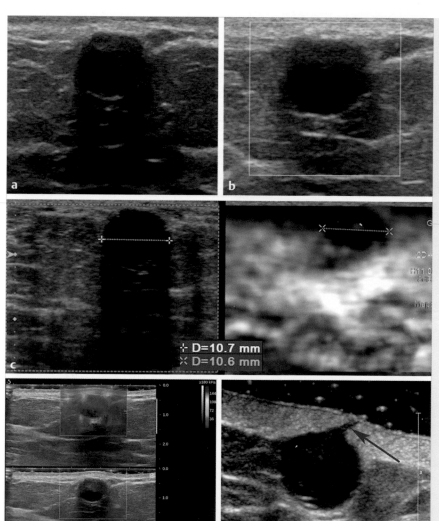

**Fig. 6.37** (a) On B-mode imaging the palpable mass is a well circumscribed anechoic lesion with a thick wall, refractive shadowing, and decreased through transmission. (b) On color Doppler imaging there is a question of a minimal amount of blood flow in the proximal wall of the lesion. (c) On strain elastography the lesion (yellow nad green arrows) is very stiff with a small soft area in the center. The E/B ratio is 0.99, suggestive of a benign lesion, but borderline. (d) On shear wave imaging the lesion has a Vs of 3.9 m/s (45 kPa) in the proximal portion of the lesion and a Vs of 2.6 m/s (20 kPa) in the anechoic portion of the lesion. Both are suggestive of a benign lesion and concordant with the strain results. (e) B-mode image of a different case not discussed in the text demonstrates the lesion positioning at the junction of the dermis and subcutaneous fat interface. In this case the opening to the skin surface is clearly identified (arrow).

lesion is at the interface between the dermis and the subcutaneous fat. The lesion has a thick wall with some internal echoes, mostly in the proximal portion of the lesion. The lesion has refractive shadowing on the sides and attenuates sound without overt posterior shadowing. On color Doppler imaging (► Fig. 6.37b) there is a question of a small amount of blood flow in the proximal portion of the lesions with echoes. The lesion was classified as BI-RADS category 3.

Strain imaging (► Fig. 6.37c) demonstrates the lesion to be stiff and have an E/B ratio of 0.99 suggestive of a benign lesion. Centrally in the elastogram of the lesion there is a small soft area. On SWE (► Fig. 6.37d) the lesion codes soft (blue) with a slightly increased Vs of 3.9 m/s (45 kPa) in the proximal portion of the lesion compared with a Vs of 2.6 m/s (20 kPa) in the anechoic portion of the lesion.

## 6.37.3 Diagnosis

Epidermal inclusion cyst. The findings were highly suggestive of an epidermal inclusion cyst or a sebaceous cyst. The patient was referred for surgical removal. The pathology on surgical removal was an epidermal inclusion cyst.

## 6.37.4 Discussion

For this discussion we include both epidermal inclusion cysts and sebaceous cysts because they are indistinguishable clinically and on imaging studies, although they have histopathological differences. Epidermal inclusion cysts arise from the hair follicle, have a wall lined by true epidermis, and contain keratinous material. Development of a squamous cell malignancy within an epidermal inclusion cyst is rare.[104] They may arise spontaneously or result from a prior trauma (including breast core biopsy).[105] These lesions can present either with a superficial palpable mass, sometimes with a whitish discharge, or as a well circumscribed lesion noted on mammography. The lesion may present as a painful lesion.

On B-mode ultrasound epidermal inclusion cysts appear as well circumscribed lesions. If the lesion has associated inflammation the wall may appear ill defined. The internal echotexture of epidermal inclusion cysts varies, ranging from cystic to more hypoechoic and heterogeneous.[105] A more complex or solid appearance is associated with variable amounts of internal keratinous debris and granulation tissue. Epidermal inclusion cysts that contain lamellated keratinous material have a characteristic internal whorled or onion-ring appearance.[106] The presence of a tiny visible opening to the skin is a helpful sign in diagnosis (► Fig. 6.37e). A whitish discharge from the opening with decompression of the cyst can occur.

As with the B-mode findings, the elastographic findings can be variable with the lesion appearing uniformly soft or uniformly stiff and any combination in between. Although no studies have been performed the soft lesions most likely have more fluid contents or may be infected with the soft area representing pus. Stiffer lesions may be representative of a mass with greater keratin content. In general the B-mode findings are more suggestive of the diagnosis, particularly if the tiny linear opening to the skin is identified. However, if the lesion has a

very stiff component (Vs > 4.5 m/s; 60 kPa), there is concern about a superficial breast cancer.

These lesions occur at the junction of the dermal–subcutaneous fat interface and are therefore located close to the transducer. To adequately visualize the lesion a standoff pad or use of a thick layer of coupling gel is helpful.

On SE the lesion may appear as stiff (black) as in this case or as a heterogeneous pattern with soft (white) and stiff (black) areas. If the lesion has a fluid component it will appear soft (white). Rarely a bull's-eye artifact can be seen if there is a significant fluid component.

On shear wave imaging the lesion will color code as soft (Vs < 4.5 m/s; < 60 kPa). The color coding may be uniform or heterogeneous. In some cases color coding may not occur.

Based on the proposed elastography classification system (similar to the BI-RADS classification) presented in Chapter 5 this lesion has an approximately 0% probability of malignancy.

# 6.38 Case 38: Epidermal Inclusion Cyst/Sebaceous Cyst

## 6.38.1 Clinical Presentation

The patient is a 70-year-old woman who was found to have a new 15 mm high-density nodule with possible microcalcifications in her left breast on routine screening mammography. A diagnostic mammogram, with spot compression views of the area, was performed with the lesion persisting. The diagnostic mammogram was classified as BI-RADS category 0, and an ultrasound was advised for further workup.

## 6.38.2 Ultrasound Findings

On B-mode imaging (► Fig. 6.38a) a lobular, taller than wider, well circumscribed hypoechoic lesion is identified. There are a few low-level internal echoes present and some through transmission. The lesion is half within the dermis and half within the subcutaneous fat. The lesion does have some internal color Doppler signal (► Fig. 6.38b). The lesion was classified as BI-RADS category 3.

On SE (► Fig. 6.38c) the lesion is stiffer than the surrounding breast tissue and has an E/B ratio of 1.4. The lesion has a score of 5 on the 5-point color scale. The strain ratio is 8.2. On SWE (► Fig. 6.38d) the lesion is stiffer with a Vs of 2.5 m/s (kPa 19) than the surrounding fatty tissue (Vs 1.1 m/s; < 10 kPa).

## 6.38.3 Diagnosis

Epidermal inclusion cyst. Based on the ultrasound finding the lesion was felt to be an epidermal inclusion cyst or sebaceous cyst. The patient was advised to return if the lesion increased in size, otherwise to return to routine screening mammography.

## 6.38.4 Discussion

For this discussion we include both epidermal inclusion cysts and sebaceous cysts because they are indistinguishable clinically and on imaging studies, although they have histopathological differences.

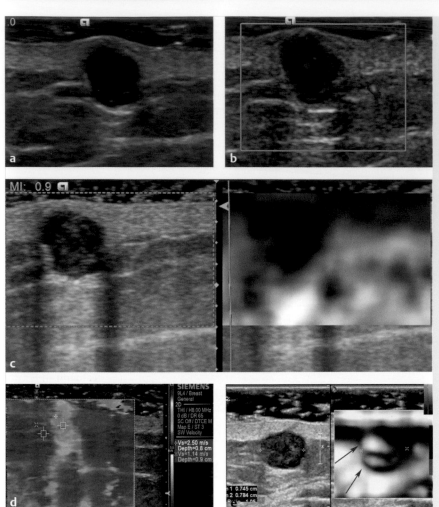

**Fig. 6.38** (a) The mass noted on screening mammography is found to be located at the dermis–subcutaneous fat junction. The lesion is hypoechoic, taller than wider, and has some internal echoes. There is a question of a small opening to the skin surface. Note that coupling gel is used to create a standoff pad to improve imaging quality. (b) On power Doppler imaging there is some internal blood flow within the lesion. (c) On strain elastography the lesion is stiffer than surrounding tissue and has an E/B ratio of 1.2. Note that with the use of the coupling gel standoff pad an adequate strain elastogram can be obtained to the skin surface. (d) On shear wave imaging the lesion has an increased Vs of 2.5 m/s (19 kPa) compared with the background tissue Vs of 1.1 m/s (7 kPa). (e) The strain findings in a different case not discussed in the text of epidermal inclusion cyst to demonstrate the marked variability of these lesions on strain imaging. In this case the lesion has two soft (white) areas located slightly eccentric in the lesion (arrows). Note the appearance of the two soft areas is suggestive of a bull's-eye artifact, but there is not a black ring surrounding the upper white spot (upper arrow).

The presentation and characteristics of epidermal inclusion cysts are discussed in Case 6.37.

On strain imaging this case is a relatively homogeneous lesion stiffer than adjacent fat. In this case only skin and subcutaneous fat are present in the elastographic FOV. Thus we do not know exactly how stiff the lesion is because the color coding dynamic range is very small. We can determine only that the lesion is stiffer than the dermis and subcutaneous fat. The E/B ratio in this case is 1.2, suggestive of a malignancy. The lesion is also taller than wider and has a lobular contour with a few angular margins. This raises the question as to whether this could be a superficial breast cancer. However, the shear wave imaging quantifies the stiffness of the lesion at Vs of 2.5 m/s (19 kPa), suggesting a benign lesion. When conflicting results occur, the most suspicious findings should outweigh the less suspicious findings unless a reason for the suspicious finding is identified (e.g., precompression increasing the stiffness of the lesion).

Because of the variable contents of epidermal inclusion cysts or sebaceous cysts their elastographic findings can be quite variable. In another patient (▶ Fig. 6.38e) on SE the lesion has two soft areas on the medial portion of the lesion. Note that the two white areas have an appearance of a bull's-eye artifact but the more superior white area does not have the surrounding black rim. The white regions represent softer components that can be liquefied material, including pus.

Based on the proposed elastography classification system (similar to the BI-RADS classification) presented in Chapter 5 this lesion would have a > 95% probability of malignancy (> 95% on SE and ~ 0% on SWE).

## 6.39 Case 39: Seroma

### 6.39.1 Clinical Presentation

A 42-year-old woman, status postbilateral breast reductions 1 year prior to presentation, presents with a palpable mass in her right breast. A well circumscribed 2.5 cm mass was identified on diagnostic mammogram. The lesion was classified as BI-RADS category 0. The patient was referred for diagnostic ultrasound.

### 6.39.2 Ultrasound Findings

On B-mode imaging (▶ Fig. 6.39a) a well circumscribed complex cystic lesion measuring 2.5 cm is identified at the dermal–subcutaneous fat junction. There is peripheral blood flow noted on color Doppler (▶ Fig. 6.39b) but no internal blood flow noted. The lesion was classified as BI-RADS category 3.

On SE (▶ Fig. 6.39c) a bull's-eye artifact is identified; however, the distal white area is not present because the debris in

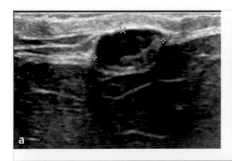
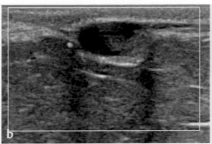
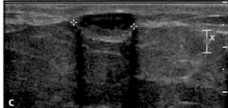
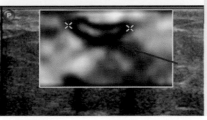

**Fig. 6.39** (a) B-mode image demonstrates a well circumscribed complex cystic lesion measuring 2.5 cm at the dermal–subcutaneous fat junction. (b) There is some adjacent blood flow on power Doppler imaging but no internal blood flow. (c) On the strain elastogram a bull's-eye appearance is identified without the distal white spot. The echogenic material in the posterior portion of the lesion is stiff and overlaps the location where the distal white spot should occur (arrow). Because the posterior portion of the lesion is stiff the internal echoes within the lesion are not freely mobile.

the posterior portion of the cyst is depicted as stiff (black) in the posterior portion of the lesion on the elastogram. Shear wave imaging is not available for this case.

### 6.39.3 Diagnosis

Seroma. The lesion was aspirated with a 20-gauge needle under ultrasound guidance. The lesion completely resolved after aspiration. Pathology was consistent with a benign seroma.

### 6.39.4 Discussion

Seroma formation is the most frequent postoperative complication seen after mastectomy and axillary surgery with an incidence of 3 to 85%.[107] Seroma after breast surgery is defined as a serous fluid collection that develops under the skin flaps or in the dead space following mastectomy and/or axillary dissection. On imaging most seromas appear identical to complicated cysts. The amount of internal debris and wall thickening can vary significantly.

The elastographic findings will be similar to those described for complicated cysts in Cases 6.2 through 6.7. The elastographic findings will vary depending on the amount of debris, nonmobile components, and wall thickening. If the lesion has minimal internal debris the lesion will have the classic bull's-eye appearance or BGR pattern on SE. On shear wave imaging these types of seromas will not color code. If the seroma has a significant amount of internal debris that is freely mobile it may still have the bull's-eye or BGR pattern on SE and will color code with a low Vs on SWE. If the fluid within the seroma is very viscous (uncommon) a bull's-eye or BGR pattern will not be identified on SE. This type of seroma will color code with a low Vs on SWE. If there is a "solid" component within the seroma, the solid (nonmobile) area will code as stiff on SE. The stiffness of the solid component will be quantitatively coded with SWE.

The ultrasound and elastographic appearance of a seroma will be identical to that of a complicated cyst. The clinical history or breast surgery in the location of the lesion will raise the question of the lesion representing a seroma. On both SE

and SWE a seroma will code with findings suggestive of a benign lesion.

Based on the proposed elastography classification system (similar to the BI-RADS classification) presented in Chapter 5 this lesion would have an ~ 0% probability of malignancy.

## 6.40 Case 40: Skin Lesion—Neurofibroma

### 6.40.1 Clinical Presentation

A 58-year-old woman with a history of neurofibromatosis type 1, dense breast tissue, and a strong family history of breast cancer presents for automated whole breast screening ultrasound.

### 6.40.2 Ultrasound Findings

The coronal view of the automated whole breast ultrasound (▶ Fig. 6.40a) demonstrates multiple hypoechoic lesions within the skin. Hand-held B-mode imaging (▶ Fig. 6.40b) of one lesion demonstrates a well circumscribed 7 mm lesion within the skin over the breast. No blood flow is identified within the lesion on color Doppler imaging (▶ Fig. 6.40c). The lesions were classified as BI-RADS category 2.

On SE (▶ Fig. 6.40d) the lesion is stiffer than the adjacent skin and underlying fatty breast tissue. The lesion appears smaller on SE. On one vendor's shear wave system (▶ Fig. 6.40e) the lesion has a low Vs of 1.5 m/s, suggestive of a benign lesion. Note the high Vs (red color coding) within the coupling gel. On another vendor's shear wave system (▶ Fig. 6.40f) the lesion has a low Vs of 1.7 m/s (8.9 kPa), whereas the fatty breast tissue has a Vs of 1.5 m/s (6 kPa). Note that in this system the coupling gel is color coded blue (a low Vs).

### 6.40.3 Diagnosis

Neurofibroma. The lesion is a neurofibroma, a dermatologic manifestation of the patient's history of neurofibromatosis.

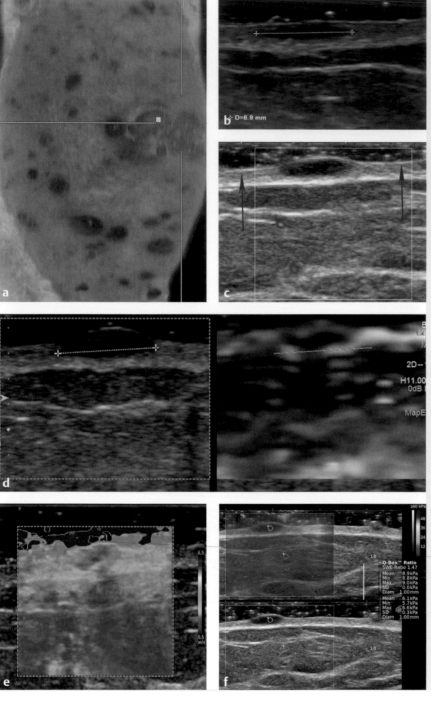

**Fig. 6.40** (a) Coronal view from an automated whole breast scanner of the superficial portion of the patient's breast demonstrates several hypo-echoic skin lesions scattered throughout the breast. (b) B-mode image of one of the skin lesions confirms the lesions to be well circumscribed hypoechoic lesions. Note the liberal use of coupling gel forming a standoff pad to allow for adequate imaging of the skin. (c) The representative lesion does not have blood flow on power Doppler imaging. (d) On strain imaging the lesion (yellow lines) is stiffer than the surrounding dermis and is smaller than in the B-mode image (E/B ratio of 0.7). Again note that with the use of a standoff pad made by ample coupling gel (arrows) good-quality elastograms can be obtained. (e) On shear wave imaging the lesion has a similar low Vs compared with surrounding tissue. The area of increased Vs (red linear structure) at the gel–skin interface is due to the bang effect and is difficult to eliminate. (f) Shear wave imaging on a different system with similar findings of a low Vs 1.7 m/s (8.9 kPa), whereas the Vs of the fatty breast tissue is 1.5 m/s (6.1 kPa).

## 6.40.4 Discussion

This example of neurofibromas as a dermatologic manifestation of neurofibromatosis is used as an example of evaluations of skin lesions using elastography. When a lesion is within the first few millimeters of the transducer it is difficult to obtain good images secondary to the focal zone of most ultrasound probes not tuned for optimal imaging in this area and artifacts from the skin transducer interface. Most SE systems will not allow placement of the FOV box within the first few millimeters of the probe–tissue interface. Therefore, to obtain better B-mode images as well as elastographic images requires the use of a standoff pad or scanning through a thick (approximately 3 mm) application of coupling gel. In this case scanning was performed through a thick application of coupling gel. In shear wave imaging an artifact of high Vs in the gel due to reflections of the ARFI push pulse from the gel–skin interface can occur as seen in (▶ Fig. 6.40e) in this case.

Superficial lesions are often encountered in breast imaging. With rare exceptions lesions that arise within the dermis are considered benign and undergo routine surveillance. Lesions that arise within the subcutaneous fat or the hypodermal layer are usually benign; however, they can occasionally represent superficial breast cancers arising from superficial terminal duct lobular units.[105] Therefore, to avoid misclassifying superficial cancers as skin lesions, it is important to recognize that a lesion originates within the subcutaneous fat rather than in the dermis.

Common dermal lesions include calcifications, epidermal inclusion cysts, and sebaceous cysts. Epidermal inclusion cysts and sebaceous cysts are not distinguishable on the basis of imaging or clinical features.[105] Lesions that can occur in the subcutaneous fat layer include lipomas, angiolipomas, fat necrosis, hemangioma, lymph node, breast cancer, peripheral papilloma, fibroadenoma, and adenosis. The elastographic features of epidermal inclusion cysts and the elastographic findings of lesions in the subcutaneous fat layer are similar to those found elsewhere in the breast and are discussed in Cases 6.37 and 6.38.

Elastography has been used to identify abscess cavities in skin lesions that may not be identified on B-mode imaging.[108] With the use of high-frequency transducers elastography has been demonstrated to help characterize skin lesions as benign or malignant.[109]

In our presented case of a neurofiboma the lesion is stiffer than underlying fatty breast tissue and dermal tissue. In the case of skin lesions we usually cannot include deeper tissues such as the pectoralis muscle to help set the dynamic range of the strain color scale; therefore the skin lesion will color code as the stiffest tissue in the FOV. As in this case the lesion will appear smaller in the elastogram, confirming it is a benign lesion. Little work has been done on breast skin lesions, but initial work on other skin lesions suggests elastography can help characterize skin lesions as benign or malignant.[109]

To obtain adequate elastograms in the near field it is necessary to create a standoff pad with coupling gel of several millimeters. Without a standoff pad the first few millimeters of the image will not produce a good elastogram. It is easier to use this technique with the no manual displacement technique. Mild or moderate displacement techniques require a firmer standoff pad that will not be displaced with the compression/release cycle.

Based on the proposed elastography classification system (similar to the BI-RADS classification) presented in Chapter 5 this lesion would have an ~ 0% probability of malignancy.

## 6.41 Case 41: Skin Lesion—Benign Skin Edema

### 6.41.1 Clinical Presentation

The patient is an 82-year-old woman presenting with an enlarged edematous left breast. The patient has a history of

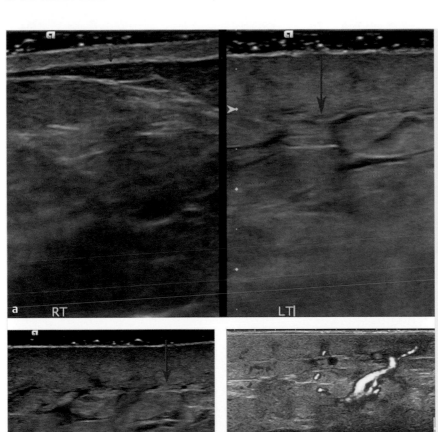

**Fig. 6.41** (a) Dual display of the patient's right and left breast comparing the skin thickness in a similar location of the breast. A red bar (or line) marks the skin thickness in both images. The skin thickness measures 2 mm in the normal breast and 8 mm in the abnormal breast. No focal lesion is identified. Edema is also noted in the fascial planes in the abnormal breast. Note the use of a standoff pad made by coupling gel to allow for good quality images of the skin. (b) B-mode image of the abnormal breast demonstrating the marked uniform skin thickening (red bar) and the edema in the fascial planes. (c) On power Doppler imaging there is generalized increased blood flow in the abnormal breast. (Continued)

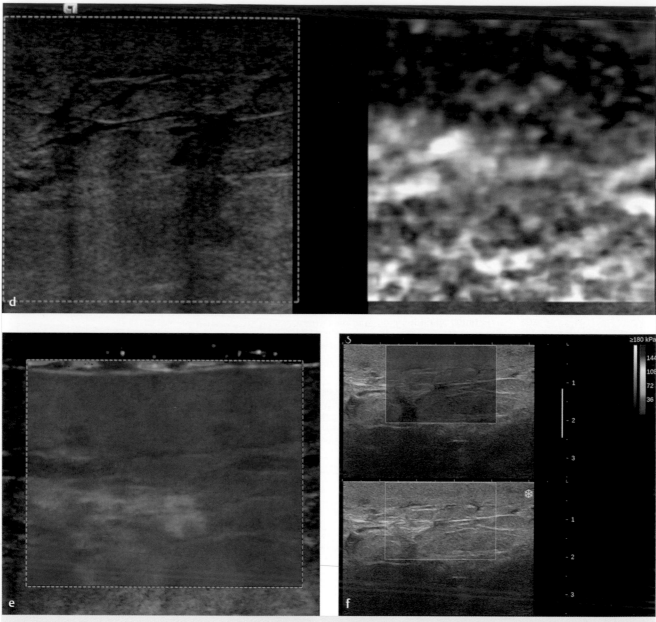

**Fig. 6.41** (*Continued*) (d) On strain imaging the skin is stiffer than the underlying fatty breast tissue. A standoff pad of coupling gel was used but cropped off the image. The strain ratio was 3.8. Because a focal lesion is not identified an E/B ratio or score on the 5-point color scale cannot be assessed. (e) On shear wave imaging the thickened skin codes soft with a Vs of 2.9 m/s (25 kPa). No focal abnormality is noted within the thickened skin. (f) Shear wave imaging on a different system provides the same results, a low Vs of the skin without focal abnormality.

congestive heart failure and mild renal insufficiency. A mammogram demonstrated diffuse skin thickening and increased density in the left breast compared with the right.

## 6.41.2 Ultrasound Findings

The skin thickness in the right breast is 2 mm, whereas it measures between 6 and 8 mm in the left breast (▶ Fig. 6.41a, b). There is diffuse edema within the fascial planes on the left. Power Doppler imaging (▶ Fig. 6.41c) demonstrates some blood flow within the edematous area.

On strain imaging the dermis is stiffer than the underlying breast tissue (▶ Fig. 6.41d) with a strain ratio (lesion to fat ratio) of 3.8. Because there is no "mass" an E/B ratio or assessment for the 5-point color scale cannot be made. Shear wave imaging (▶ Fig. 6.41e, f) demonstrates the thickened skin has low Vs of 2.9 m/s (25 kPa).

## 6.41.3 Diagnosis

Benign skin thickening. The patient underwent a skin biopsy, which demonstrated edema and lymphatic enlargement but no evidence of malignancy

### 6.41.4 Discussion

Skin thickening can have many causes, and its imaging appearance is nonspecific. Skin thickening can be focal or diffuse, unilateral or bilateral. Skin thickening can be seen in both benign and malignant lesions. Benign causes include aseptic mastitis, bacterial mastitis, nonspecific inflammation, vascular obstruction (congestive heart failure, superior vena cava syndrome, and anasarca), psoriasis, lymphatic obstruction, and systemic disease (scleroderma, dermatomyositis, congenital absence of the lymphatics). Skin thickening can be due to inflammatory cancer. Thickened skin usually accompanies inflammatory breast carcinoma, a highly aggressive manifestation of breast cancer with poor prognosis. In inflammatory breast cancer, tumor invades the dermal lymphatics. The thickened skin accentuates the pores and has the classic appearance that suggests the skin of an orange (peau d'orange). Skin thickening can also be seen in noninflammatory breast cancers that have been ignored by the patient and have spread to the skin. Diffuse skin thickening associated with noninflammatory cancer is a late change indicating advanced disease.

Based on the proposed elastography classification system (similar to the BI-RADS classification) presented in Chapter 5 this lesion would have an ~ 0% probability of malignancy.

## 6.42 Case 42: Radial Scar

(Case courtesy of Dr. Fredrick Schaefer from KSH, Kiel, Germany.)

### 6.42.1 Clinical Presentation

The patient is a 76-year-old woman who has a new mass identified in her left breast on mammography. Ultrasound was advised for further workup.

### 6.42.2 Ultrasound Findings

On B-mode imaging (▶ Fig. 6.42a,b) there is a 6 mm taller than wider hypoechoic mass with indistinct borders. On power Doppler imaging (▶ Fig. 6.42c) there is a small amount of blood flow noted within the lesion.

SE is not available in this case. On shear wave imaging (▶ Fig. 6.42d–f) the lesion has a high Vs of 7 m/s (147 kPa). The lesion was classified as BI-RADS category 5. The lesion was removed surgically.

### 6.42.3 Diagnosis

Radial scar. The lesion was surgically removed. On pathological evaluation the lesion was a radial scar without evidence of associated atypia or malignancy.

### 6.42.4 Discussion

Radial scar, also known as complex sclerosing lesion, is a benign lesion characterized by a fibroelastotic core with entrapped ducts and surrounding radiating ducts and lobules. The exact pathogenesis of radial scar is unknown. It has been postulated that these lesions arise as a result of unknown injury, leading to fibrosis and retraction of surrounding breast tissue, thus imparting a stellate configuration. Accumulating evidence indicates that they are associated with atypia and/or malignancy and may be an independent risk factor for the development of carcinoma in either breast.[110]

Radial scars of the breast are common benign lesions, which are often radiographic occult. On mammography radial scar is identified as an area of architectural distortion. The mammographic features of a radial scar have been thoroughly described and are best summarized by Tabar and Dean.[111] Calcifications are common[112] and found in areas of adenosis or epithelial hyperplasia. Lesions may be multifocal and bilateral, and clustering of scars may occur.[113] Although epithelial atypia is not a diagnostic feature, these lesions are not infrequently associated with atypical hyperplasia (ductal or lobular) and in situ or invasive carcinoma.[110]

The sonographic features of radial scars have been reported as irregular hypoechoic masses with ill-defined borders and posterior acoustical shadowing.[114]

The radial scar or complex sclerosing lesion of the breast represents a management dilemma on diagnosis at breast core needle biopsy because the risk of associated malignancy is identified only upon surgical excision. Radial scar or complex sclerosing lesion diagnosed at core needle biopsy still warrants surgical excision because of the significant percentage (9%) of cases with associated malignancy.[115]

Based on the proposed elastography classification system (similar to the BI-RADS classification) presented in Chapter 5 this lesion would have a probability of > 95% of malignancy.

## 6.43 Case 43: Atypical Ductal Hyperplasia

### 6.43.1 Clinical Presentation

The patient is a 61-year-old woman who presents with a new palpable mass in the left breast. The patient's recent screening mammogram was classified as BI-RADS category 1 with scattered fibroglandular tissue.

### 6.43.2 Ultrasound Findings

On B-mode imaging (▶ Fig. 6.43a) a 1.2 cm lobular hypoechoic mass is identified. The lesion has a small amount of peripheral blood flow (▶ Fig. 6.43b). The lesion was classified as BI-RADS category 3.

On SE (▶ Fig. 6.43c) the lesion is stiffer than surrounding tissue, with an E/B ratio of 0.7 suggestive of a benign lesion. The lesion has a score of 3 on the 5-point color scale. The lesion has a strain ratio (lesion to fat ratio) of 3.8, also suggestive of a benign lesion (▶ Fig. 6.43d). On VTi (▶ Fig. 6.43e) the lesion is slightly stiffer than surrounding breast tissue. On shear wave imaging (▶ Fig. 6.43f) the lesion has a Vs of 2.4 m/s (17 kPa), whereas the adjacent fatty tissue has a Vs of 1.9 m/s (12 kPa).

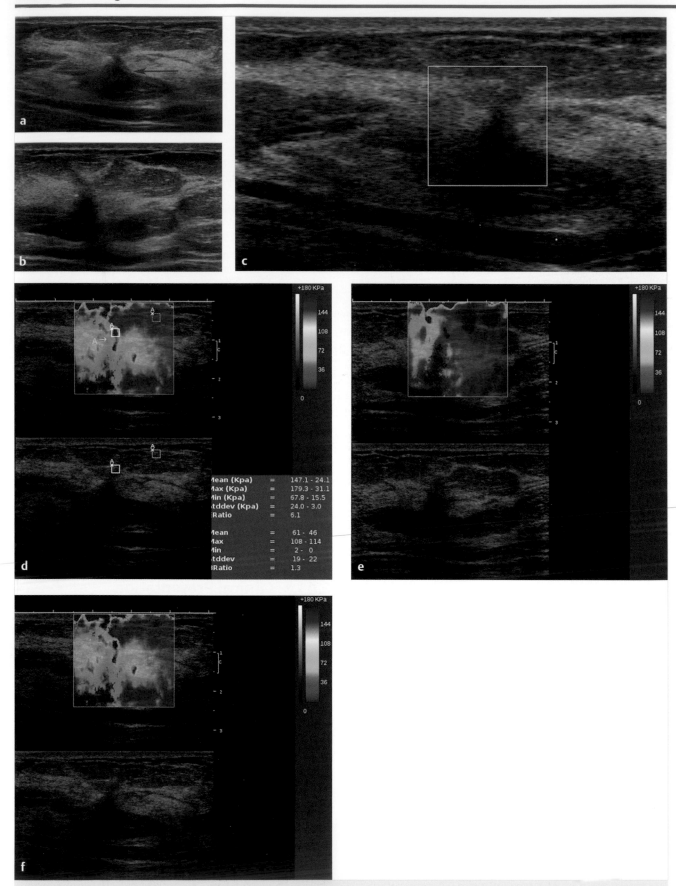

**Fig. 6.42** (a) B-mode imaging of the palpable mass demonstrates a 6 mm ill defined hypoechoic mass (arrows). (b) B-mode image in a different location confirms the presence of the ill defined hypoechoic mass. There is a question of a small adjacent calcification in this image (arrows). (c) On power Doppler imaging there is a small amount of blood flow noted within the lesion. (d) On shear wave imaging there is a high Vs of 7 m/s (147 kPa) within the lesion. The area of stiffness on the shear wave elastogram is larger in size than the abnormality on B-mode imaging. The Vs of the adjacent fatty tissue is 4.6 m/s (61 kPa), which is elevated for normal fatty tissue, suggesting there may have been some precompression applied when obtaining this image. (e) A repeat shear wave image now has a lower Vs of the fatty tissue than in (c), suggesting that precompression was applied in the previous image. The lesion still has a similar high Vs surrounding the lesion. (f) Repeat shear wave elastogram confirms the finding in (d).

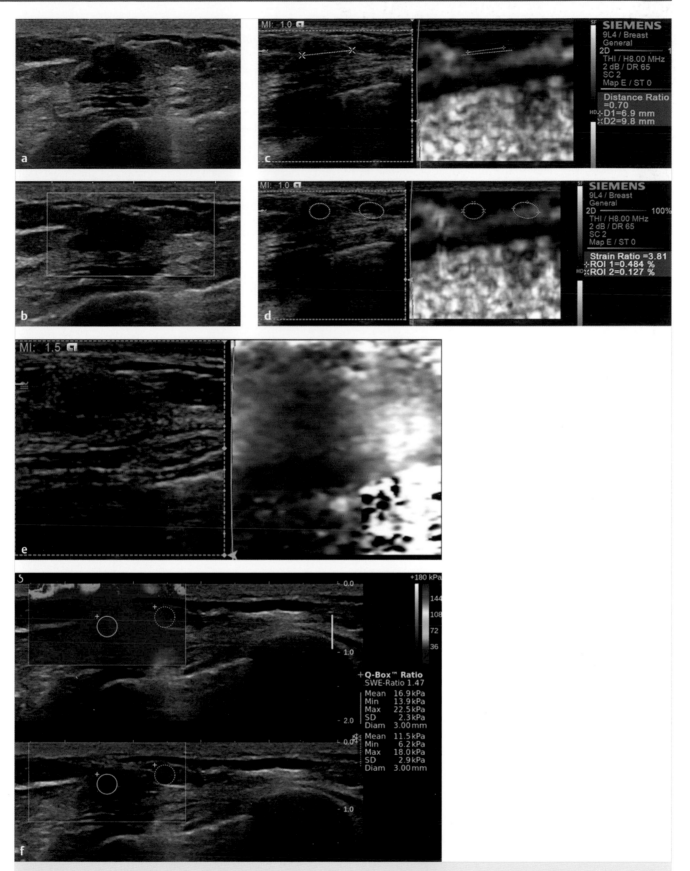

**Fig. 6.43** (a) The new palpable mass is a lobular hypoechoic slightly heterogeneous 1.2 cm mass on B-mode imaging. (b) The lesion does not have blood flow noted on power Doppler imaging. (c) On strain elastography the lesion is stiffer than surrounding tissue. The lesion measures 9.8 mm (yellow line) and 6.9 mm (green line) on elastography with an E/B ratio of 0.7, suggestive of a benign lesion. (d) The strain ratio (lesion to fat ratio) is 3.8, again suggestive of a benign lesion. (e) On Virtual Touch imaging (VTi, Siemens) (strain imaging using acoustic radiation force impulse [ARFI]) the lesion is ill defined and has a slightly higher stiffness than surrounding tissue. (f) On shear wave imaging the lesion is soft with a Vs of 2.4 m/s (17 kPa), with adjacent fatty tissue having a Vs of 1.9 m/s (12 kPa).

### 6.43.3 Diagnosis

Atypical ductal hyperplasia. The lesion was biopsied under ultrasound guidance using a 12-gauge vacuum-assisted core-biopsy needle. The pathology was atypical ductal hyperplasia.

### 6.43.4 Discussion

Atypical ductal hyperplasia (ADH) is a lesion with significant malignant potential. ADH is a premalignant lesion with a moderately increased risk (four to five times that of age-matched control subjects) of having invasive carcinoma develop.[116] It is defined histopathologically as a ductal proliferation with some but not all of the features of DCIS. Because of the potential for undersampling of DCIS or invasive cancers associated with neighboring ADH on core biopsy, excisional biopsy is advised. A recent study[117] reported upgrading on surgical resection to DCIS or invasive carcinoma in 20% of cases diagnosed with ADH by core biopsy.

Only small studies have been performed on the use of elastography to evaluate ADH. It is unclear if elastography will be useful in distinguishing which lesions may be upgraded at surgery. In a series of 18 ADH lesions[118] no difference was found in the 5-point color scale or lesion to fat ratio between ADH lesions that were not upgraded at surgery and those that were upgraded at surgery. For biopsy, elastography can be used to select the stiffest portion of the lesion. Although there is no proof this will improve the detection of cancerous lesions that would otherwise be classified as ADH, it is a reasonable assumption.

In this case the conventional ultrasound findings are of a BI-RADS category 4B lesion. The E/B ratio and the strain ratio (lesion to fat ratio) are predictive of a benign lesion. On SWE the lesion has a stiffness value well within the benign range. It is not known whether using serial follow-up elastography of ADH lesions will be able to predict the conversion to a cancerous lesion.

Based on the proposed elastography classification system (similar to the BI-RADS classification) presented in Chapter 5 this lesion would have an ~ 0% probability of malignancy.

# 7 Clinical Cases: Malignant Lesions

## 7.1 Case 1: Ductal Carcinoma in Situ

### 7.1.1 Clinical Presentation

A 67-year-old woman with a history of invasive ductal carcinoma of her right breast presents for yearly routine mammography. The patient is 5 years from lumpectomy, chemotherapy, and radiation therapy. New suspicious calcifications without a mass were identified in her left breast on mammogram. The mammogram was classified as Breast Imaging–Reporting and Data System (BI-RADS) category 4C. The breast was small in size, and a stereotactic biopsy was felt to be difficult to perform. Ultrasound was recommended for further evaluation and to determine if ultrasound-guided biopsy of the calcifications could be performed.

### 7.1.2 Ultrasound Findings

On B-mode imaging (▶ Fig. 7.1a) an 8 mm isoechoic, ill-defined mass is associated with the microcalcifications. On color Dop-

pler (▶ Fig. 7.1b) there is moderate blood flow associated with the mass. The lesion was classified as BI-RADS category 4B on ultrasound

On strain elastography (SE) (▶ Fig. 7.1c) the mass is stiffer than surrounding glandular tissue and has an elastogram/B-mode (E/B) ratio of 1.2 (▶ Fig. 7.1d). The lesion has a score of 5 on the 5-point color scale. The strain ratio (lesion to fat ratio) is 6.1 (▶ Fig. 7.1e). On shear wave elastography (SWE) (▶ Fig. 7.1f) the lesion has a maximum shear wave velocity (Vs) of 4.22 m/s (54 kPa). The adjacent normal breast tissue has a Vs of 2 m/s (12 kPa).

### 7.1.3 Diagnosis

Ductal carcinoma in situ. The patient underwent an ultrasound-guided vacuum-assisted core biopsy of the mass. The pathology was ductal carcinoma in situ. The patient had a lumpectomy with a histology of ductal carcinoma in situ; intermediate grade Estrogen Receptor (ES) (+) 75% Progesterone Receptor (PR) (−). No evidence of invasive cancer was identified.

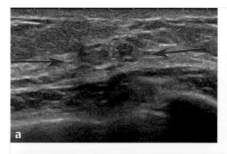
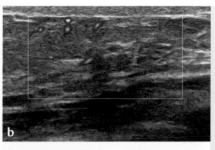
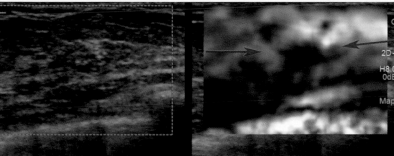
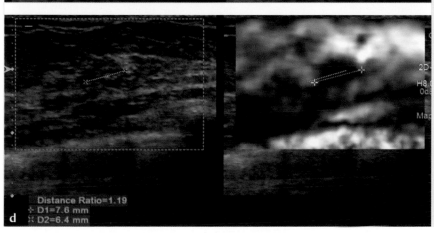

**Fig. 7.1** (a) In the area of the suspicious calcifications on mammography there is an 8 mm vague hypoechoic lesion (arrows) with some associated calcifications. (b) On power Doppler imaging there is generalized increased blood flow in the area with some blood flow within the lesion. (c) On strain elastography the lesion (arrows) is stiffer than adjacent tissue with an E/B ratio of 1.2. This lesion has a score of 5 on the 5-point color scale. (d) The lesion measures 6.4 mm on B-mode (yellow line) and 7.6 mm on SE (green line) with an E/B ratio of 1.2. (*Continued*)

Distance Ratio=1.19
D1=7.6 mm
D2=6.4 mm

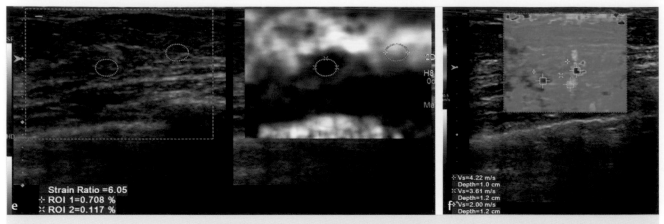

**Fig. 7.1** (*Continued*) (e) The lesion has a strain ratio (lesion to fat ratio) of 6.1 on strain imaging, suggestive of a malignant lesion. (f) On shear wave imaging the lesion has a maximum Vs of 4.2 m/s (52 kPa), which is close to the cutoff value for a malignant lesion.

## 7.1.4 Discussion

Ductal carcinoma in situ (DCIS) is the most common type of noninvasive breast cancer. Ductal carcinoma refers to the development of cancer cells within the milk ducts of the breast. The cells are confined to the duct and have not extended to any surrounding tissue. DCIS is noninvasive breast cancer that encompasses a wide spectrum of diseases ranging from low-grade lesions that are not life threatening to high-grade lesions that may harbor foci of invasive breast cancer. DCIS is classified according to architectural pattern (solid, cribriform, papillary, and micropapillary), tumor grade (high, intermediate, and low grade), and the presence or absence of comedo histology.

DCIS rarely produces symptoms or a palpable mass and is mostly found on screening mammography.[119] DCIS has become one of the most commonly diagnosed breast conditions, now accounting for 20% of breast cancers and precancers that are detected through screening mammography.[120] DCIS is usually identified on mammography as microcalcifications.

Surgical excision removing all of the abnormal duct elements is a common treatment. Radiation after surgery further reduces the risk that the DCIS will recur. Biomarkers can identify which women diagnosed with DCIS are at high or low risk of subsequent invasive cancer.[121,122] Hormonal therapy is recommended for some women with estrogen-receptor-positive DCIS to help prevent invasive breast cancer.

Unless treated, approximately 60% of low-grade DCIS lesions will become invasive at 40 years follow-up.[123] High-grade DCIS lesions that have been inadequately resected and not given radiotherapy have a 50% risk of becoming invasive breast cancer in 7 years. Approximately half of low-grade DCIS detected at screening will represent overdiagnosis, but overdiagnosis of high-grade DCIS is rare.[123]

Although DCIS is detected through microcalcifications at mammography, those without calcifications cannot be detected by mammography, and 6 to 23% of cases of DCIS are felt to remain undetected.[124–126] Izumori et al[127] examined 150 cases with DCIS using ultrasound and retrospectively classified them into a cystic or solid mass, ill-defined hypoechoic mass, microlobulated mass, duct dilatation, and calcification. Among these, in 37 (79%) of 47 cases with ultrasound findings alone, a cystic or solid mass was observed. Most were ovoid in shape, and the margins were circumscribed or microlobulated, making it difficult to differentiate from benign lesions. Moreover, approximately half of these cases had heterogeneous internal echoes.

Based on the proposed elastography classification system (similar to the BI-RADS classification) presented in Chapter 5 the lesion would have a > 95% probability of malignancy. (> 95% on SE; 2–95% on SWE).

## 7.2 Case 2: Ductal Carcinoma in Situ—Fibroadenoma with Foci of DCIS

### 7.2.1 Clinical Presentation

A 43-year-old woman presents with a new mass containing suspicious calcifications on screening mammogram. The lesion was classified as BI-RADS category 0, and an ultrasound was requested for further workup.

### 7.2.2 Ultrasound Findings

On B-mode (▶ Fig. 7.2a) the mass noted on mammography is a lobular well circumscribed mass with several echogenic foci within the mass representing the calcifications noted on mammography. The lesion has significant blood flow on power Doppler (▶ Fig. 7.2b). The lesion was classified as BI-RADS category 3.

On strain imaging (▶ Fig. 7.2c) the lesion is stiffer than the surrounding glandular tissue. The mass is larger on SE than on B-mode imaging with an E/B ratio of 1.2. The lesion has a score of 2 on the 5-point color scale. On shear wave imaging (▶ Fig. 7.2d) the elasticity of the lesion is heterogeneous with scattered foci of a high Vs up to 4.5 m/s (60 kPa). The background Vs of the lesion is 2.8 m/s (24 kPa). The background breast tissue has a Vs of 2.3 m/s (17 kPa).

### 7.2.3 Diagnosis

Fibroadenoma with foci of DCIS. The lesion was biopsied using a 12-gauge vacuum-assisted core needle under ultrasound

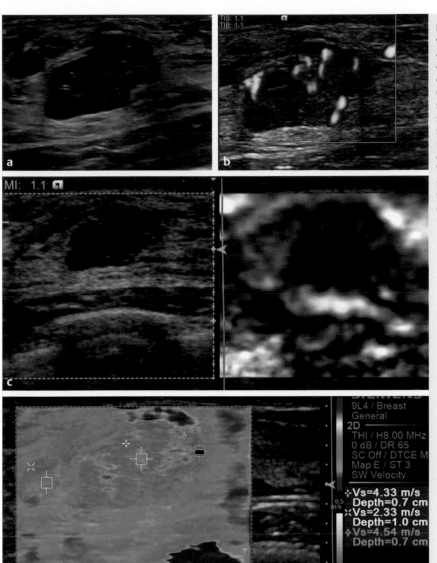

**Fig. 7.2** (a) The palpable mass is a lobular 1.6 cm well defined lobular lesion with some punctate areas of hyperechogenicity suggestive of micro-calcifications. (b) The lesion has marked increased blood flow on power Doppler imaging. (c) On strain imaging the lesion is stiffer than surrounding tissue and has an E/B ratio of 1.2, suggestive of a malignant lesion. This lesion has a score of 5 on the 5-point color scale. The strain ratio (lesion to fat ratio) was not calculated in this case. (d) On shear wave imaging the lesion has a Vs of 4.5 m/s, suggestive of a malignancy. The shear wave imaging color coding demonstrates the lesion has components of varying stiffness (3.5–4.5 m/s; 38–60 kPa)

guidance. The areas of increased Vs were targeted on the biopsy. The pathology demonstrated a fibroadenoma with foci of DCIS. The patient underwent a lumpectomy with the pathology an intermediate-grade DCIS, multifocal, cribriform, and solid patterns, arising in fibroadenoma.

## 7.2.4 Discussion

Fibroadenoma may be associated with fibrocystic changes, proliferative epithelial changes, and, extremely rarely, with noninvasive and invasive cancer. The incidence of carcinoma within fibroadenoma is reported between 0.1 and 0.3% in a screened population, with a peak age of occurrence between 42 and 44 years.[128–131] The biological behavior of carcinoma occurring within fibroadenoma does not differ from that of breast carcinoma not related to fibroadenoma.[130–132] Preoperative clinical criteria and radiological criteria are usually insufficient to suggest that malignant change has occurred in a fibroadenoma, especially in cases with DCIS.[133]

In this case the stiffness within the lesion is heterogeneous, ranging from 2.3 m/s (17 kPa) to 4.5 m/s (60 kPa). On pathology the lesion was a benign fibroadenoma with scattered foci of DCIS. Although direct comparison of the imaging to pathology was not performed, the areas of increased stiffness most likely represent the areas of DCIS. It is important to use the elastographic finding to guide an image-guided core biopsy. Although no studies have been performed, targeting the areas with the highest stiffness values could allow for more accurate pathological correlation of core biopsies with surgical specimens.

The maximum Vs in this case was 4.5 m/s (60 kPa), which is a borderline value for the cutoff value for benign and malignant. On SE the E/B ratio was 1.2. The maximum stiffness value and the E/B ratio have been suggested to correlate with the tumor grade. The higher the Vs or E/B ratio the greater the probability of a higher-grade tumor.[28] Low-grade lesions such as DCIS or mucinous carcinoma can have an E/B ratio of 1; therefore, we always biopsy lesions with an E/B ratio of 1 or greater.

Based on the proposed elastography classification system (similar to the BI-RADS classification) presented in Chapter 5 this lesion would have a probability of > 95% of malignancy.

## 7.3 Case 3: Invasive Ductal Carcinoma—Borders Ill Defined, Grade 1

### 7.3.1 Clinical Presentation

A 47-year-old woman with a recent negative mammogram but a density 4 breast presents with a BI-RADS category 4C lesion on a screening automated whole breast ultrasound. The mammogram was classified as BI-RADS category 2, the automated whole breast ultrasound was classified as BI-RADS category 0, and a handheld ultrasound was advised for further workup.

### 7.3.2 Ultrasound Findings

A selected image (▶ Fig. 7.3a) from an automated whole breast ultrasound demonstrates a 1.5 cm irregular, hypoechoic mass. On handheld B-mode ultrasound (▶ Fig. 7.3b) the lesion is again noted with irregular borders, marked hypoechogenicity, and shadowing. On color Doppler imaging (▶ Fig. 7.3c) the lesion has significant blood flow. The lesion was classified as BI-RADS category 5.

On SE (▶ Fig. 7.3d) the lesion is much stiffer than the surrounding breast tissue. It is difficult to calculate an accurate E/B ratio because the borders of the lesion are not defined on B-mode. The lesion has a lesion to fat ratio of 10.5 (▶ Fig. 7.3e). On Virtual Touch imaging (VTi, Siemens Ultrasound, Mountain View, CA) the lesion is much stiffer than the surrounding breast tissue. The lesion appears of similar size to the B-mode image. On shear wave imaging (▶ Fig. 7.3f) the lesion has a max Vs of 9.7 m/s (> 180 kPa).

### 7.3.3 Diagnosis

Invasive ductal carcinoma, grade 1. The lesion was biopsied under ultrasound guidance using a 12-gauge vacuum-assisted core needle. The pathology was an invasive ductal carcinoma, well differentiated, grade 1. The patient had a lumpectomy where the maximum size of the tumor on surgical resection was 2.5 cm. The patient was node negative.

### 7.3.4 Discussion

The morphology of breast cancer is heterogeneous because breast cancer is not one disease. The histopathological features of a breast cancer are needed for appropriate management. Breast cancer can be classified into types including lobular, tubular, medullary, mucinous, and no special type (NST).[134] Tumor staging is the most useful means for predicting survival. The TNM staging system is the mainstay for prognostication of breast cancer. Histologic grading is usually performed using the Scarff, Bloom, and Richardson (SBR) system. This system is a composite of degrees of glandular formation, nuclear pleomorphism, and mitotic activity. Each of these parameters is assigned a numerical score from 1 to 3 based on specific criteria. Scores from each category are then summed; a score of 3 to 5 is

equivalent to grade 1, a score of 6 or 7 is equivalent to grade 2, and a score of 8 or 9 is equivalent to grade 3.

This patient had a screening mammogram interpreted as BI-RADS category 2 with breast density 4. The patient had an automated whole breast screening ultrasound that detected a 1.5 cm irregular spiculated hypoechoic mass (▶ Fig. 7.3a). The examination was classified as a BI-RADS 0, and a whole breast ultrasound was requested. At this time a standard of interpretation of automated whole breast scanning has not been implemented. At our institution, automated whole breast scans are interpreted similar to screening mammography where an abnormality is read as a BI-RADS 0, and a handheld ultrasound is requested for further workup. At the handheld examination the lesion can be better evaluated with transducer position changes, color or power Doppler, and elastography. A BI-RADS category score of 2 to 5 can then be issued and appropriate follow-up then advised.

In this case the handheld ultrasound confirmed the presence of a 1.5 cm irregular, hypoechoic mass (▶ Fig. 7.3b) with significant blood flow (▶ Fig. 7.3c). The SE images confirm that the lesion is much stiffer than adjacent breast tissue (▶ Fig. 7.3d) with a strain ratio of 10.5 (▶ Fig. 7.3e). An accurate E/B ratio cannot be determined because the lesion borders are difficult to assess on B-mode. Note that the posterior margin of the mass is well defined in the elastogram compared with the B-mode image where there is significant shadowing. On VTi (strain imaging with acoustic radiation force impulse [ARFI]) the lesion is stiffer than surrounding tissue and appears to have an E/B ratio of approximately 1. Note that the surrounding glandular tissue is white (▶ Fig. 7.3f, arrows). Therefore the dynamic range of stiffness values set by the machine is quite large with the malignancy being very stiff, setting the upper portion of the scale. Therefore the glandular tissue is relatively "whiter" than if a malignancy were not present. Because of this scaling process SE images with a cancer often appear black and white with very few gray coding areas.

The lesion has a very high Vs of 9.7 m/s on shear wave imaging (▶ Fig. 7.3g). In this case the blue portion of the tumor had poor-quality shear waves in this area on the quality map. However, the area with high Vs had good-quality shear waves. Because of the poor shear wave generation in many breast malignancies the central portion of the tumor is either not color coded or has a poor-quality map in this region. However, the peripheral portions of the tumor will have a high Vs, thus often giving the appearance of a "ring" of high Vs surrounding the lesion.

Based on the proposed elastography classification system (similar to the BI-RADS classification) presented in Chapter 5 we would consider this lesion to have a > 95% probability of malignancy.

## 7.4 Case 4: Invasive Ductal Carcinoma—Grade 2

### 7.4.1 Clinical Presentation

An 82-year-old woman with bilateral palpable breast masses presented for a diagnostic mammogram. A 1 cm new mass was identified in the retroaureolar region of

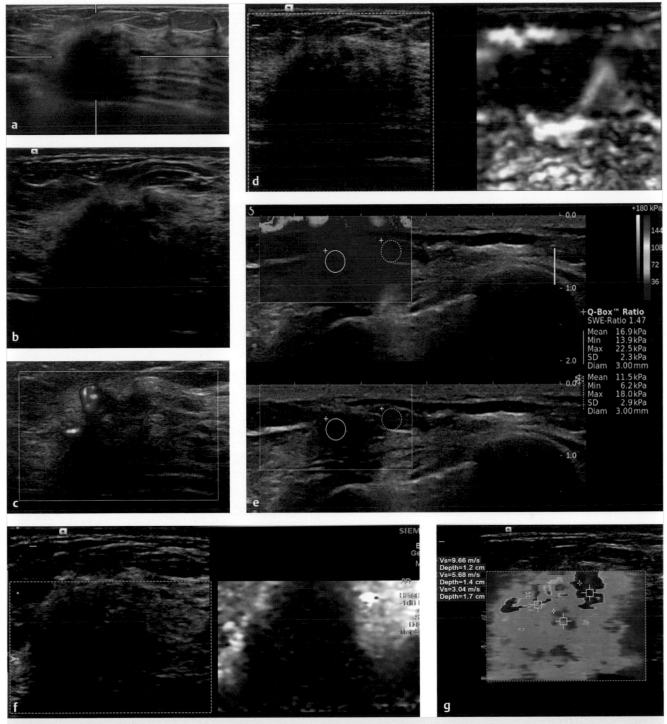

**Fig. 7.3** (a) Selected image from an automated whole breast ultrasound demonstrating a 1.5 cm irregular mass with a hyperechoic rim. (b) Handheld ultrasound of the lesion in (a) confirms the presence of a 1.5 cm irregular hypoechoic mass with a hyperechoic rim and shadowing (Harmonic imaging used). (c) There is moderate blood flow adjacent to the lesion on power Doppler imaging. (d) On strain elastography the lymph node is stiffer than surrounding tissue and has an E/B ratio of 1.1 suggestive of a malignancy. (e) On shear wave imaging the lesion has a Vs of > 7.7 m/s (> 180 kPa), highly suggestive of a malignancy. (f) The quality map confirms adequate shear waves are generated for an accurate Vs measurement to use for interpretation. (g) On shear wave elastography the lesion has heterogeneous stiffness with a maximum Vs of 9.7 m/s, suggestive of a malignant lesion.

the left breast. The lesion was classified as BI-RADS category 0 and ultrasound recommended for further evaluation.

## 7.4.2 Ultrasound Findings

On B-mode ultrasound (▶ Fig. 7.4a) a 1.5 cm irregular, hypoechoic, heterogeneous mass is identified. On color Doppler imag-

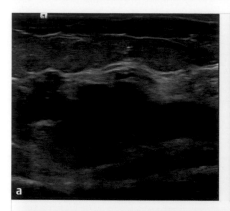
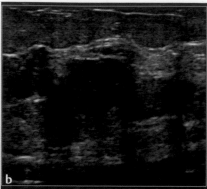

**Fig. 7.4** (a) B-mode image demonstrates an irregular hypoechoic mass with a question of some internal punctate calcifications. (b) There is a small amount of blood flow adjacent to the lesion on power Doppler imaging. (c) On strain elastography (SE) imaging the lesion is stiffer than adjacent tissue. The lesion measures 13.6 mm (yellow line) and 16.1 mm (green line) with an E/B ratio of 1.2 and a score of 5 on the 5-point color scale, both suggestive of a malignant lesion. (d) The strain ratio (lesion to fat ratio) on SE is 5.8, also suggestive of a malignant lesion. (*Continued*)

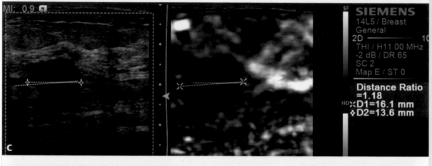

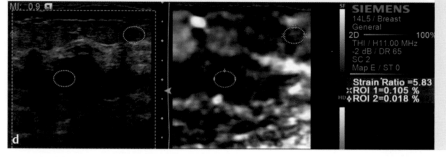

ing (▶ Fig. 7.4b) there is some peripheral blood flow. The lesion was classified as BI-RADS category 4C.

On strain imaging (▶ Fig. 7.4c) the lesion is stiffer than surrounding breast tissue and has an E/B ratio of 1.2. The lesion has a lesion to fat ratio of 5.8 (▶ Fig. 7.4d). On the 5-point color scale this lesion would be given a score of 5. Similar finding are identified on VTi (▶ Fig. 7.4e). On shear wave imaging (▶ Fig. 7.4f) the lesion has a max Vs of 4.7 m/s (68 kPa). On shear wave imaging on a different system (▶ Fig. 7.4g) the lesion has a max Vs of 5.7 m/s (96 kPa).

### 7.4.3 Diagnosis

Invasive ductal carcinoma, grade 2. The lesion was biopsied using a 12-gauge vacuum-assisted core needle under ultrasound guidance. The pathology was an Invasive Moderately Differentiated Ductal Cancer, grade 2 with mucinous features with associated low grade Ductal Carcinoma-in-situ.

### 7.4.4 Discussion

This case has concordant findings on SE and SWE. The lesion is stiffer than surrounding breast tissue on SE with an E/I ratio of 1.2, a strain ratio (lesion to fat ratio) of 5.8, a score of 5 on the 5-point color scale. Similar finding are found with VTi (strain imaging with ARFI). Both shear wave systems demonstrate a Vs of > 4.5 m/s (> 60 kPa) suggestive of a malignancy. As is a common feature of shear wave elastography the central portion of the malignancy is color-coded softer than the periphery. On the quality map this area has poor quality shear wave. However the ring of higher Vs surrounding the lesion is the major finding to suggest this is a malignancy. The ring may be due to neoplastic tissue that allows for good shear wave generation or may be due to reflections from the soft to hard interface between the malignancy and adjacent sort tissue (RG Barr, personal communication 1 October 2013). Further studies are needed to clarify the exact cause of the ring.

This case was classified as a BI-RADS 4C on conventional ultrasound and merits biopsy based on those findings. The addition of elastography is helpful to determine the stiffest portion of the mass to guide biopsy. Although not yet proven it is expected that better correlation with pathology finds will occur when elastography is used to guide biopsies.

Based on the proposed elastography classification system (similar to the BI-RADS classification) presented in Chapter 5 this lesion would have a > 95% probability of malignancy.

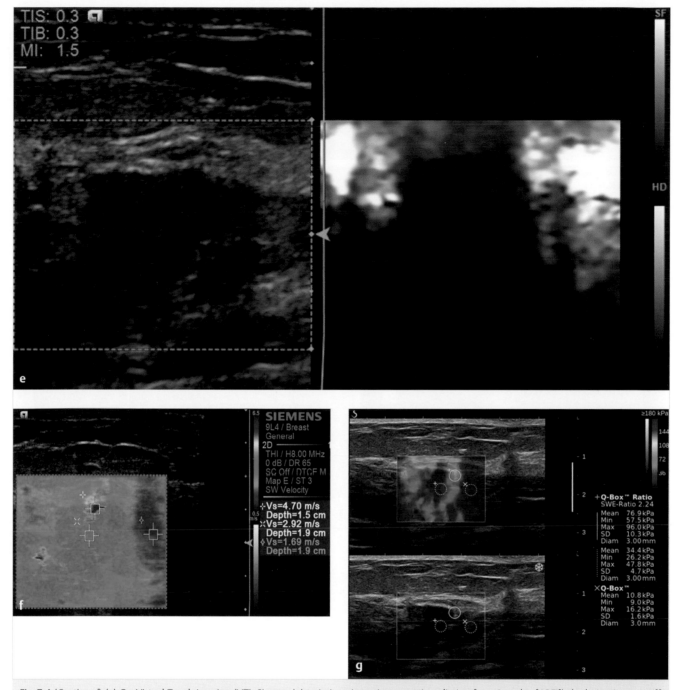

**Fig. 7.4** (*Continued*) (e) On Virtual Touch imaging (VTi, Siemens) (strain imaging using acoustic radiation force impulse [ARFI]) the lesion is very stiff with a similar appearance to SE using the manual displacement technique (c). (f) On shear wave elastography (SWE) the stiffness of the lesion is heterogeneous with the maximum Vs of 4.7 m/s (68 kPa), suggestive of a malignancy. (g) SWE obtained on a different system demonstrates the central portion of the lesion to have a lower Vs, but there is a ring of high Vs in the periphery of the lesion, also suggestive of a malignancy.

## 7.5 Case 5: Invasive Ductal Carcinoma—Grade 1

### 7.5.1 Clinical Presentation

A 50-year-old woman with bilateral breast implants was found to have a new mass in her left breast on screening mammography. The lesion was classified as BI-RADS category 0, and an ultrasound was recommended for further evaluation.

### 7.5.2 Ultrasound Findings

On B-mode imaging (▶ Fig. 7.5a) a 1.7 cm lobular, wider than taller, hypoechoic mass is identified. On color Doppler imaging (▶ Fig. 7.5b) there is marked blood flow within the lesion. The lesion was classified as BI-RADS category 4A.

On SE (▶ Fig. 7.5c) the lesion is stiffer than the surrounding breast tissue and has an E/B ratio of 1.2. The lesion to fat ratio was 14.9 (▶ Fig. 7.5d). Similar findings are identified on VTi

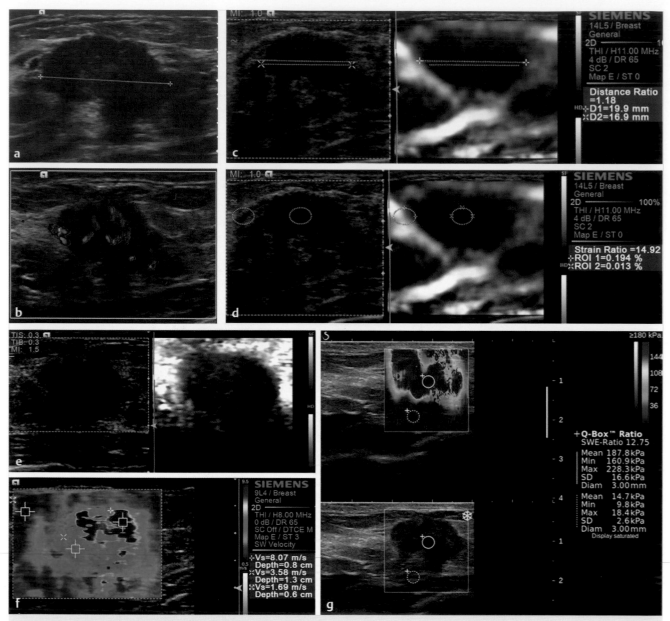

**Fig. 7.5** (a) On B-mode imaging the lesion has a lobular border with the posterior portion of the lesion not well defined. (b) On color Doppler imaging the lesion (green line) has a moderate amount of internal blood flow. (c) On strain elastography the lesion is stiffer than adjacent tissue. The lesion measures 16.9 mm (yellow line) on B-mode image and 19.9 mm (green line) on SE with an E/B ratio of 1.2. The lesion has a score of 5 on the 5-point color scale, both suggestive of a malignant lesion. (d) The strain ratio (lesion to fat ratio) is 14.9, suggestive of a malignant lesion. (e) On Virtual Touch imaging (VTi, Siemens) the lesion is stiffer than the adjacent breast tissue and has an E/B ratio of 1.2, suggestive of a malignant lesion. (f) On shear wave elastography (SWE) the lesion has a Vs of 8.1 m/s (>180 kPa), highly suggestive of a malignant lesion. (g) SWE on a different shear wave system has similar findings, with a Vs of 7.8 m/s (188 kPa).

(▶ Fig. 7.5e). On shear wave imaging (▶ Fig. 7.5f) the max Vs is 8.1 m/s (>180 kPa). On a different shear wave system (▶ Fig. 7.5g) the lesion has a uniformly high Vs with a max Vs of >9 m/s (228 kPa).

## 7.5.3 Diagnosis

Invasive ductal carcinoma, grade 1. The lesion was biopsied with a 12-gauge vacuum-assisted core needle under ultrasound guidance. The pathology was an invasive ductal carcinoma, grade 1.

## 7.5.4 Discussion

There is an emerging molecular classification of breast cancer. Breast cancer is now considered as consisting of at least five different molecular subtypes, which are each characterized by distinct gene expression profiles.[135–137] The patients with varying subtypes have different clinical outcomes, and each responds differently to treatment. Breast cancer subtypes defined by gene profile are listed in ▶ Table 7.1.[135,138–142] Another emerging molecular subtype is Luminal C, which corresponds to the histopathological

**Table 7.1** Breast cancer subtypes defined by gene profile

| Subtype | % of cancers | Distant disease-free survival | Overall survival | Gene profile |
|---|---|---|---|---|
| Luminal A | 51–61 | 75 | 90 | ER +, PR +, HER2- |
| Luminal B | 14–16 | 47 | 40 | ER +, and/or PR +, HER2 + |
| HER2 | 7–9 | 34 | 31 | ER-, PR-, HER2 + |
| Basal | 11–20 | 18 | 0 | ER-, PR-, HER2- Cytokeratin 5/6 and EGRF + |
| Unclassified | 2–6 | NA | NA | - for all markers |

subtype of infiltrating lobular carcinoma. The molecular subtypes based on gene expression profiling dictate prognosis.

This case of an invasive ductal carcinoma has all of the positive features of elastography. On SE the lesion is stiffer than adjacent tissue and has an E/B ratio of 1.2, a strain ratio (lesion to fat ratio) of 14.9, a score of 5 on the 5-point color scale. The VTi (strain imaging with ARFI) are similar. The lesion has high Vs through the lesion with a good-quality map throughout the lesion. The Vs is 8 m/s (> 180 kPa). All findings are concordant and highly suspicious for a malignancy. Note is made that the E/B ratio is slightly above 1, but the stiffness based on the strain ratio (lesion to fat ratio) (SE) and the Vs (SWE) suggests a markedly stiff lesion. The correlation between the E/B ratio and the strain ratio has not been evaluated.

The lesion was a BI-RADS category 4A lesion on conventional ultrasound. The elastographic findings are significantly more suspicious.

Based on the proposed elastography classification system (similar to the BI-RADS classification) presented in Chapter 5 this lesion would have a > 95% probability of malignancy.

## 7.6 Case 6: Invasive Ductal Carcinoma—Grade 2

### 7.6.1 Clinical Presentation

An 82-year-old woman presents with a palpable mass. Mammography was not performed.

### 7.6.2 Ultrasound Findings

On B-mode ultrasound (▶ Fig. 7.6a) an irregular 3.5 cm hypoechoic mass is identified. On color Doppler imaging (▶ Fig. 7.6b) there is some peripheral blood flow. The lesion was classified as BI-RADS category 4C.

On strain imaging (▶ Fig. 7.6c) the lesion is stiffer than the surrounding breast tissue and has an E/B ratio of 1.04. The lesion to fat ratio is 12.3 (▶ Fig. 7.6d). Similar findings are found with VTi (▶ Fig. 7.6e). On shear wave imaging (▶ Fig. 7.6f) the max Vs is 4.6 m/s (65 kPa). On three-dimensional (3D) shear wave imaging (▶ Fig. 7.6g) there is increased Vs in the proximal portion of the lesion with a Vs of 7.7 m/s (180 kPa).

## 7.6.3 Diagnosis

Invasive ductal carcinoma, grade 3 with extensive tumor necrosis.

## 7.6.4 Discussion

On B-mode imaging the lesion borders are ill defined but are better identified on SE. Shadowing also interferes with the determination of the posterior border of the lesion. The posterior border of the lesion is well defined on SE. The strain elastographic findings of an E/B ratio of 1.04, strain ratio of 12.3, score of 5 on the 5-point color scale, and similar VTi (strain with ARFI) findings are all suggestive of a malignant lesion. The shear wave images are also suggestive of a malignancy with a Vs of > 4.5 m/s. The use of 3D elastography is helpful to evaluate the entire lesion to determine the site of the highest Vs. This case is one where the center of the cancer color codes blue, which is most likely an artifact of the algorithm. With improved algorithms this "blue" area will not be color coded, confirming that the shear waves in this region were of poor quality and should not be used in interpretation.

Based on the proposed elastography classification system (similar to the BI-RADS classification) presented in Chapter 5 this lesion would have a > 95% probability of malignancy.

## 7.7 Case 7: Invasive Ductal Carcinoma—SE and SWE Not Concordant, Grade 3

### 7.7.1 Clinical Presentation

A 59-year-old woman presents with a palpable mass near right axilla.

### 7.7.2 Ultrasound Findings

On B-mode imaging (▶ Fig. 7.7a) there is a 1 cm oval, hypoechoic lesion with ill-defined borders. On color Doppler imaging (▶ Fig. 7.7b) there is a small amount of blood flow in the lesion. The lesion was classified as BI-RADS category 4A.

On SE (▶ Fig. 7.7c) the lesion is stiffer than the surrounding fatty breast tissue and has an E/B ratio of 3.5. On shear wave imaging (▶ Fig. 7.7d) the lesion has a Vs of 2.5 m/s (19 kPa). On the quality map (▶ Fig. 7.7e) there is some yellow in the lesion, although the majority of the lesion has green (good shear wave quality). On a different shear wave system (▶ Fig. 7.7f) the lesion has a max Vs of 2 m/s (13 kPa).

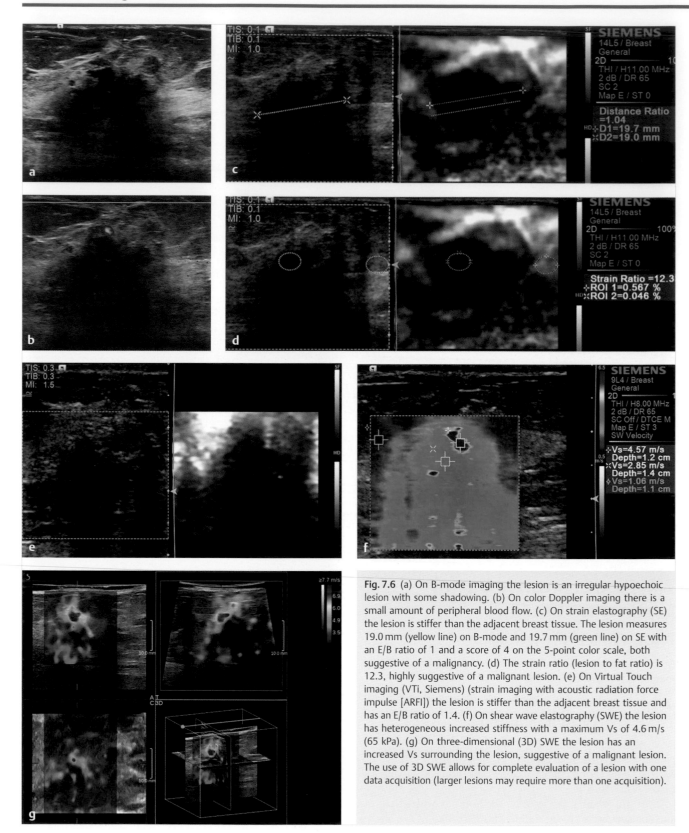

**Fig. 7.6** (a) On B-mode imaging the lesion is an irregular hypoechoic lesion with some shadowing. (b) On color Doppler imaging there is a small amount of peripheral blood flow. (c) On strain elastography (SE) the lesion is stiffer than the adjacent breast tissue. The lesion measures 19.0 mm (yellow line) on B-mode and 19.7 mm (green line) on SE with an E/B ratio of 1 and a score of 4 on the 5-point color scale, both suggestive of a malignancy. (d) The strain ratio (lesion to fat ratio) is 12.3, highly suggestive of a malignant lesion. (e) On Virtual Touch imaging (VTi, Siemens) (strain imaging with acoustic radiation force impulse [ARFI]) the lesion is stiffer than the adjacent breast tissue and has an E/B ratio of 1.4. (f) On shear wave elastography (SWE) the lesion has heterogeneous increased stiffness with a maximum Vs of 4.6 m/s (65 kPa). (g) On three-dimensional (3D) SWE the lesion has an increased Vs surrounding the lesion, suggestive of a malignant lesion. The use of 3D SWE allows for complete evaluation of a lesion with one data acquisition (larger lesions may require more than one acquisition).

## 7.7.3 Diagnosis

Poorly differentiated ductal carcinoma. The lesion was biopsied with a 12-gauge vacuum-assisted needle under ultrasound guidance. The pathology was poorly differentiated ductal carcinoma.

## 7.7.4 Discussion

This case was classified as a BI-RADS category 4A lesion but may have been classified as a BI-RADS 3 lesion by some reviewers. The SE findings are suggestive of a malignancy. If the lesion was classified as BI-RADS category 3 lesion the SE finding

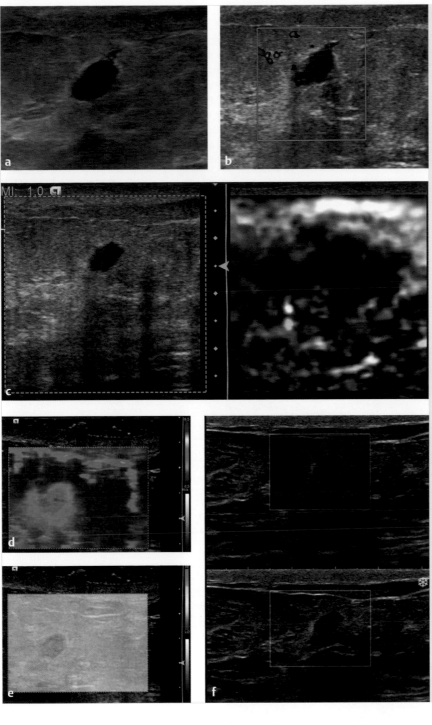

**Fig. 7.7** (a) B-mode imaging demonstrates a 10 mm hypoechoic lesion with an indistinct border and the question of a small echogenic halo. (b) On color Doppler imaging the lesion has a small amount of internal blood flow. (c) On strain elastography the lesion is stiffer than the surrounding breast tissue, with an E/B ratio of 3.5 and a score of 5 on the 5-point color scale. (d) On shear wave elastography (SWE) the lesion has a Vs within the benign range. (e) The corresponding quality map of image (d) demonstrates that all of the shear waves are of poor quality and should not be used in interpretation. (f) SWE with another system also has a Vs within the benign range. With newer improved algorithms the lesion would not color code incorporating the quality map into one image.

would upgrade this lesion to a BI-RADS category 4A lesion and merits a biopsy.

The lesion has a markedly evaluated E/I ratio of 3.5 suggestive of a high-grade malignancy despite the < 10% probability of a malignancy on the conventional ultrasound findings.

In this case the SE and SWE findings are not concordant. The SWE findings are not suggestive of a malignancy in both systems; however, the quality map demonstrates poor-quality shear waves throughout the field of view (FOV). This lesion was close to the skin surface, and a coupling gel standoff pad was made to obtain the images. Poor transmission of the ARFI pulse through the gel may be one reason for the poor-quality shear waves. Good-quality shear waves have been obtained in many cases using this technique. Another possible case is that this high-grade malignancy has caused changes in the surrounding tissue that interfere with good shear wave propagation.

Based on the proposed elastography classification system (similar to the BI-RADS classification) presented in Chapter 5 the lesion would have a > 95% probability of malignancy. (> 95% on SE and ~ 0% on SWE).

## 7.8 Case 8: Invasive Ductal Carcinoma—SE and SWE Not Concordant, Grade 3

### 7.8.1 Clinical Presentation

A 72-year-old woman with a history of left breast cancer 5 years prior, status postlumpectomy, chemotherapy, and radiation therapy presents with a new 1 cm mass on the screening right mammogram. The mammogram was classified as BI-RADS 0, and ultrasound was requested for further workup.

### 7.8.2 Ultrasound Findings

On B-mode imaging (► Fig. 7.8a) an 0.8 cm, taller than wider, hypoechoic lesion with indistinct borders is identified in the 1:00 position 6 cm from the nipple. No blood flow is noted in the lesion on color Doppler imaging (► Fig. 7.8b). The lesion was classified as BI-RADS category 4B.

On strain imaging (► Fig. 7.8c) the lesion is stiffer than the surrounding breast tissue with an E/B ratio of 1.8. The strain ratio (lesion to fat ratio) was 6.5, and the lesion had a score of 5 on the 5-point color scale. Similar findings are identified on VTi (► Fig. 7.8d). All of the SE image findings are suggestive of a malignancy. On shear wave imaging (► Fig. 7.8e) the lesion has a Vs of 4.3 m/s (58 kPa) on one system and similar findings on a different shear wave system (► Fig. 7.8f).

A second 9 mm lesion was identified in the 11:00 position of the right breast 5 cm from the nipple, which had an E/B ratio of 1.6, a score of 5 on the 5-pont color scale, and a strain ratio (lesion to fat ratio) of 5.9 (► Fig. 7.8g). On SWE (► Fig. 7.8h) the Vs was 4.7 m/s (65 kPa).

### 7.8.3 Diagnosis

1:00: Invasive ductal carcinoma, grade 2 with DCIS; 11:00: DCIS, solid papillary type. Right breast 1:00: invasive, moderately differentiated ductal carcinoma and DCIS, intermediate grade, cribriform and papillary type. Right breast 11:00: low

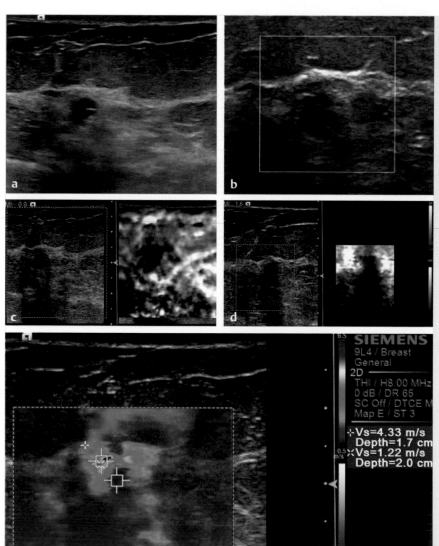

**Fig. 7.8** (a) On B-mode imaging the lesion is an 8 mm hypoechoic lesion with an internal septation and ill-defined borders. (b) On power Doppler imaging no blood flow is identified within the lesion. (c) On strain elastography the lesion is stiffer than the surrounding tissue and has an E/B ratio of 1.8, a score of 5 on the 5-point color scale, and a strain ratio (lesion to fat ratio) of 6.5, all suggestive of a malignant lesion. (d) On Virtual Touch imaging (VTi, Siemens) (strain imaging using acoustic radiation force impulse [ARFI]) the lesion is stiffer than the adjacent tissue, with an E/B ratio of 1.2. (e) On shear wave elastography (SWE) the lesion has a Vs of 4.3 that is borderline for a malignant lesion. (*Continued*)

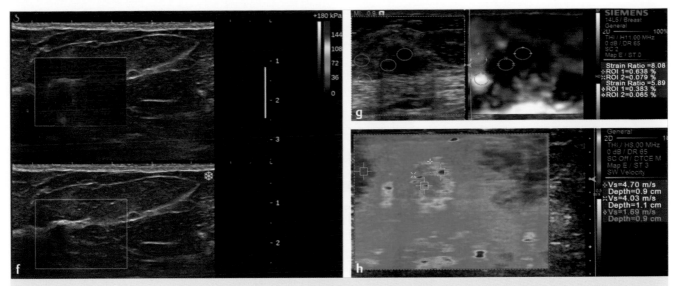

**Fig. 7.8** (*Continued*) (f) On another SWE system the lesion does not color code centrally but has a ring of increased Vs of 4.5 m/s (60 kPa), also borderline for a malignant lesion. (g) The second lesion in this case was a 9 mm lesion that had a strain ratio of 5.9, consistent with a malignant lesion. (h) The second lesion was stiff on SWE with a Vs of 4.7 m/s (65 kPa), suggestive of a malignant lesion.

grade DCIS, solid/papillary type with small focus of stromal microinvasion.

## 7.8.4 Discussion

The lesion in the 1:00 position of the right breast had findings suggestive of a malignancy on SE imaging but borderline findings in SWE. In cases of discordance the more suggestive findings should be used to classify the lesion unless there is a confident cause of the discordance. This lesion had an E/I ratio 1.8, a score of 5 on the 5-point color scale, and a strain ratio (lesion to fat ratio) of 6.5, all suggestive of a malignancy; however, the SWE findings are borderline with a "ring" of higher Vs surrounding the lesion but not to the level suggestive of a malignancy.

It is of note that the second lesion in this case that was DCIS gave concordant findings of a malignancy. Our experience is that DCIS rarely gives the blue or soft cancer finding on SWE. The finding of artificial softness in some invasive cancers (which are very stiff) is secondary to some unique histology of invasive ductal cancers. The finding of a paradoxically soft mass on SWE, to the author, is not identified in other neoplasms (RG Barr, personal observation, October 1, 2013).

Based on the proposed elastography classification system (similar to the BI-RADS classification) presented in Chapter 5 this lesion would have a probability of > 95% malignancy. (> 95% on SE; 2–95% on SWE).

## 7.9 Case 9: Invasive Ductal Carcinoma—No Color Coding on SWE, Grade 2

### 7.9.1 Clinical Presentation

A 60-year-old woman presented with a palpable mass in her right breast. The patient had had a remote lumpectomy in a dif-

ferent quadrant of her right breast. A diagnostic mammogram and ultrasound at an outside institution did not identify an abnormality to account for the mass. Magnetic resonance imaging (MRI) was performed for further workup. On MRI a lobular mass > 2 cm with washout characteristics was identified at the site of the palpable abnormality. A second-look ultrasound with elastography was requested to determine if it could guide a biopsy.

### 7.9.2 Ultrasound Findings

On B-mode imaging (► Fig. 7.9a) a > 3 cm ill-defined area with shadowing and irregular borders is identified. No flow is identified in the lesion or adjacent to the lesion (► Fig. 7.9b). The lesion was classified as BI-RADS category 4C given the MRI results.

On strain imaging (► Fig. 7.9c) the lesion is stiffer than the surrounding breast tissue. The lesion is more defined on SE than on B-mode. It is not possible to calculate an accurate E/B ratio or a score on the 5-point color scale because the lesion borders are not identified on B-mode imaging. The strain ratio (lesion to fat ratio) is 5.2. On shear wave imaging (► Fig. 7.9d,f) both systems do not color code the mass. The quality map (► Fig. 7.9e) is yellow and red, confirming that adequate shear waves were not present in the lesion. In the area of increased Vs in the periphery the quality map is green (good quality).

### 7.9.3 Diagnosis

Invasive ductal carcinoma, grade 2. The patient had a surgical resection of the lesion. The lesion was an invasive ductal carcinoma, grade 2.

### 7.9.4 Discussion

The lesion in this case is difficult to identify on ultrasound. The initial diagnostic mammogram and diagnostic ultrasound could

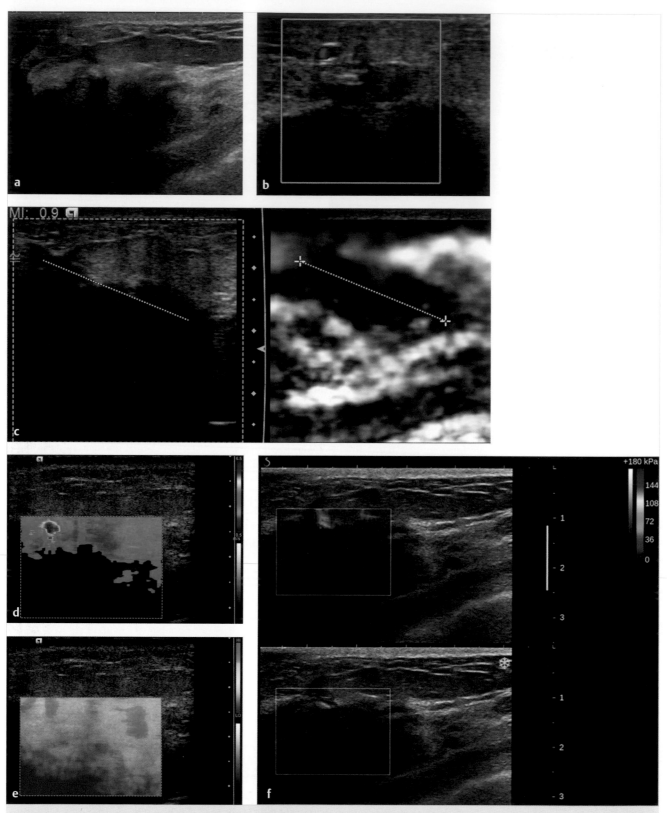

**Fig. 7.9** (a) On B-mode imaging there is an ill-defined hypoechoic mass. (b) On color Doppler imaging there is a small amount of adjacent blood flow. (c) On strain elastography the lesion (yellow line) is better defined than in the corresponding B-mode image. The lesion is stiffer than the adjacent breast tissue. The posterior border of the lesion is now identified; the posterior border on B-mode imaging is poorly visualized due to shadowing. (d) On shear wave elastography (SWE) the lesion does not color code, but there is an increased Vs anterior to the lesion. (e) The quality map of image (d) confirms that the shear waves within the lesion and adjacent to the lesion are of poor quality and should not be used in interpretation. (f) Similar findings to (e) are identified on another SWE system.

not account for the palpable mass. A 2 cm mass was identified on MRI. A second-look ultrasound was requested to determine if the lesion could be biopsied under ultrasound. On the B-mode image an area of ill-defined hypoechogenicity is identified at the site of the MRI abnormality. However, with SE the mass is clearly defined, but it is difficult to calculate an E/B ratio or assign a score on the 5-point scale because the lesion size is not known on B-mode imaging. However, a strain ratio can be calculated, which was 5.2, suggestive of a malignancy. On SWE the lesion has a poor-quality map on one system and is not color coded in the other system (also due to poor-quality shear waves). Therefore, an assessment based on SWE cannot be made. However, in general when a solid mass does not generate adequate shear waves (and is not too deep) the lesion is most likely a malignancy. The use of SE allowed for identification of the lesion so that an ultrasound-guided biopsy could be performed.

Based on the proposed elastography classification system (similar to the BI-RADS classification) presented in Chapter 5 this lesion has a probability of > 95% of malignancy.

# 7.10 Case 10: Invasive Ductal Carcinoma—Grade 2 with High-Grade DCIS

## 7.10.1 Clinical Presentation

A 61-year-old woman presents with an abnormal screening mammogram. The mammogram was classified as BI-RADS category 0, and ultrasound was recommended for further workup.

## 7.10.2 Ultrasound Findings

A 4 mm angular hypoechoic lesion with an echogenic halo is identified on B-mode imaging (▶ Fig. 7.10a). There is an echogenic halo around the lesion and architectural distortion with ligaments being pulled to the lesion. There is significant blood flow in the lesion on color Doppler (▶ Fig. 7.10b). The lesion was classified as BI-RADS category 4C.

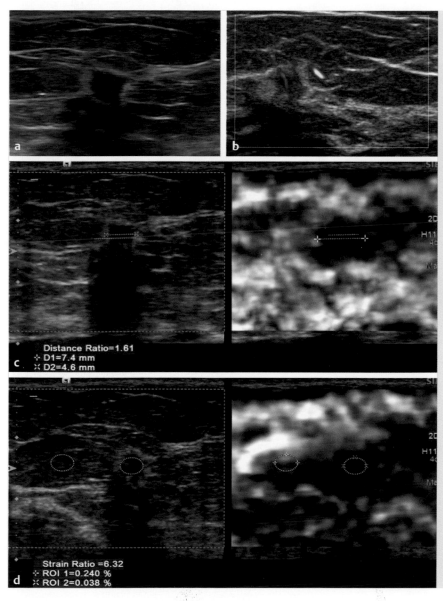

**Fig. 7.10** (a) On B-mode imaging there is a taller than wider, 4 mm hypoechoic lesion with an echogenic halo and retraction of tissue to the lesion. (b) On power Doppler imaging there is significant blood flow within the lesion. (c) On strain elastography (SE) the lesion is stiffer than the adjacent tissue. The lesion measures 4.6 mm (yellow line) on B-mode and 7.4 mm (green line) on SE with an E/B ratio of 1.6 and a score of 5 on the 5-point color scale, both suggestive of a malignancy. (d) The strain ratio (lesion to fat ratio) is 6.3, consistent with other SE findings suggestive of a malignancy. (*Continued*)

Distance Ratio=1.61
÷ D1=7.4 mm
✕ D2=4.6 mm

Strain Ratio =6.32
÷ ROI 1=0.240 %
✕ ROI 2=0.038 %

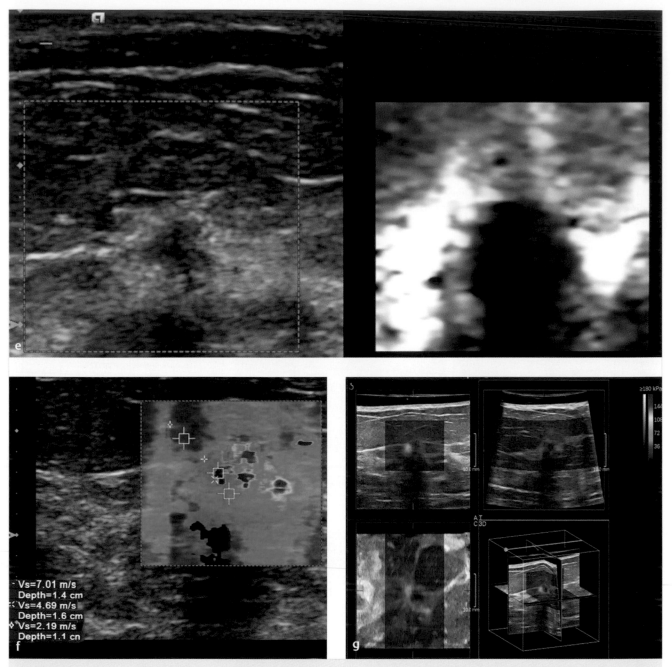

**Fig. 7.10** (*Continued*) (e) On Virtual Touch imaging (VTi, Siemens) (strain imaging with acoustic radiation force impulse [ARFI]) the lesion is significantly stiffer than the surrounding tissue, with an E/B ratio of 1.8 suggestive of a malignancy and concordant with the manual displacement technique (c, d). (f) On shear wave elastography (SWE) the lesion has a Vs of 7 m/s (168 kPa) consistent with the SE finding, consistent with a malignancy. (g) On three-dimensional SWE the lesion has a ring of high Vs, suggestive of a malignant lesion.

On strain imaging (▶ Fig. 7.10c) the lesion is significantly stiffer than the surrounding breast tissue with an E/B ratio of 1.6. The lesion to fat ratio is 6.3 (▶ Fig. 7.10d). On VTi (strain imaging using ARFI) the marked increased lesion stiffness compared with surrounding breast tissue and the increased size of the lesion on elastography are appreciated (▶ Fig. 7.10e). On shear wave imaging (▶ Fig. 7.10f) the lesion has a Vs of 7 m/s (140 kPa). The lesion size based on the abnormal Vs is also larger than on B-mode. On 3D SWE (▶ Fig. 7.10g) the increased Vs is noted around the lesion.

## 7.10.3 Diagnosis

Invasive ductal carcinoma, grade 2 with a minor component of high-grade DCIS. ER +, PR +, Her 2–. The lesion was biopsied using a 12-gauge vacuum-assisted needle under ultrasound guidance. The pathology was an invasive ductal carcinoma, grade 2 with a minor component of high-grade DCIS; ER(+), PR(+), Her 2(–).

### 7.10.4 Discussion

This case has concordant findings with both SE and SWE findings suggestive of a malignancy. On SE imaging the lesion has an E/B ratio of 1.6, a score of 5 on the 5-point color scale, and a strain ratio (lesion to fat ratio) of 6.3. On the VTi (strain imaging with ARFI) the lesion is very black compared with the background tissue, including the glandular tissue. This appearance is seen with stiff tumors on SE because the dynamic range of the coding scale is large, with the stiff tumor marking the upper setting and fat the lower setting. As can be seen in the diagram of Vs of various breast tissues in ▶ Fig. 2.5 the stiffness of the glandular tissue is close to that of the fatty tissue and very much softer than a breast malignancy, leading to this "black and white" image with very little mid- to dark-gray coding.

In cases where there is an echogenic halo the measurement on the B-mode image should be taken only of the hypoechoic mass because that is how all published papers have determined the cutoff value. It is not known if the increased size on the elastogram is due to breast cancer that is not identified on the B-mode image or an influence on the surrounding tissue (body's defense mechanism against the cancer). Investigations are under way to determine the exact cause of the increased size of malignant lesions on elastography. It is felt unlikely that this effect is due only to desmoplastic reaction because that does not explain why benign lesions appear smaller on elastography. There is no "antidesmoplastic" reaction to account for the benign findings.

Based on the proposed elastography classification system (similar to the BI-RADS classification) presented in Chapter 5 this lesion would have a > 95% probability of malignancy.

## 7.11 Case 11: Invasive Ductal Carcinoma—Grade 3 with Central Necrosis

### 7.11.1 Clinical Presentation

The patient is a 60-year-old woman presenting with focal pain in the right breast and a palpable mass. A mammogram was

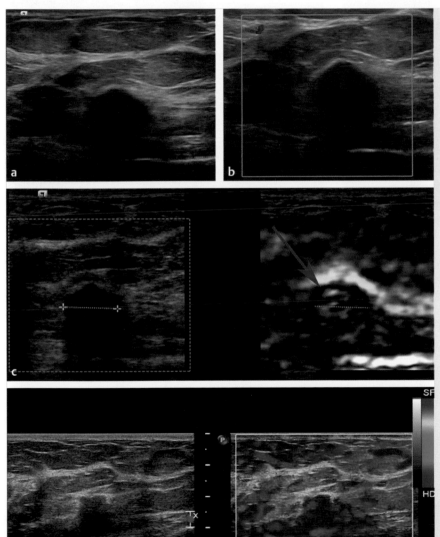

Fig. 7.11 (a) On B-mode imaging the lesion is a 1 cm hypoechoic lesion with ill-defined borders, has a questionable hypoechoic rim, and is taller than wider. The lesion displaces the pectoralis muscle but did not appear to invade the muscle. (b) No blood flow is identified within the lesion on power Doppler imaging. (c) On strain elastography (SE) imaging the lesion (yellow line) has a soft central area (arrow) with a thin rim of increased stiffness. The E/B ratio is 1 and the lesion has a score of 2 on the 5-point color scale. (d) SE image using a blue is stiff color scale with findings similar to (c). (Continued)

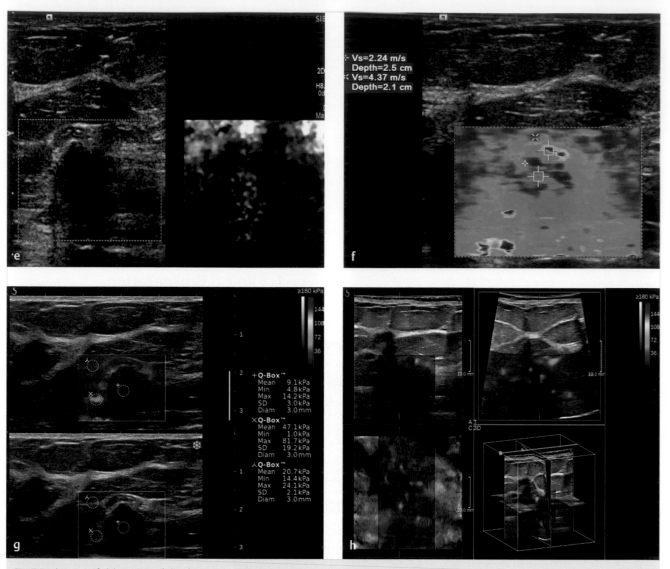

**Fig. 7.11** (*Continued*) (e) On Virtual Touch imaging (VTi, Siemens) (strain imaging with acoustic radiation force impulse [ARFI]) the lesion has similar findings to the manual displacement technique with a soft center and a thin stiff rim. (f) On shear wave elastography (SWE) the lesion is centrally soft (Vs of 2.2 m/s; 15 kPa) with the rim having borderline stiffness of malignancy of 4.4 m/s (57 kPa). (g) SWE on a different system has similar findings of a soft central area with a stiff rim similar to (f). (h) Similar SWE findings are obtained using three-dimensional SWE.

performed and interpreted as normal with scattered fibroglandular densities and unchanged from prior exams. Because of the palpable abnormality the mammogram was classified as BI-RADS category 0, and ultrasound was advised for further workup.

## 7.11.2 Ultrasound Findings

There is a 1 × 1 cm hypoechoic lesion with slightly ill defined borders in the right breast 7:00 position, 8 cm from the nipple (▶ Fig. 7.11a). There is a question of a hyperechoic rim. The pectoralis muscle was slightly displaced secondary to the mass, but there did not appear to be invasion of the muscle. The lesion corresponds to the patient's area of pain. Color Doppler evaluation (▶ Fig. 7.11b) does not demonstrate blood flow within the lesion or adjacent to the lesion. The lesion was classified as BI-RADS category 4B.

On SE (▶ Fig. 7.11c) the lesion is softer than the surrounding tissue with a thin rim of stiff tissue. In this case the lesion was measured (yellow line) and was "shadowed" onto the elastogram to confirm the position of the lesion. The use of a copy or shadow function is helpful in correlating findings between the B-mode image and the elastogram. This lesion would have a score of 2 on the 5-point color scale (▶ Fig. 7.11d). Using VTi (ARFI to generate stress and analysis as strain) demonstrates a pattern similar to the manual compression strain (▶ Fig. 7.11e).

With SWE (▶ Fig. 7.11f, g) the lesion color codes blue (soft). Using regions of interest (ROIs) an exact measurement of the shear wave velocity (expressed either in m/s or kPa) can be obtained. In this case the lesion has a mean kPa value of 9 (Vs 1.7 m/s), whereas the adjacent breast tissue has kPa values between 20 and 47 (Vs 2.6–3.9 m/s). A 3D SWE image is provided in ▶ Fig. 7.11h.

### 7.11.3 Diagnosis

Invasive ductal carcinoma, grade 3 with prominent perineural invasion. The lesion was biopsied with a 12-gauge vacuum-assisted core biopsy under ultrasound guidance. Pathology demonstrated invasive poorly differentiated ductal carcinoma. The patient underwent a lumpectomy yielding the same diagnosis with prominent perineural invasion.

### 7.11.4 Discussion

This case has an interesting finding of a soft central area on *both* SE and SWE. In the previous cases of "blue" or "soft" cancer on SWE presented here, the SE images always had a stiff central area despite the SWE images suggesting a soft center (with a poor-quality map in most cases). The confidence of a soft central area is significantly increased when the finding is concordant with SE and SWE. The appearance here is similar to the cases of mastitis presented in Cases 6.23 and 6.24. In our experience of elastography in over 400 cases of breast cancer the finding of a soft center is rare. This case and Case 7.12 are the only cases of breast malignancy we have identified with a soft central area. In this case the soft center was due to necrotic tumor. Most breast cancers have avascular fibrotic centers and not soft necrotic centers.

When a soft central area is identified within a lesion, confirmed on both SE and SWE with good quality, a lesion other than breast cancer should be considered. Other possibilities include mastitis (see Cases 6.23 and 6.24), and nonbreast adenocarcinoma (see Case 8.5), and fat necrosis (see Cases 6.23 and 6.24) should be considered. As discussed in detail in Case 8.6, if we see an adenocarcinoma with a soft necrotic center and it is a triple negative cancer additional markers are requested to determine if the lesion is not of breast origin.

Based on the proposed elastography classification system (similar to the BI-RADS classification) presented in Chapter 5 this lesion would have an ~ 0% probability of malignancy.

## 7.12 Case 12: Invasive Ductal Carcinoma—Grade 3

### 7.12.1 Clinical Presentation

An 84-year-old woman presents with a new palpable mass since the last screening mammogram (BI-RADS category 2).

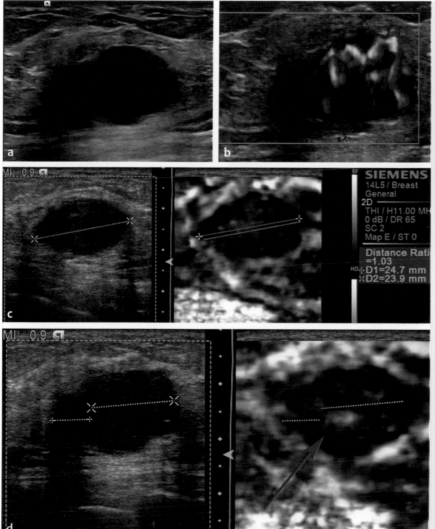

**Fig. 7.12** (a) On B-mode imaging the lesion is a 2.7 cm oval hypoechoic mass that has an ill-defined medial border. (b) The lesion has significant blood flow on power Doppler imaging. (c) On strain elastography (SE) the lesion has a softer central area (arrow) with a thick, stiffer rim. The lesion measures 23.9 mm (yellow line) and 24.7 mm (green line) and the E/B ratio is 1 with a score of 2 on the 5-point color-scale. (d) On both B-mode imaging and SE there is a question of a second lesion on the medial portion of the lesion (smaller dotted line). On SE the medial portion is softer (arrow) than the thick rim on the lateral portion of the lesion. (*Continued*)

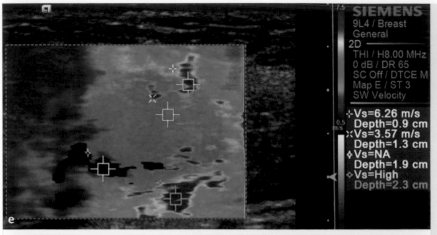

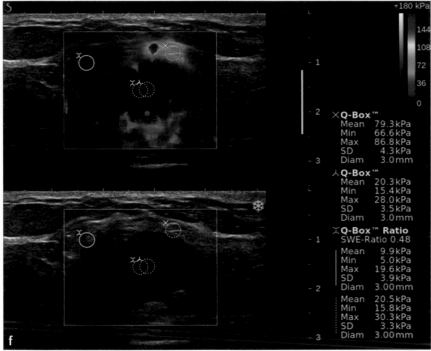

**Fig. 7.12** (*Continued*) (e) On shear wave elastography (SWE) the lesion has a Vs of > 7.7 m/s (180 kPa). The medial portion of the lesion noted above is softer or does not color code. (f) On a different SWE system the lesion is color coded blue, but there is a ring of higher stiffness with a Vs of 7.7 m/s (180 kPa).

New mammography was not performed, and an ultrasound was requested.

## 7.12.2 Ultrasound Findings

B-mode imaging (► Fig. 7.12a) shows a 2.7 cm oval hypoechoic mass that is wider than taller and has an ill-defined medial border. There is marked blood flow in the lesion on power Doppler imaging (► Fig. 7.12b). The lesion was classified as BI-RADS category 4A.

On strain imaging (► Fig. 7.12c) the lesion is stiffer than the surrounding breast tissue and has an E/B ratio of 1.03. In another position (► Fig. 7.12d) there is a question of a second adjacent lesion on the medial border, which is also stiffer than the surrounding breast tissue. There is also a soft area centrally within the mass. The lesion would have a score of 5 on the 5-point color scale. On shear wave imaging (► Fig. 7.12e) the max Vs is > 7.5 m/s (> 180 kPa). On a different shear wave system (► Fig. 7.12f) the increased Vs is noted in the proximal portion of the lesion.

## 7.12.3 Diagnosis

Invasive ductal carcinoma, grade 3. The lesion was biopsied using a 12-gauge vacuum-assisted needle under ultrasound guidance. The biopsy of the lesion on the medial border was dark brown on visual inspection, whereas that of the lateral portion of the mass was yellow-white. The pathology was invasive poorly differentiated ductal carcinoma, with prominent focal necrosis and lyphoplasmacytic inflammation.

## 7.12.4 Discussion

This case of invasive ductal carcinoma has a soft central area of liquefactive necrosis that is discussed in detail in Case 7.11.

The appearance of this lesion can be seen in a fibroadenoma, both in conventional imaging and in elastography. Some reviewers may have classified this mass as a BI-RADS category 3 lesion. The classification of BI-RADS 4A was given due to the border irregularity on the medical portion of the lesion. On SE the area with border irregularity appears stiffer than the remainder of the lesion.

The elastographic finding in this case increases confidence that a biopsy is the appropriate follow-up for this lesion.

Based on the proposed elastography classification system (similar to the BI-RADS classification) presented in Chapter 5 the lesion would have a > 95% probability of malignancy.

# 7.13 Case 13: Invasive Ductal Carcinoma—No Color Coding on SWE, Grade 2

## 7.13.1 Clinical Presentation

A 72-year-old woman was found to have a new 10 mm irregular mass in the right breast on screening mammography. The lesion was confirmed on spot compression views. No associated microcalcifications were identified. The mammogram was classified as BI-RADS category 0, and an ultrasound was advised for further workup.

## 7.13.2 Ultrasound Findings

On B-mode imaging (▶ Fig. 7.13a) a 1 cm hypoechoic lesion that is taller than wider with indistinct borders and shadowing is identified. On color Doppler imaging (▶ Fig. 7.13b) there is some blood flow within the lesion. The lesion was classified as BI-RADS category 4C.

On strain elastography (▶ Fig. 7.13c) the lesion is much stiffer than the adjacent glandular tissue and has an E/B ratio of 2.4. The lesion has a strain ratio (lesion to fat ratio) of 4.3 (▶ Fig. 7.13d). The lesion has a score of 5 on the 5-point color scale. On shear wave imaging (▶ Fig. 7.13e) the lesion does not color code, and there is no ring of high Vs around the lesion.

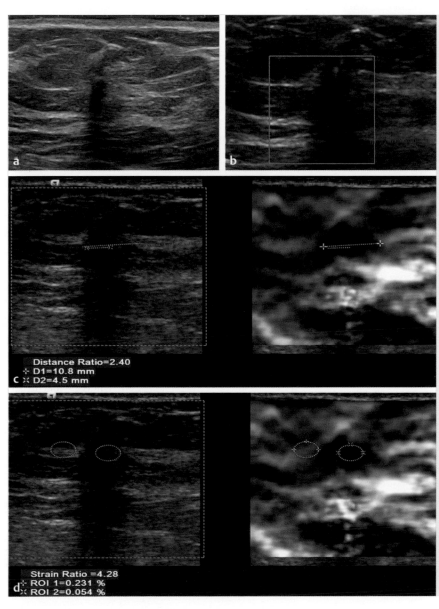

**Fig. 7.13** (a) On B-mode imaging there is a taller than wider hypoechoic lesion measuring 1 cm with indistinct borders. (b) The lesion has some proximal blood flow on power Doppler imaging. (c) On strain elastography the lesion is stiffer than the adjacent tissue. The lesion measures 4.5 mm (yellow line) on B-mode and 10.8 mm (green line) on SE with an E/B ratio of 2.4 and a score of 5 on the 5-point color scale, both suggestive of a malignant lesion. (d) The strain ratio (lesion to fat ratio) is 4.3, borderline for a malignancy. (Continued)

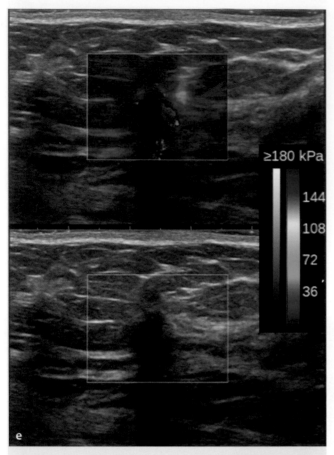

**Fig. 7.13** (*Continued*) (e) On shear wave elastography the lesion does not color code. Because the lesion is solid this finding is suspicious for a malignancy. There is a ring of increased stiffness adjacent to the lesion (arrow), also suggestive of a malignancy.

### 7.13.3 Diagnosis

Invasive ductal carcinoma, grade 2. The lesion was biopsied under ultrasound guidance using a 12-gauge vacuum-assisted needle. The diagnosis on pathology was an invasive, moderately differentiated ductal carcinoma. The lesion was ER (+, >90%), PR (+, >90%), Her-2 (−).

### 7.13.4 Discussion

This lesion has suspicious findings for malignancy on all of the SE measures; the E/I ratio is 2.4, the lesion has a score of 5 on the 5-point color scale, and the strain ratio (lesion to fat ratio) is 4.3. On SWE the lesion does not color code secondary to poor-quality shear waves. This is the appearance of previous "soft" or "blue" cancers seen with older SWE algorithms. In cases where there is no color coding of the lesion the lesion can either be a simple cyst with simple fluid that does not support shear wave propagation or a solid lesion with a high probability of being a malignant lesion.[65]

Often refractive shadowing from ligaments will have an appearance similar to this lesion. The appearance may give concern of a lesion similar to this. The refractive artifact can often be eliminated by angling the probe to correct for the critical angle of the ultrasound beam to the ligament. Elastography can also be helpful in this situation. If the lesion is an artifact it will code soft, whereas if it is a solid lesion it will usually code stiffer than adjacent tissue and code very stiff if a malignancy.

Based on the proposed elastography classification system (similar to the BI-RADS classification) presented in Chapter 5 this lesion would have a > 95% probability of malignancy.

## 7.14 Case 14: Invasive Ductal Carcinoma—Grade 3 with Extensive Necrosis

### 7.14.1 Clinical Presentation

An 83-year-old woman presents with a new mass identified on screening mammography. The mammogram was classified as BI-RADS category 0, and ultrasound was recommended for further workup.

### 7.14.2 Ultrasound Findings

On B-mode imaging (▶ Fig. 7.14a) a 3.5 cm irregular, heterogeneous mass is identified. There is marked color Doppler flow in the lesion (▶ Fig. 7.14b). The lesion was classified as a BI-RADS category 4C lesion.

On strain imaging (▶ Fig. 7.14c) the lesion is significantly stiffer than the surrounding breast tissue. Determining an accurate E/B ratio is difficult because the lesion is difficult to measure on B-mode. On the 5-point color scale this would be given a score of 4 or 5. The strain ratio (lesion to fat ratio) is 13.5 (▶ Fig. 7.14d). On VTi (strain imaging using ARFI) the lesion is stiffer than the adjacent breast tissue with a similar finding to SE (▶ Fig. 7.14e). On shear wave imaging the lesion has a Vs of 7.6 m/s (180 kPa) on one system (▶ Fig. 7.14f) and a Vs of 7.5 m/s (170 kPa) on another system (▶ Fig. 7.14g).

### 7.14.3 Diagnosis

Invasive ductal carcinoma, grade 3 with extensive necrosis. The lesion was biopsied with a 12-gauge vacuum-assisted needle under ultrasound guidance. The lesion was an invasive ductal carcinoma, poorly differentiated with extensive tumor necrosis on pathology.

### 7.14.4 Discussion

This lesion appears as a very heterogeneous mass on B-mode imaging. It is difficult to determine if the lesion is one large abnormal mass or a lesion that is infiltrating adjacent tissue with areas of normal tissue maintained. However, on both SE and SWE the lesion is stiff throughout, suggesting there are no intervening components of nonneoplastic breast tissue. Both the SE and the SWE findings are suggestive of a malignancy.

This case demonstrates the differences that are sometimes identified between the two shear wave systems. One system

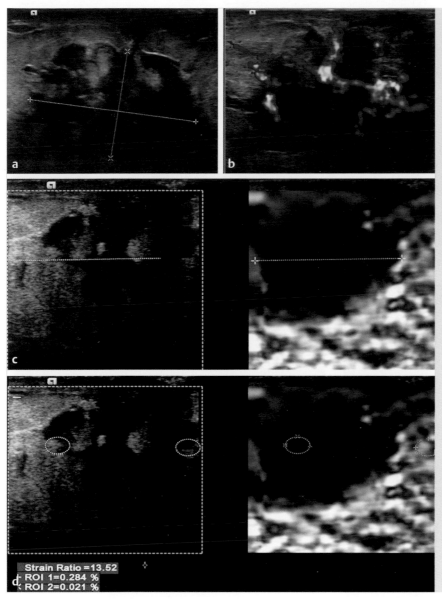

**Fig. 7.14** (a) On B-mode imaging there is an irregular, heterogeneous 3.5 cm mass (lines). (b) On power Doppler imaging there is a significant amount of internal blood flow. (c) On strain elastography the lesion (lines) is stiffer than the surrounding tissue. The E/B ratio is difficult to calculate because the lesion margins are not well appreciated on B-mode imaging. The lesion would have a score of 4 or 5 on the 5-point color scale. (d) The lesion has a strain ratio (lesion to fat ratio) of 13.5, highly suggestive of a malignancy. (e) On Virtual Touch imaging (VTi, Siemens) (strain imaging with acoustic radiation force impulse [ARFI]) the lesion is stiffer than the adjacent tissue and appears similar in size to the lesion on B-mode imaging. (f) On shear wave elastography (SWE) the lesion has a Vs of 7.6 m/s (180 kPa), highly suspicious for malignancy. (g) SWE on a different system has a Vs of 7.6 m/s (170 kPa), similar to the findings in (f). The findings using this system are more prominent in the lesion–normal tissue interface. (*Continued*)

has more color coding of red within the lesion, whereas the other has more color coding of red in the periphery of the lesion. This difference has not been studied but may be due to the differences in the two methods of SWE. One system uses a series of ARFI pulses to generate a single image (not real-time imaging) while the other uses a series of ARFI pulses to generate a mach wave in which real-time SWE can be performed. In the latter case reflections of the mach wave off the interface between soft and very stiff tissue may account for the more prominent "ring" of high Vs and less red color coding centrally. The same findings are found less often in the former technique. When interpreting SWE findings the color coding of the lesion as well as surrounding tissue should be evaluated. Both systems provide the ability to characterize a lesion as benign or malignant.

Based on the proposed elastography classification system (similar to the BI-RADS classification) presented in Chapter 5 this lesion would have a > 95% probability of malignancy.

## 7.15 Case 15: Invasive Lobular Carcinoma

### 7.15.1 Clinical Presentation

The patient is a 90-year-old woman with a 1.5 cm speculated mass with suspicious calcifications on screening mammography. The mammogram was classified as BI-RADS category 5, and ultrasound-guided biopsy was recommended.

### 7.15.2 Ultrasound Findings

On B-mode imaging (▶ Fig. 7.15a) a 1.5 cm markedly hypoechoic lesion with shadowing is identified. The lesion has speculated margins. On power Doppler imaging (▶ Fig. 7.15b) no blood flow is identified in the mass or surrounding tissue. The lesion was classified as BI-RADS category 5.

On strain imaging (▶ Fig. 7.15c) the lesion is much stiffer than the surrounding breast tissue. The E/B ratio is 1.3. The lesion to

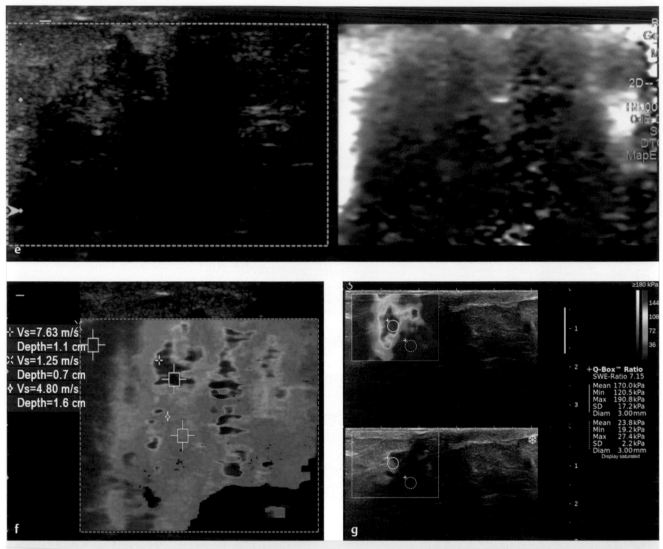

**Fig. 7.14** (*Continued*) (e) On Virtual Touch imaging (VTi, Siemens) (strain imaging with acoustic radiation force impulse [ARFI]) the lesion is stiffer than the adjacent tissue and appears similar in size to the lesion on B-mode imaging. (f) On shear wave elastography (SWE) the lesion has a Vs of 7.6 m/s (180 kPa), highly suspicious for malignancy. (g) SWE on a different system has a Vs of 7.6 m/s (170 kPa), similar to the findings in (f). The findings using this system are more prominent in the lesion–normal tissue interface.

fat ratio is 16 (▶ Fig. 7.15d). The strain findings are highly suggestive of a malignancy. On shear wave imaging (▶ Fig. 7.15e) the lesion has a Vs of 9.7 m/s (> 180 kPa) compared with the background tissue, which has a Vs of 2.1 m/s (14 kPa). On a different shear wave system (▶ Fig. 7.15f) the tissue surrounding the lesion has a Vs of 4.8 m/s (79 kPa). Both shear wave systems are suggestive of a malignancy.

### 7.15.3 Diagnosis

Invasive lobular carcinoma, grade 1 with lobular carcinoma in situ. The lesion was biopsied using a 12-gauge vacuum-assisted needle. The pathology was invasive lobular carcinoma, grade 1 with lobular carcinoma in situ.

### 7.15.4 Discussion

Invasive lobular carciinoma (ILC) accounts for 6 to 9% of breast cancers.[143,144] ILC spreads as sheets of a single-cell layer along Cooper ligaments often referred to as Indian filing. Because of this infiltrative growth pattern, ILC is more difficult to detect at clinical examination and with mammography than invasive ductal carcinoma.[145–147] ILC is therefore usually large at diagnosis and often multifocal.[143,148] Lymph node metastasis is less common with ILC than with invasive ductal carcinoma for lesions of equal size, however,[147] so the stage at diagnosis for ILC is overall similar to that for invasive ductal carcinoma despite the larger size at diagnosis.[149]

The most common clinical findings of ILC are palpable thickening and skin or nipple retraction.[150] The clinical examination findings are often more prominent than are the imaging findings. The mammogram often underestimates tumor size relative to the physical examination findings.[143] ILC also has a propensity for metastatic spread to the peritoneum, retroperitoneum, and gynecologic organs[151,152]; therefore, consider the diagnosis of ILC in women presenting with ascites, hydronephrosis, or pelvic masses.[148]

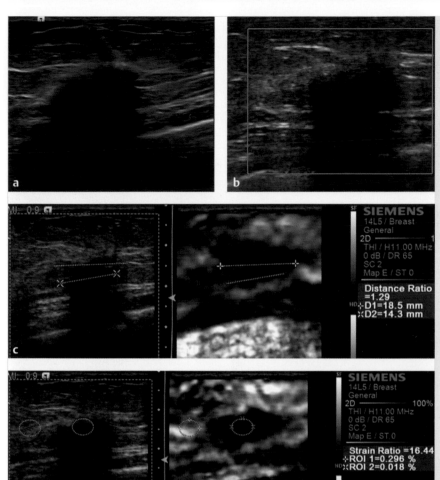

**Fig. 7.15** (a) The mass identified on screening mammography is a 1.5 cm speculated irregular hypoechoic mass with a hyperechoic halo. (b) On color Doppler imaging there is no significant blood flow within or adjacent to the lesion. (c) On strain imaging the lesion is stiffer than the surrounding tissue. The mass measures 14.3 mm (yellow line) on B-mode and 18.5 mm (green line) on SE with an E/B ratio of 1.3. On the 5-point color scale the lesion is a score of 5. Note that the posterior aspect of the lesion is well defined on elastography. In this case the shadowing is not intense enough to completely prohibit signals in the area of shadowing to be identified. (d) The strain ratio (lesion to fat ratio) of the mass is 16.4, highly suggestive of a malignancy. (*Continued*)

The most frequent mammographic manifestation of ILC is architectural distortion with or without a central mass[153] or a focal asymmetry.[149] Calcifications are a very uncommon feature of ILC.[149,153] Mammography often greatly underestimates the size of ILC as seen at histologic examination.[147] When ILC is large, the affected breast may appear to be decreasing in size on the mammogram; this has been termed the shrinking breast.[154] The decreased size of the breast on mammography is probably due to the sheets of tumor cells causing decreased compressibility of the breast so that the breast tissue does not spread out as well during mammographic compression. The shrinking breast is a mammographic and not a clinical finding of ILC. The physical size of the breast at clinical inspection is not different.

On ultrasound, the numerous sheets of tumor cells will frequently cause architectural distortion and posterior acoustic shadowing and, as at mammography, often without a discrete mass. It may occasionally be difficult to distinguish the mild posterior acoustic shadowing that may be seen with fibrocystic changes from that of ILC. The appearance of the shadowing can be more prominent when harmonic imaging is used. In the case of a benign fibrocystic change, application of firm pressure with a transducer will often remove the mild shadowing. Survey scanning by using compound imaging reduces shadowing, which may be the primary ultrasound finding of ILC.[148]

Management of a lesion manifesting as architectural distortion without a central mass is controversial because the differential diagnosis includes radial sclerosing lesion (radial scar). Surgical excision is often recommended rather than core biopsy because 7 to 30% of radial sclerosing lesions may be associated with small foci of invasive ductal carconima or DCIS.[110] However, 29% of lesions suspected of being radial sclerosing lesions at imaging are actually carcinomas at biopsy.[155] Core biopsy prior to excision is therefore often helpful in surgical planning.

ILC is more frequently associated with positive margins at excision[156] and is more frequently treated with mastectomy.[147] This is likely due to the large size of ILC at diagnosis and the underestimation of the disease extent at conventional imaging. Ultrasound or MRI may be useful for assessing the extent of the disease.[146,157] In 39% of women with ILC, MRI depicts more extensive disease than is suspected with conventional imaging.[157] On MRI scans, ILC may manifest as an enhancing solitary mass with irregular margins, multiple enhancing lesions, or only enhancing septa.[158] It is unknown if the elastographic size of the lesion will correlate more accurately with the pathological size of the cancer.

In this case all of the SE and SWE findings are concordant and highly suggestive of a malignancy. Given the BI-RADS category 5 findings on conventional ultrasound the elastographic results

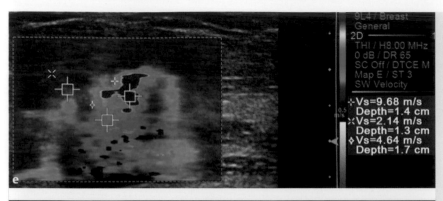

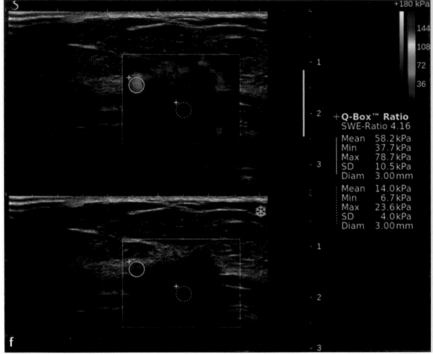

Fig. 7.15 (*Continued*) (e) On shear wave imaging the mass has a maximum Vs of 9.7 m/s (>180 kPa) highly suggestive of a malignancy. (f) On a different shear wave system the lesion has a lower Vs with a ring of higher Vs. This is a case where the newer algorithm would reject the shear waves in the mass due to significant noise. With the new algorithm the mass would not be color coded.

do not add significantly to this case. With the high probability of malignancy of BI-RADS category 5 lesions on conventional ultrasound it is unlikely that any elastographic finding would downgrade the lesion away from biopsy.

Based on the proposed elastography classification system (similar to the BI-RADS classification) presented in Chapter 5 this lesion has a probability of >95% of being malignant.

# 7.16 Case 16: Invasive Lobular Carcinoma

## 7.16.1 Clinical Presentation

A 78-year-old woman with a remote history of breast bilateral implants presents with a new mass on screening mammography in the right breast. The lesion was classified as BI-RADS 0, and ultrasound was advised for further workup.

## 7.16.2 Ultrasound Findings

On B-mode (▶ Fig. 7.16a) imaging a 4.2 mm lesion is identified adjacent to the breast implant. The lesion had moderate inter-

nal blood flow on color Doppler imaging (▶ Fig. 7.16b). The lesion was classified as BI-RADS category 4A.

On SE (▶ Fig. 7.16c) the lesion is stiffer than the surrounding breast tissue and has an E/B ratio of 1.1. The lesion has a score of 5 on the 5-point color scale. The strain ratio (lesion to fat ratio) is 6.4 (▶ Fig. 7.16d). On shear wave imaging the lesion has a max Vs of 6.1 m/s (115 kPa) on one system (▶ Fig. 7.16e) and a max Vs of 7.1 m/s (153 kPa) on a different system (▶ Fig. 7.16f). A second similar lesion was identified (not shown).

## 7.16.3 Diagnosis

Invasive lobular carcinoma. Because the lesion was adjacent to the breast implant a 25-gauge needle was advanced under the lesion with ultrasound guidance, and 3 mL of buffered lidocaine was injected to increase the distance of the lesion from the implant (▶ Fig. 7.16g). The lesion was then biopsied with a 25-gauge needle under constant ultrasound guidance using a fine-needle aspiration (FNA) technique. The second lesion was biopsied in the same fashion. The pathology of both FNAs was ILC. The patient went to surgery where the implant and masses were removed. On pathology the ILC was growing along the implant.

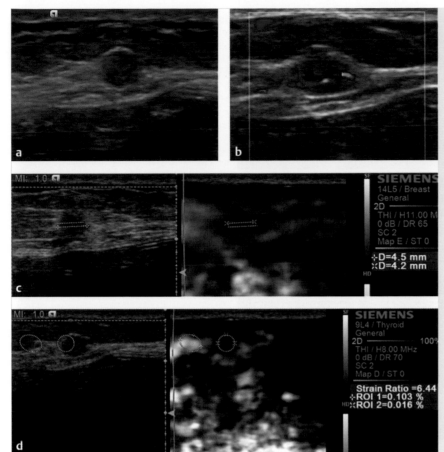

**Fig. 7.16** (a) On B-mode imaging the mass identified on mammography is a 4.2 mm well circumscribed isoechoic mass just superior to the breast implant. Not shown here is a second similar lesion approximately 3 cm from this lesion. (b) On color Doppler imaging the mass as significant internal vascularity. (c) On strain imaging the lesion is stiffer than surrounding tissue. The lesion measures 4.2 mm (yellow line) on B-mode and 4.5 mm (green line) on SE with an E/B ratio of 1.1. The lesion has a score of 5 on the 5-point color scale, both suggestive of a malignancy. (d) On strain imaging the strain ratio (lesion to fat ratio) is 6.44, also suggestive of a malignancy. (*Continued*)

## 7.16.4 Discussion

The SE findings in this case are all suggestive of malignancy: an E/I ratio of 1.1, a strain ratio (lesion to fat ratio) of 6.4, and a score of 5 on the 5-point color scale. The SWE findings are also suggestive of a malignancy with Vs > 7 m/s. Both SWE systems have a high Vs throughout the lesion, confirming that adequate shear waves are generated throughout this malignancy. It is interesting that the E/I ratio is only slightly greater than 1 but the stain ratio is significantly elevated at 6.4. The relationship of the E/I ratio to lesion stiffness is not known, although the E/I ratio appears to correlate with lesion grade.[28]

Based on the proposed elastography classification system (similar to the BI-RADS classification) presented in Chapter 5 this lesion would have a > 95% probability of malignancy.

## 7.17 Case 17: Invasive Papillary Carcinoma

### 7.17.1 Clinical Presentation

The patient is a 77-year-old woman with a mass increasing in size on screening mammography. The lesion was classified as BI-RADS 0, and an ultrasound was recommended for further workup.

## 7.17.2 Ultrasound Findings

A 2.5 cm well circumscribed complex cystic and solid lesion is identified on B-mode imaging (▶ Fig. 7.17a). Through transmission is noted. The appearance of the lesion did not change on repositioning of the patient. On color Doppler imaging there is some peripheral blood flow but no blood flow within the echogenic portions of the lesion (▶ Fig. 7.17b). The lesion was classified as BI-RADS category 4B.

On strain imaging (▶ Fig. 7.17c) the fluid component of the lesion is soft without a bull's-eye artifact, suggesting the fluid is viscous. The echogenic portion of the lesion is stiffer (black) than the surrounding breast tissue, with a strain ratio (lesion to fat ratio) of 4.5. The lesion would have a score of 5 on the 5-point color scale. On shear wave imaging (▶ Fig. 7.17d) the anechoic portion codes very soft, with a Vs value of 1.2 m/s (7 kPa). The solid component codes stiffer than surrounding breast tissue, with a value of Vs of 4 m/s (48 kPa).

## 7.17.3 Diagnosis

Invasive intraductal papillary carcinoma, grade 1 and DCIS. The lesion was biopsied with a 12-gauge vacuum-assisted needle under ultrasound guidance. The pathology was invasive ductal carcinoma, grade1. The patient underwent a lumpectomy with the same diagnosis, predominantly intraductal papillary carcinoma.

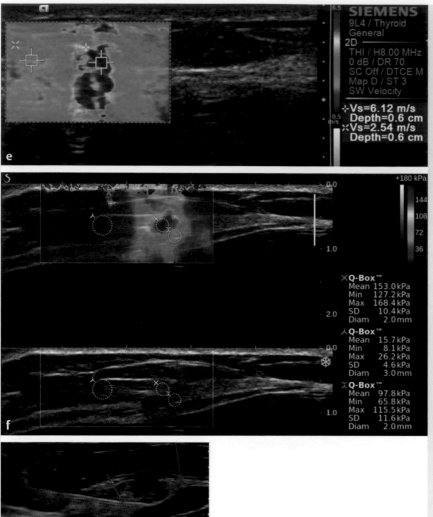

**Fig. 7.16** (*Continued*) (e) On shear wave imaging the lesion has a high Vs of 6.1 m/s (115 kPa). The area of increased stiffness extends to the breast implant. (f) Shear wave imaging on a different system has similar findings, with the mass having a Vs of m/s (153 kPa). (g) The mass was biopsied using a 22-gauge needle with a fine-needle aspiration technique. Initially 5 mL of buffered lidocaine was placed under the lesion to raise the lesion from the implant (arrow). Continued visualization of the needle was maintained during the procedure to document that the implant was not punctured.

### 7.17.4 Discussion

Papillary carcinoma accounts for about 1% of breast cancers[144] and often manifests as an intraductal or intracystic mass.[159] Women with papillary carcinoma often present with nipple discharge or a palpable central mass. The mammographic appearance is typically a round, relatively circumscribed, equal- or high-density mass.[160] On ultrasound scans, papillary carcinoma often manifests as a cyst with an intracystic mass or a more complex cystic mass.

Intracystic carcinomas account for less than 1% of breast cancers and are usually papillary carcinomas. Aspiration of these lesions often yields bloody fluid. Traditionally, these lesions have been surgically excised due to the concern that the mass will resolve with aspiration, hampering the ability to accurately excise the lesion.

The clinical and imaging findings of papillary carcinoma can be similar to those of benign intraductal papillomas, which likewise frequently manifest with nipple discharge and are most common in the central breast.

Based on the proposed elastography classification system (similar to the BI-RADS classification) presented in Chapter 5 the lesion would have a 2 to 95% probability of malignancy.

## 7.18 Case 18: Mucinous Carcinoma

### 7.18.1 Clinical Presentation

An 82-year-old woman presents with a new 2 cm well circumscribed lesion on screening mammography. The lesion was classified as BI-RADS category 0, and ultrasound was requested for further evaluation.

### 7.18.2 Ultrasound Findings

On B-mode ultrasound (▶ Fig. 7.18a) the lesion is a 2.3 cm hypoechoic, well-circumscribed lobular mass. Color Doppler imaging (▶ Fig. 7.18b) demonstrates a small amount of blood flow in the lesion. The lesion was classified as BI-RADS category 4A.

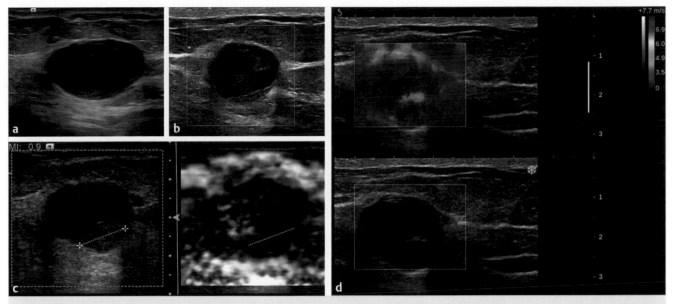

**Fig. 7.17** (a) The mass noted on mammography is a complex cystic and solid mass on B-mode imaging. The lesion is well circumscribed with thick septation and an area of thickened wall. There is some through transmission. (b) On power Doppler imaging there is a small amount of peripheral flow but no flow within the lesion. (c) On strain imaging the lesion has a stiff rim and the "solid" component (line) is also stiff. The anechoic portion of the lesion is soft without a bull's-eye artifact. This suggests the "fluid" within the lesion is viscous or semisolid. (d) On shear wave imaging the anechoic portion of the lesion codes with a low Vs of 1.2 m/s (7 kPa), whereas the wall and solid components code with a higher Vs of 4 m/s (48 kPa). The findings are similar to the strain findings.

On strain imaging (▶ Fig. 7.18c) the lesion is stiffer than the surrounding glandular tissue, and the lesion has an E/B ratio of 1.4 (▶ Fig. 7.18d). The strain ratio (lesion to fat ratio) is 5.7. The lesion has a score of 5 on the 5-point color scale. On shear wave imaging (▶ Fig. 7.18e) the lesion has a Vs of 6.2 m/s (115 kPa). On a different shear wave imaging system (▶ Fig. 7.18f) the central portion of the lesion has a Vs of 1.8 m/s (10 kPa), but the proximal portion of the lesion has a Vs of 4.9 m/s (73 kPa).

### 7.18.3 Diagnosis

Mucinous carcinoma. The lesion was biopsied with a 12-gauge vacuum-assisted core needle under ultrasound guidance. The pathology was a well differentiated mucinous carcinoma.

### 7.18.4 Discussion

Mucinous carcinoma accounts for about 2% of breast cancers.[144] Its prevalence is age related. A prevalence of as much as 7% is found among women 75 years or older, whereas the prevalence is only 1% in women younger than 35 years.[161,162] Mucin is a dominant feature at histologic examination. Mucinous carcinoma can be divided into pure mucinous carcinoma and mixed mucinous carcinoma, depending on the mucinous content of the carcinoma. Pure and mixed carcinomas have different prognoses. Pure mucinous carcinoma is reported to be associated with a better prognosis[163] and a lower incidence of axillary lymph node metastasis.[164]

These cancers tend to manifest as soft masses because of the large amount of mucin within the lesion. Because of the pre-dominance of mucin, this carcinoma typically manifests as a low-density, relatively well defined or microlobulated oval or lobular mass at mammography.[148,161] The margins of the lesion are usually ill defined rather than sharply defined. On ultrasound scans, mucinous carcinomas are often heterogeneous in echogenicity and may have mixed solid and cystic components.[161] Posterior acoustic enhancement is common; posterior acoustic shadowing is very uncommon. On MRI scans, mucinous carcinomas are one of the few cancers that have very high signal intensity on T2-weighted images,[165] due to the fluid nature of mucin.

Because mucinous cancers are softer than other breast cancers there is a concern that the elastographic features may be different than for other malignancies. Also given that the lesion may contain a large amount of semisolid mucin would the lesion produce a bull's-eye artifact? In our experience mucinous cancers are stiff enough to produce elastographic features similar to other breast malignancies. The E/B ratio is often 1 or close to 1. This is one reason we prefer to use an E/B ratio of ≥ 1 as our cutoff for distinction between benign and malignant. DCIS is the other malignant lesion that may have an E/B close to 1. One study found an E/B ratio of 1.2 provides increased specificity; however, this study did not include mucinous cancers or many cases of DCIS.[10] The mucin is very viscous and does not produce a bull's-eye artifact.[48]

This case has all SE and SWE findings suggestive of malignancy. The SE and SWE findings are concordant.

Based on the proposed elastography classification system (similar to the BI-RADS classification) presented in Chapter 5 the lesion would have a > 95% probability of malignancy.

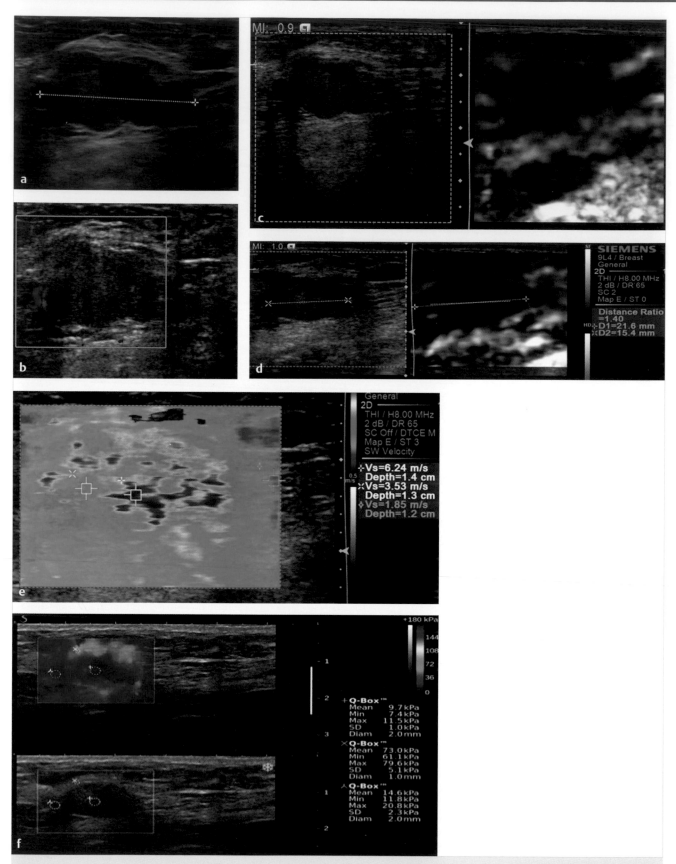

**Fig. 7.18** (a) The lesion noted on the screening mammogram is a 2.3 cm lobular, well circumscribed, isoechoic, slightly heterogeneous mass on B-mode imaging (dotted line). (b) Color Doppler imaging demonstrates a small amount of blood flow with the lesion. (c) On strain imaging the lesion is stiffer than the surrounding tissue. (d) The lesion measures 15.4 mm (yellow line) on B-mode imaging and 21.6 mm (green line) on SE. The lesion has an E/B ratio of 1.4 on strain imaging. The lesion has a score of 5 on the 5-point color scale. (e) The lesion has a high Vs on shear wave imaging with a maximum Vs of 6.2 m/s (115 kPa), highly suggestive of a malignancy. (f) On a different shear wave system the lesion has a ring of high Vs (4.9 m/s; 73 kPa), although the central portion of the lesion has a lower Vs of 1.8 m/s (10 kPa).

## 7.19 Case 19: Mucinous Carcinoma—Mucinous Carcinoma with Adjacent Invasive Ductal Carcinoma, Grade 2

### 7.19.1 Clinical Presentation

A 56-year-old woman presents with a palpable mass in the right breast. On mammography a new 2 cm lobular mass is identified. The lesion is classified as BI-RADS category 0, and an ultrasound is recommended for further evaluation.

### 7.19.2 Ultrasound Findings

On B-mode imaging (▶ Fig. 7.19a) a 2.2 cm hypoechoic, irregular mass is identified. On color Doppler imaging (▶ Fig. 7.19b) no internal blood flow is identified. The lesion was classified as BI-RADS category 4C.

On strain imaging (▶ Fig. 7.19c) the lesion is stiffer than the surrounding fatty breast tissue and the E/B ratio is 1.3. The lesion has a strain ratio (lesion to fat ratio) of 5.5. The lesion has a score of 5 on the 5-point color scale. On further scanning a second 0.5 cm lesion is identified approximately 1 cm from the larger lesion (▶ Fig. 7.19d). This satellite lesion has an E/B ratio of 1.2, strain ratio (lesion to fat ratio) of 5.2 and a score of 5 on the 5-point color scale (▶ Fig. 7.19e). On shear wave imaging (▶ Fig. 7.19f) the larger lesion has a Vs of 6.5 m/s (125 kPa), whereas the smaller lesion has a Vs of 4.5 m/s (60 kPa).

### 7.19.3 Diagnosis

Large lesion—colloid (mucinous) carcinoma; satellite lesion—invasive ductal carcinoma, grade 2. Both lesions were biopsied under ultrasound guidance with a 12-gauge vacuum-assisted core needle. The pathology of the larger lesion was colloid carcinoma, moderately differentiated, whereas the smaller lesion was invasive, moderately differentiated ductal carcinoma.

### 7.19.4 Discussion

The pathophysiology of mucinous (colloid) cancer is presented in Case 7.18.

The large lesion that was identified on mammography has all the SE and SWE features of a malignancy. The second lesion was not identified on the diagnostic mammogram. The satellite lesion also has SE and SWE features of a malignancy similar to those of the large lesion. On the stress elastogram there is a bridge of soft, normal-appearing breast tissue, raising the question that there are two separate lesions, although extension of the larger lesion is still possible. Both lesions were biopsied given the normal tissue between the lesions.

Although mucinous (colloid) cancers are felt to be softer than invasive ductal carcinoma, in this case the mucinous cancer has stiffer elastographic characteristics compared with invasive ductal carcinoma. This may be due to the size difference between the two lesions. On SWE the entire central portion of the lesion has a high Vs. It is possible that if there is a portion of the lesion that is mostly mucin the Vs may be lower in that portion of the lesion.

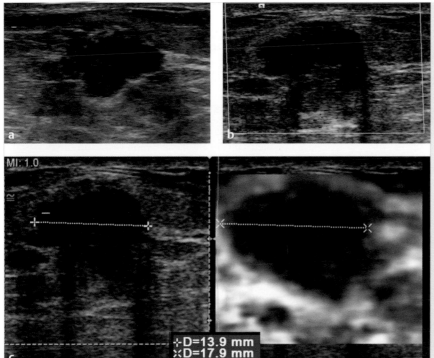

Fig. 7.19 (a) The palpable mass is an irregular heterogeneous well defined mass on B-mode imaging. There is a question of a surrounding echogenic halo, particularly in the distal portion of the mass. (b) There is questionable small amount of blood flow in the lesion on power Doppler. (c) On strain imaging the lesion is stiffer than the surrounding tissue. The leasion measures 13.9 mm (yellow line left images) on B-mode and 17.9 mm (yellow line right image) with an E/B ratio of 1.3. The lesion has a score of 5 on the 5-point color scale. (*Continued*)

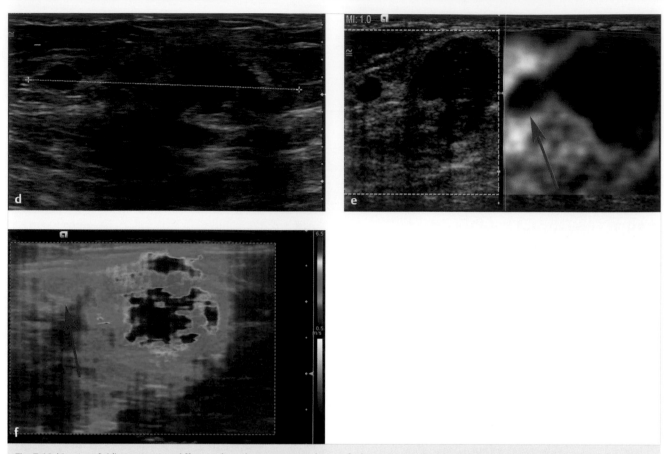

**Fig. 7.19** (*Continued*) (d) Imaging in a different plane demonstrates a cluster of adjacent hypoechoic lesions. (e) On strain imaging the smaller satellite lesion (arrow) is also stiffer than the surrounding tissue and has an E/B ratio of 1.3. The satellite lesion has a score of 5 on the 5-point color scale. There is an approximately 1 cm area of normal-appearing breast tissue between the two lesions. (f) On shear wave imaging the larger lesion has a significantly high Vs of 6.5 m/s (125 kPa), whereas the smaller lesion (arrow) has a Vs of 4.5 m/s (60 kPa).

Based on the proposed elastography classification system (similar to the BI-RADS classification) presented in Chapter 5 both lesions have a > 95% probability of malignancy.

# 7.20 Case 20: Inflammatory Breast Carcinoma

(Case courtesy of Professor Alexander Mundinger, Osnabrunk, Germany.)

## 7.20.1 Clinical Presentation

This 57-year-old patient presented with a palpable, nonmobile mass in the left breast. The mass was identified on a diagnostic mammogram.

## 7.20.2 Ultrasound Findings

On B-mode imaging (▶ Fig. 7.20a) there is a 12.5 mm mass that is taller than wider, irregular, and extending into the adjacent skin.

On shear wave imaging (▶ Fig. 7.20b,c) the mass and the surrounding skin have a markedly elevated Vs of > 7.7 m/s (180 kPa). Strain imaging was not performed in this case.

## 7.20.3 Diagnosis

Inflammatory breast cancer.

## 7.20.4 Discussion

Inflammatory breast cancer is a rare and very aggressive disease in which cancer cells block lymph vessels in the skin of the breast. This type of breast cancer is called inflammatory because the breast often looks swollen and red, or inflamed. In addition to the swelling and redness the skin has a pitted appearance similar to the skin of an orange (peau d'orange). The symptoms are caused by the buildup of fluid in the skin due to blocked lymph vessels in the skin. Other symptoms of inflammatory breast cancer include a rapid increase in the size of the breast and a sensation of heaviness, burning, or tenderness. Inflammatory breast cancer accounts for 1 to 5% of all breast cancers diagnosed in the United States. Most inflammatory breast cancers are invasive ductal carcinomas.

Inflammatory breast cancer progresses rapidly, often in a matter of weeks or months. Inflammatory breast cancer is either stage III or IV at diagnosis, depending on whether cancer cells have spread only to nearby lymph nodes or to other tissues as well.

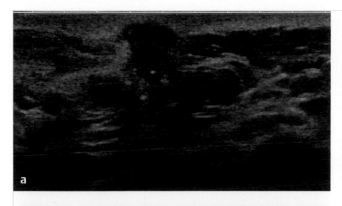

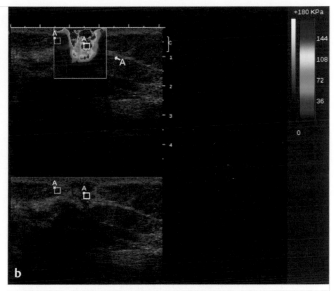

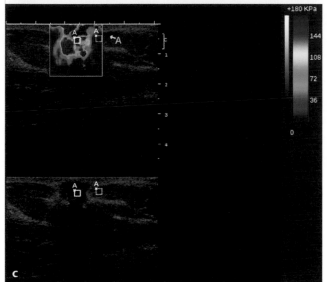

**Fig. 7.20** (a) On B-mode imaging there is an irregular hypoechoic mass that extends into the skin with associated skin thickening. (b) On shear wave imaging the mass and adjacent skin have an increased Vs, consistent with malignancy. (c) A repeat shear wave image confirms the high Vs in both the mass and the adjacent skin.

Compared with other types of breast cancer, inflammatory breast cancer tends to be diagnosed at younger ages (median age of 57 years, compared with a median age of 62 years for other types of breast cancer). It is more common and diagnosed at younger ages in African American women than in white women. The median age at diagnosis in African American women is 54 years, compared with a median age of 58 years in white women. Inflammatory breast tumors are frequently hormone receptor negative, which means that hormone therapies that interfere with the growth of cancer cells fueled by estrogen may not be effective against these tumors.[166]

Minimum criteria for a diagnosis of inflammatory breast cancer include the following:

(1) A rapid onset of erythema (redness), edema (swelling), and a peau d'orange appearance and/or abnormal breast warmth, with or without a lump that can be felt; (2) the aforementioned symptoms have been present for less than 6 months; (3) the erythema covers at least a third of the breast; and (4) initial biopsy samples from the affected breast show invasive carcinoma.[167,168]

This case demonstrates a breast mass that invades the skin. The elastographic features on SWE are highly suggestive of a malignancy that has extended into the skin. This case of invasive ductal carcinoma with skin involvement has a very high Vs of the skin compared with the case of skin thickening due to a benign cause presented in Case 6.41.

Based on the proposed elastography classification system (similar to the BI-RADS classification) presented in Chapter 5 the lesion has a > 95% probability of malignancy.

# 8 Clinical Cases of Other Lesions

## 8.1 Case 1: Lymph Nodes—Benign Intramammary Lymph Node

### 8.1.1 Clinical Presentation

A 79-year-old woman presents with a 1 cm well circumscribed new mass in the right upper outer breast on mammography. The mammogram was classified as Breast Imaging–Reporting and Data System (BI-RADS) 0, and an ultrasound was advised for further workup.

### 8.1.2 Ultrasound Findings

On B-mode ultrasound (▸ Fig. 8.1a) a 10 mm oval well circumscribed hypoechoic lesion with a central area of increased echogenicity is identified. On color Doppler (▸ Fig. 8.1b) there is significant blood flow with some vessels appearing to enter the cortex and not at the hilum. The lesion was classified as BI-RADS category 4A.

On strain elastography (SE) (▸ Fig. 8.1c) the cortex of the lesion is stiffer than surrounding tissue and the central area is soft (white). The lesion is smaller on elastography. The strain ratio (lesion to fat ratio), using the cortex as lesion is 3.8 (▸ Fig. 8.1d). On shear wave elastography (SWE) (▸ Fig. 8.1e) the lesion has a Vs of 1.7 m/s (9 kPa).

### 8.1.3 Diagnosis

Benign intramammary lymph node. The lesion was biopsied with an 18-gauge core needle under ultrasound guidance. The pathology was a benign intramammary lymph node.

### 8.1.4 Discussion

Normal and abnormal axillary lymph nodes are commonly identified on mammography. Normal axillary lymph nodes are frequently identified and are typically small and oval with a lucent center due to hilar fat. Abnormal lymph nodes are characterized by high density, absence of hilar fat, and a round, irregular, ill-defined shape with or without intranodal calcifications on the Medial Lateral Oblique (MLO) view.[169,170] The spectrum of calcifications within lymph nodes comprises microcalcifications, punctate or amorphous calcifications, and coarse calcifications.

Ultrasonography of the axillary region is an imaging method that can be used when an abnormal lymph node is detected on a negative mammogram. On ultrasound, a normal lymph node has a thin hypoechogenic cortex in the periphery and an echogenic hilum. Abnormal nodes tend to become more rounded. Eccentric enlargement with focal thickening of the cortex is a strong indicator of malignant transformation. Indentation of the hilum, and especially obliteration of the hilum, is highly suggestive of malignancy.[171]

Peripheral flow and transcapsular vessels seen on color Doppler favor malignancy compared with central flow in normal axillary lymph nodes. For an accurate diagnosis, needle aspiration or biopsy should be performed under ultrasound guidance.

Enlargement of lymph nodes can be due to a variety of benign and malignant causes. The most common malignant cause of abnormal axillary lymph nodes is breast cancer; however, when lymph nodes enlarge because of metastatic breast cancer, the primary tumor within the breast is usually visualized mammographically. Occult breast cancer presenting as axillary metastasis is uncommon, accounting for less than 1% of all patients with primary breast cancer at diagnosis.[172,173]

In addition to metastatic breast cancer, another malignant cause of lymph node enlargement with a negative mammogram is metastases from other primary tumors (e.g., lymphoma, malignant melanoma, or lung or ovarian carcinomas). Benign causes of abnormal axillary lymph nodes include systemic inflammatory processes (sarcoidosis), infectious diseases (bacterial lymphadenitis, tuberculosis), collagen vascular diseases, and several miscellaneous causes (silicone implants, tattooing).

This lymph node has the elastographic features of a benign lymph node. The fatty hilum is soft, and the cortex of the lymph node is stiffer than surrounding tissue. The lymph node has an E/B ratio of < 1, and the strain ratio (lesion to fat ratio) of the cortex is usually less than 4. On SWE the lymph node usually has a Vs of < 3.2 m/s (30 kPa). The elastographic features of an abnormal lymph node include an E/B ratio of ≥ 1, a strain ratio of > 4.5, and a focal area of stiffness (stiffer than the normal lymph node cortex).

Based on the proposed elastography classification system (similar to the BI-RADS classification) presented in Chapter 5 the lesion has an ~ 0% probability of malignancy.

## 8.2 Case 2: Lymph Nodes—Benign Axillary Lymph Node

### 8.2.1 Clinical Presentation

An 84-year-old woman with a history of breast cancer with mastectomy now presents with a left axillary mass on physical exam. Mammography was not performed.

### 8.2.2 Ultrasound Findings

B-mode imaging (▸ Fig. 8.2a) shows a normal-appearing 1.8 cm lymph node. On color Doppler (▸ Fig. 8.2b) no blood flow is identified. The lesion was classified as BI-RADS 3.

On strain imaging (▸ Fig. 8.2c) the cortex of the lesion is stiffer than surrounding tissue, with the hilum of the lymph node soft and of similar stiffness to the adjacent fat. The elastogram/B-mode (E/B) ratio is 0.95, and the strain ratio is 3.8. On shear wave imaging (▸ Fig. 8.2d) the lymph node has uniform stiffness with a Vs of 2.6 m/s (20 kPa).

### 8.2.3 Diagnosis

Mature lymphocytes consistent with lymph node origin. The lesion was biopsied with a 20-gauge needle using a fine-needle aspiration (FNA) technique. The pathology was mature lymphocytes consistent with lymph node origin.

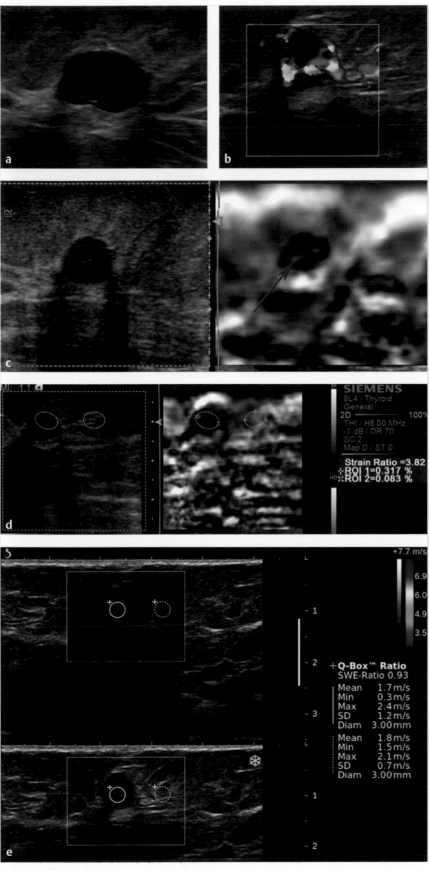

**Fig. 8.1** (a) The mass identified on mammography is a well circumscribed, hypoechoic mass with a central area that is hyperechoic. (b) On color Doppler imaging there is significant blood flow in the lesion with a large feeding vessel and draining vein. (c) On strain elastography the mass has a soft central area with a thick rim that is stiffer than surrounding breast tissue. The lesion is smaller on elastography than in B-mode imaging. The lesion would be classified with a score of 2 or 3 in the 5-point color scale. (d) The strain ratio (lesion to fat ratio) is 3.8 on strain imaging, suggestive of a benign lesion. (e) On shear wave imaging the lesion has a Vs of 1.7 m/s (9 kPa), suggestive of a benign lesion.

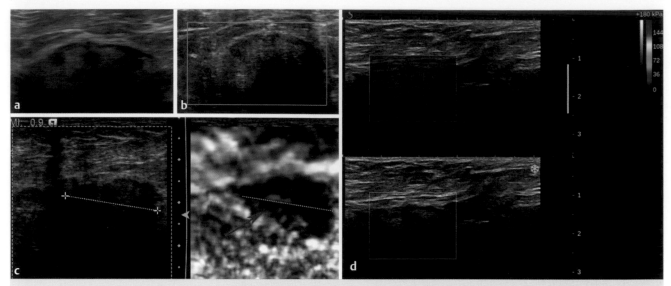

**Fig. 8.2** (a) On B-mode imaging the mass is a 1.8 cm lesion with the appearance of a lymph node. The cortex of the lymph node is relatively uniform in size, and the central echogenic fat is maintained. (b) On power Doppler no blood flow is identified in the lesion. (c) On strain imaging the cortex of the lymph node is stiffer than the adjacent breast tissues, whereas the central fatty hilum (arrow) is soft as expected. The lesion (dotted line) is similar in size on the B-mode image and elastogram. (d) On shear wave imaging the lymph node has a low Vs of 2.6 m/s (20 kPa) consistent with a benign lesion.

## 8.2.4 Discussion

Inflammation of lymph nodes by bacterial or granulamotous infections such as tuberculosis is known as lymphadenitis. The most common causes of axillary lymphadenitis are bacterial agents that are located in the normal flora of the skin. Focal lymphadenitis is prominent in streptococcal infection, tuberculosis, nontuberculous mycobacterial infection, tularemia, plague, and cat-scratch disease. Multifocal lymphadenitis is common in infectious mononucleosis, cytomegalovirus infection, toxoplasmosis, brucellosis, secondary syphilis, and disseminated histoplasmosis.[170,171] Tuberculous lymphadenitis (or tuberculous adenitis) is a chronic specific granulomatous inflammation with caseation necrosis of the lymph nodes. On physical examination, tenderness, redness, swelling, fluctuation, or abscess formation are detected as a result of bacterial lymphadenitis, whereas tuberculosis lymphadenitis may result in cold abscesses, which develop so slowly that there are no signs of inflammation unless it becomes complicated.

In this case a larger than normal (1.8 cm) axillary lymph node is identified. No other conventional sonographic abnormality is identified. On SE the hilar fat is identified as soft central tissue. The cortex is stiffer than adjacent tissue with an E/B ratio of 0.95. The strain ratio of the cortex is 3.8. On SWE the lymph node has a Vs of 2.5 m/s (19 kPa). The SE findings are benign as are the SWE findings.

Based on the proposed elastography classification system (similar to the BI-RADS classification) presented in Chapter 5 the lesion has an ~ 0% probability of malignancy.

## 8.3 Case 3: Lymph Nodes—Metastatic Adenocarcinoma to Axillary Lymph Node

### 8.3.1 Clinical Presentation

A 63-year-old woman with a history of left invasive ductal breast cancer presents with a new palpable mass in her left breast. On mammography a 1.5 cm irregular, hypoechoic mass is identified, and a lobular mass is also identified in the axilla. The mammogram was classified as BI-RADS 0, and an ultrasound was advised for further workup.

### 8.3.2 Ultrasound Findings

On B-mode imaging (▶ Fig. 8.3a) there is a lobular mass in the axilla. The normal lymph node appearance is not identified. The mass has marked increased blood flow on power Doppler imaging (▶ Fig. 8.3b) and color Doppler imaging (▶ Fig. 8.3c) with blood vessels noted entering the cortex of the lymph node. The breast mass is not presented here.

On SE (▶ Fig. 8.3d) the abnormal lymph node is stiffer than adjacent tissue with an E/B ratio of 1.1 and a strain ratio of 4.7. The lesion has a score of 5 on the 5-point color scale. On SWE (▶ Fig. 8.3e) the lymph node has a Vs of > 7.7 m/s (> 180 kPa), highly suggestive of a malignancy. The quality map (▶ Fig. 8.3f) of the lesion confirms good-quality shear waves

### 8.3.3 Diagnosis

Metastatic adenocarcinoma to axillary lymph nodes. The breast mass and the abnormal lymph nodes were biopsied with a 12-

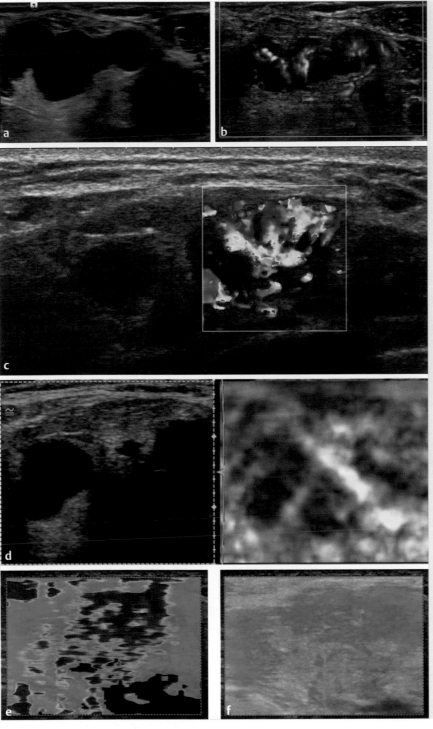

**Fig. 8.3** (a) B-mode image of the axilla demonstrated several well circumscribed masses. The lesions did not have a normal lymph node appearance with absence of the central fat. (b) The power Doppler image demonstrates a large amount of internal blood flow. Some blood vessels enter through the cortex of the lymph node. (c) The color Doppler image demonstrates similar findings as (b). (d) On strain elastography the lymph node is stiffer than surrounding tissue and has an elastogram/B-mode (E/B) ratio of 1.1, suggestive of a malignancy. (e) On shear wave imaging the lesion has a Vs of > 7.7 m/s (> 180 kPa), highly suggestive of a malignancy. (f) The quality map confirms adequate shear waves are generated for accurate interpretation.

gauge vacuum-assisted needle. The breast mass was an invasive ductal carcinoma, grade 3, and the lymph node was replaced with metastatic disease.

## 8.3.4 Discussion

Nori et al[174] evaluated axillary lymph nodes for hilar and cortical thickening and ratio between the sinus diameter and the total longitudinal diameter. Lymph nodes with hilar diameters equal to or greater than 50% of the longitudinal diameter were considered normal. Of the 102 patients evaluated, 77 (75.7%) had normal axillary nodes according to the ultrasound criteria adopted. Negativity was confirmed by histology in 56 cases (72.7%, true-negative); 21 (27.3%, false-negative) were found to be positive, in contrast with the sonographic appearance. The false-negative cases were due to lymph node micrometastasis that probably did not cause morphological alterations perceptible at ultrasound. The remaining 25 patients (24.5%) had axillary lymph nodes classified as suspicious. In 13 cases of (52%, true-positive) there was agreement with histology, whereas in

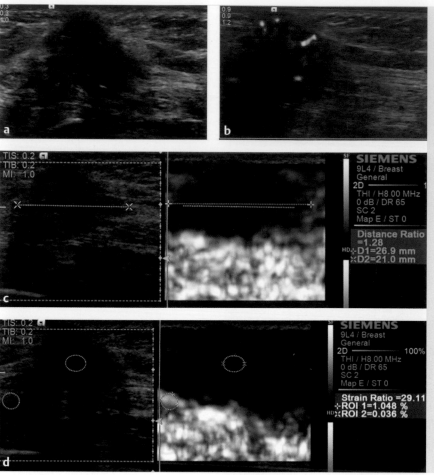

**Fig. 8.4** (a) B-mode image of the painful axillary mass identifies a 2 cm irregular hypoechoic mass. (b) On power Doppler imaging there is marked blood flow within the mass. (c) On strain elastography the mass is much stiffer than the adjacent tissues. The lesion measures 21.0 mm (yellow line) on B-mode and 26.9 mm (green line) on SE with an elastogram/B-mode (E/B) ratio of 1.3. The lesion has a score of 3 on the 5-point color scale. (d) The strain ratio (lesion to fat ratio) is 29.1. All of the strain measurements are suggestive of a malignancy. (*Continued*)

12 cases (48%, false-positive) the ultrasound suspicion was not confirmed at surgery. The most important sonographic alteration was the gradual reduction in hilar echogenicity (seen in 100% metastatic nodes); conversely, hilar denting or irregularities, as well as dimensional criteria, proved to be poorly specific.

In this case the B-mode findings of the lymph nodes are highly suspicious. There is lack of the normal hilar fat, the lymph nodes are rounded, and blood flow is noted entering the cortex of the lymph nodes. The SE findings are abnormal, with an E/B ratio of 1.1, no hilar softness, and a strain ratio (lesion to fat ratio) of 4.7. The SWE findings are also abnormal with a Vs > 7.7 m/s (> 180 kPa).

Based on the proposed elastography classification system (similar to the BI-RADS classification) presented in Chapter 5 the lesion has a > 95% probability of malignancy.

# 8.4 Case 4: Lymph Nodes—Metastatic Adenocarcinoma to Axillary Lymph Node

## 8.4.1 Clinical Presentation

A 74-year-old woman with a history of left breast cancer, status postmastectomy, chemotherapy, and radiation therapy 12 years prior presented with a painful left axillary mass. Mammography was not performed.

## 8.4.2 Ultrasound Findings

On B-mode imaging (▶ Fig. 8.4a) a 2 cm irregular hypoechoic mass is identified. There is significant blood flow on color Doppler imaging (▶ Fig. 8.4b). The lesion was classified as BI-RADS category 4C.

On strain imaging (▶ Fig. 8.4c) the mass is stiffer than the adjacent tissue, and the E/B ratio is 1.3. The lesion to fat ratio is 29.1 (▶ Fig. 8.4d). Similar findings are identified on Virtual Touch imaging (VTi, Siemens) (▶ Fig. 8.4e). On shear wave imaging the mass is markedly stiff with a Vs of > 7.7 m/s (180 kPa). Similar findings are seen with a different shear wave system (▶ Fig. 8.4g).

## 8.4.3 Diagnosis

Invasive ductal carcinoma. The lesion was biopsied with an 18-gauge Tru-cut needle under ultrasound guidance. The pathology was a lymph node replaced with invasive poorly differentiated adenocarcinoma, consistent with breast origin.

## 8.4.4 Discussion

In this case advanced metastatic disease to the axillary lymph node is present. The lymph node does not have the appearance of a lymph node but an irregular mass. The SE findings of E/I ratio of 1.3, loss of hilar softness, and strain ratio (lesion to fat

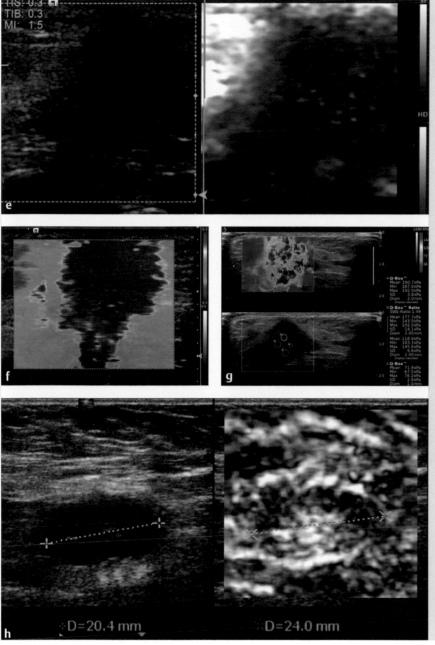

**Fig. 8.4** (*Continued*) (e) On Virtual Touch imaging (VTi, Siemens) (strain imaging using acoustic radiation force impulse [ARFI]) demonstrates a mass with an E/B ratio > 1 and significantly stiffer than surrounding tissue. (f) On shear wave imaging the mass has a Vs of > 7.7 m/s (> 180 kPa), highly suggestive of a malignancy. (g) On a different shear wave system similar findings suggestive of a malignancy are obtained with a Vs of Vs > 7.7 m/s (191 kPa). (h) Strain elastogram from a different patient demonstrates a stiff area (red circle) that was persistent. The exam is from a patient with a 2.5 cm BI-RADS category 5 mass. The persistent stiff area was biopsied under ultrasound guidance and was confirmed to be a focal metastatic lesion.

ratio) of 29.1 are all highly suggestive of malignancy. The shear wave imaging findings with Vs of > 6.5 m/s (125 kPa) are highly suspicious for malignancy.

Based on the proposed elastography classification system (similar to the BI-RADS classification) presented in Chapter 5 the lesion has a > 95% probability of malignancy.

▶ Fig. 8.4h is from a different patient and demonstrates the opposite end of the spectrum of metastatic disease to the lymph nodes. This patient presented with a 2.5 cm BI-RADS 5 mass that was subsequently biopsied and was an invasive ductal cancer. In this case there is a focal area of persistent stiffness in the cortex of the lymph node (circle). This persisted on multiple views. This area was biopsied under elastographic guidance and was a focus of metastatic disease. Any area of stiffness greater than the adjacent cortex of a lymph node or deformity of the cortex seen only on elastog-raphy should be considered a possible metastatic foci and biopsied.

# 8.5 Case 5: Lymphoma

## 8.5.1 Clinical Presentation

An 85-year-old woman with a history of non-Hodgkin lymphoma presents with bilateral breast masses on screening mammogram. The mammogram was classified as BI-RADS 0, and ultrasound was recommended for further workup.

## 8.5.2 Ultrasound Findings

On B-mode imaging (▶ Fig. 8.5a) a 1.8 cm well circumscribed lobular hypoechoic lesion is identified. The lesion had internal

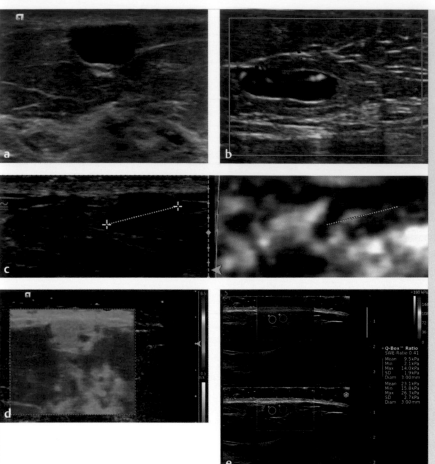

**Fig. 8.5** (a) The B-mode image of one of the two palpable masses demonstrates a hypoechoic well circumscribed lesion. The second lesion in the contralateral breast had a similar appearance (not presented). (b) The power Doppler image of the lesion demonstrates significant internal blood flow. The lesion in the contralateral breast had similar findings (not presented). (c) On strain elastography the mass (yellow line) is of mixed soft and stiff signal. The lesion has a score of 2 on the 5-point color scale. The elastogram/B-mode (E/B) ratio is hard to calculate but is < 1. Both methods of analysis are suggestive of a benign lesion. The lesion in the contralateral breast had similar findings (not presented). (d) On shear wave elastography the lesion has a higher Vs than surrounding fatty tissue measuring 2.7 m/s (23 kPa), also suggestive of a benign lesion. Findings in the lesion in the contralateral breast were similar (not presented). (e) Shear wave imaging on a different system has a similar appearance with a Vs maximum of 2.7 m/s (23 kPa). Similar results were obtained from the lesion in the contralateral breast (not presented).

blood flow on power Doppler imaging (► Fig. 8.5b). The second lesion in the other breast had identical imaging characteristics. The lesions were classified as BI-RADS category 4A.

On strain imaging (► Fig. 8.5c) the lesion is soft and similar in stiffness to adjacent fatty tissue. The E/B ratio was less than 1. The lesion to fat ratio was not performed. On the 5-point color scale this lesion has a score of 2. On shear wave imaging (► Fig. 8.5d,e) the lesion is soft, with a Vs of 2.8 m/s (23 kPa). The lesion in the other breast had identical elastographic features.

### 8.5.3 Diagnosis

Lymphoma. Both lesions were biopsied with a vacuum-assisted 12-gauge core needle. Both lesions were diffuse large B cell lymphoma similar to the patient's previous diagnosis.

### 8.5.4 Discussion

Breast cancer accounted for 230,000 of the cancer diagnoses in 2011.[175] Although most metastases to the breast are from contralateral breast carcinomas, approximately 0.4 to 1.3% of breast cancers are metastases from extramammary cancers.[176,177] Of these, the most common primary cancers, in decreasing order,

are leukemia/lymphomas, malignant melanomas, lung cancers, renal cell carcinomas, and ovarian tumors.[176,177]

Diffuse B-cell non-Hodgkin lymphoma is the most common type of lymphoma found in the breast; it is still a rare diagnosis, encompassing approximately 0.15% of all malignant breast cancers.[178–180] In a series of 106 cases of lymphomas of the breast, Talwalkar et al[178] reported that diffuse large B-cell lymphoma was the most common type of lymphoma overall, but that follicular lymphoma was the most prevalent nonprimary lymphoma of the breast. The differentiation from primary breast cancer and metastatic disease of the breast is a very important clinical distinction because it changes outcome and treatment. Our patient had a previous history of lymphoma, which in addition to the radiographic findings increased the clinical suspicion for nonprimary breast cancer.

Metastatic lymphomas to the breast most often present on mammogram as a noncalcified mass with indistinct margins. Most often they do not present with skin edema or skin thickening.[181] On ultrasound, Zack et al described a case of metastatic lymphoma as a well circumscribed mass with a hyperechogenic border and hypoechoic center.[182] Yang et al, in a case of 32 lymphomas metastatic to the breast, found that most masses on ultrasound were lobular (52%) and with indistinct margins (72%).[180]

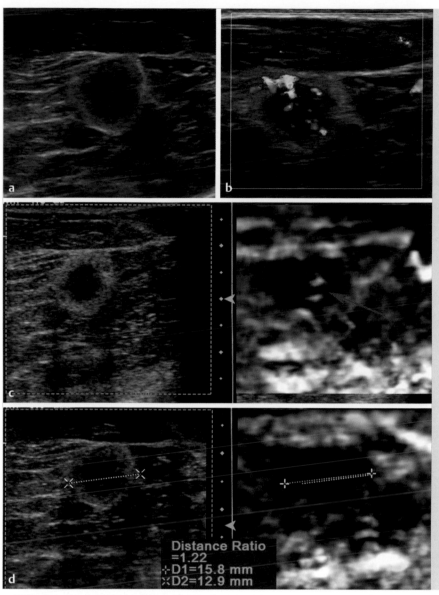

Fig. 8.6 (a) B-mode image of the mass noted on mammography identifies an irregular mass with a thick echogenic halo (arrows). The lesion does not distort the surrounding breast tissue. (b) The lesion has significant blood flow in both the central portion of the mass as well as the echogenic halo on color Doppler evaluation. (c) On strain elastography the lesion has a soft central area and a thick stiff rim. The appearance of the central portion of the lesion has the appearance of a bull's-eye artifact (arrow). The lesion is larger on elastography with an elastogram/B-mode (E/B) ratio of 1.2. The lesion would have a score of 2 on the 5-point color scale. (d) The lesion measures 12.9 mm (yellow line) on B-mode and 15.8 mm (green line) on SE with an E/B ratio of 1.2. (*Continued*)

The differentiation of metastatic cancer to the breast from primary breast cancer is often complicated. Although Yang et al and Ha et al have reported that most metastatic lymphomas of the breast were irregular, hypoechoic, and hypervascular with indistinct margins,[180,181] it has also been reported that breast lymphomas can appear hyperechoic.[182,183] This unpredictability leads to the fact that conventional radiographic findings do not always help to differentiate primary and metastatic lesions. In fact, several studies have shown that on mammography and conventional ultrasound the two are indistinguishable from one another.[177,184] Sonoelastography has recently been used to diagnose malignant breast cancers. Primary breast cancer is routinely stiffer than the surrounding tissue on sonoelastography[25,26,30,58]; this was not the case for lymphoma metastatic to the breast.

Based on the proposed elastography classification system (similar to the BI-RADS classification) presented in Chapter 5 this lesion (and the contralateral lesion) has an ~ 0% probability of malignancy.

## 8.6 Case 6: Adenocarcinoma Metastatic (Nonbreast)—Adenocarcinoma of Lung Origin

### 8.6.1 Clinical Presentation

A 55-year-old woman diagnosed with a history of lung adenocarcinoma presented for follow-up computed tomography (CT). A 6 mm mass was identified in her breast. On a follow-up CT 2 months later the mass had increased to 10 mm. A mammogram confirmed a 14 mm high-density, round mass with indistinct borders.[185] The mammogram was classified as BI-RADS category 0, and ultrasound was advised for further workup.

### 8.6.2 Ultrasound Findings

B-mode imaging (▶ Fig. 8.6a) identifies a 14 mm hypoechoic mass with a thick echogenic rim. There was moderate blood

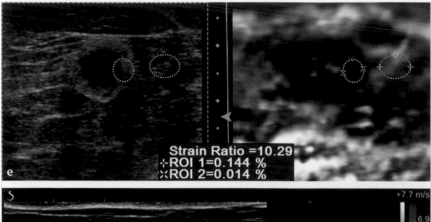

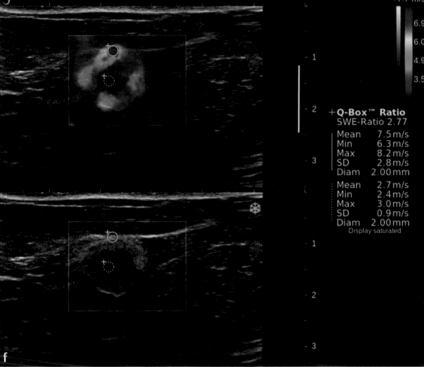

**Fig. 8.6** (*Continued*) (e) The strain ratio of the lesion rim is very stiff with a strain ratio (lesion to fat ratio) of 10.3. The central portion of the lesion has a strain ratio of 1. (f) On shear wave imaging the rim of the lesion has a Vs maximum of 7.5 m/s (165 kPa), whereas the central portion has a Vs of 2.7 m/s (21 kPa).

flow in the lesion on color Doppler (▶ Fig. 8.6b). The lesion was classified as BI-RADS category 5.

On strain elastography (▶ Fig. 8.6c) the elasticity imaging/B-mode (EI/B-mode) ratio was 1.2 (▶ Fig. 8.6d), suggestive of a malignancy. The thick rind was stiff with a strain ratio of 10 (▶ Fig. 8.6e). The center of the lesion was very soft. On shear wave imaging (▶ Fig. 8.6f) the thick echogenic rim had a stiffness of 175 kPa (7.5 m/s), whereas the central area had a stiffness of 21 kPa (2.7 m/s).

### 8.6.3 Diagnosis

Adenocarcinoma, lung primary. Moderately to poorly differentiated adenocarcinoma with lymphatic invasion. The lesion was triple negative. Immunohistochemical strains were consistent with a primary lung cancer.

### 8.6.4 Discussion

Breast cancer is the most common cancer of women in the United States; in 2011 there were approximately 230,000 new cases of breast cancer and 40,000 deaths from breast cancer.[175] However, cancer that metastasizes to the breast is uncommon. Most of these are metastases from contralateral breast carcinoma,[176] and, according to the literature, only 0.4 to 1.3% of all breast cancer cases are metastatic from extramammary sites.[176,177] In these instances, the cancer is most often secondary to leukemia/lymphoma, malignant melanoma, lung cancers, renal cell carcinoma, and ovarian tumors.[176,177,186] Even though most of these cancers can be readily found in both genders, the overwhelming majority of patients who presented with metastasis to the breast from an extramammary primary cancer were women.[176,177,187]

Diagnosis of metastatic cancer to the breast versus a primary breast cancer can be complicated. Many studies and case reports have identified that on mammography and ultrasound these masses will be indistinguishable from a primary breast cancer.[177,184,186] One study, which looked only at metastatic disease to the breast, reported that, of 11 masses found on ultrasound, 9 of them (81.8%) had an ill-defined margin. At the same time, 4 (36.3%) showed an echogenic boundary around the mass. In total, metastatic disease to the breast was reported to be most often unilateral lesions (80%) with multiple masses (86.7%).[188] In one case report of pulmonary adenocarcinoma metastatic to the breast, mammography demonstrated an asymmetrical lesion without calcifications in the upper outer quadrant of the breast.[184] In a report of two patients with adenocarcinoma of the lung that had metastasized to the breast, CT scanning demonstrated solitary lesions in the contralateral breast in both patients.[186]

Our patient's mass was similar to the aforementioned extramammary metastatic cancers in that it was unilateral with an irregular and echogenic border on ultrasound. On mammogram it was also similar to other extramammary metastatic tumors in that it presented as a single mass with an indistinct margin. Although the conventional imaging findings are similar, the elastographic findings for lymphoma are significantly different from other metastatic lesions to the breast. Lymphoma is a soft lesion and codes soft (benign appearing),[185] whereas other metastatic lesions are hard. Elastography can identify a soft necrotic center as in our case. This is a rare occurrence in primary breast cancer[185] but can be seen in nonbreast adenocarcinoma metastatic to the breast as noted in our case.

The outer rim of our patient's lesion had a stiffness value of 97 kPa, suggestive of a malignancy. With SWE of the breast the central portion of the mass may not propagate shear wave and either not provide a number or appear soft.[63] A quality measure of the shear wave is helpful to determine if an adequate shear wave was present. In this case the central area of the mass had a low kPa and a high-quality factor suggesting the central area is soft and consistent with the strain findings. Central necrosis demonstrated by a very soft center on SE or SWE is an unusual finding in primary breast cancer (Barr RG, personal observation, 6/1/2013). This finding can be seen in breast abscesses where the soft abscess is surrounded by a thick hard wall.[18]

Pathologically, the mass itself or a FNA of the mass is often enough to diagnose a metastasis to the breast based on cytology and architectural findings alone. Sneige et al[189] reported a series of 20 FNAs of extramammary metastatic disease to the breast, of which the results of 11 FNAs alone were sufficient to diagnose metastatic disease. Another 8 out of 20 could have been confused with primary breast cancer, but a clinical history of previous cancer prompted further evaluation by electron microscope and immunohistochemistry. One adenocarcinoma of the lung was misdiagnosed as a primary breast cancer due to lack of clinical history and microscopic appearance that resembled primary breast adenocarcinoma.[189] One study of 32 FNAs of extramammary metastatic disease to the breast showed that 81% of the cases had a known history of primary cancer. Two of these cases were lung adenocarcinoma that was undistinguishable on histology, but due to the clinical history of previous cancer further workup was performed to make the correct diagnosis.[178] Cytology and clinical history are often sufficient for pathologists to diagnose a mass as primary or metastatic in nature. Adenocarcinoma of the lung, however, has been noted to appear similar to primary breast cancer and can be misdiagnosed as such.[178,189]

In addition to the normal histological examination, immunohistochemistry has become important in the diagnosis of this rare occurrence of extramammary metastatic disease to the breast. Specifically, Thyroid Transcription Factor 1 (TTF-1) is positive in 75 to 80% of lung adenocarcinomas and always negative in primary breast adenocarcinomas.[190,191] Napsin A is expressed in 84.5% of primary lung adenocarcinomas but not in adenocarcinoma of other primary sites. Additionally, breast cancers are one of the few cancers that routinely express estrogen receptors.[192] Our patient's core biopsy failed to identify any estrogen receptors, which is consistent with extramammary metastatic disease. The lesion might have been interpreted as a triple negative breast adenocarcinoma had clinical history and radiographic suspicion not been present. This raises the question of whether or not some tumors interpreted as triple negative breast cancers might actually be metastatic adenocarcinoma of a nonbreast primary.

Based on the proposed elastography classification system (similar to the BI-RADS classification) presented in Chapter 5 the lesion has a > 95% probability of malignancy.

# 9 Future Perspective and Conclusions

## 9.1 Present Status

Some form of elastography is now available on most ultrasound systems. Elastography is an area of active research not only for the breast but for other organs as well. There are several techniques available for breast elastography, as summarized in ▸ Table 3.1. These can be grouped into two main categories, strain elastography (SE) and shear wave elastography (SWE). Within these two main groups there are several techniques used to generate elastograms. There have been minimal studies comparing the various techniques. All these techniques have high sensitivity and specificity for characterization of breast masses as benign or malignant. Although the techniques are easy to perform, they require attention to details to obtain optimal images for interpretation. Each of the techniques has advantages and disadvantages (▸ Table 5.1). These techniques are now maturing, but continued work on standardizing elastography techniques is required. Further comparative studies are needed to determine which technique or combination of techniques is most appropriate for various clinical problems.

No comparative studies have been performed to suggest one method is better than another. Although a meta-analysis or direct study comparing the various SE interpretation techniques has not been reported, most papers using E/B ratio have a sensitivity of > 98% and specificity of > 85%. These are higher than the reports using the 5-point color scale or the strain ratio (lesion to fat ratio). We do not know if this is a function of the interpretation technique or the variability of the acquisition technique (equipment specific). There are presently two techniques used to generate SWE in the breast. No direct comparative studies have been performed. Our observation is that there are subtle differences between the two techniques with interpretation of one system having a more prominent "ring" of high Vs surrounding the lesion as the more diagnostic feature.

Although most studies are reported as using a "light touch," very few studies have controlled the amount of precompression with a consistent method. This may lead to the differences of cutoff values in SWE. On SE precompression does not affect the E/B ratio but leads to poor-quality elastograms. Precompression can significantly affect the strain ratio (lesion to fat ratio) on SE.

The bull's-eye artifact seen with SE has been shown to be extremely helpful in characterization of cystic lesions.[48] We have been able to eliminate a large number of breast biopsies using this technique. The ability to characterize a lesion as a benign complicated cyst with almost perfect accuracy has led to decreased biopsy and need for short-term follow-up. The increased confidence has also led to less patient anxiety and decreased requests for biopsy or surgical removal of these lesions. Further confirmation of the accuracy of this artifact in characterizing a lesion as a benign complicated cyst will hopefully lead to addition of this artifact as a special case in the ultrasound Breast Imaging–Reporting and Data System (BI-RADS).

Guidelines for elastography in the breast have been presented.[15,16] The guidelines all recommend the use of elastography in characterization of breast lesions as benign or malignant. The guidelines do not recommend one method over another. The guidelines suggest that elastography may be used to upgrade or downgrade the BI-RADS category score but do not provide detailed specific guidance on when this should be used.

Additional studies are needed to determine cutoff values for the various techniques and interpretation methods. The studies need to have better control of technique, especially controlling the amount of precompression. Based on the studies published to date, guidance in interpretation based on the probability of malignancy can be provided. ▸ Fig. 5.2 presents these data on a scale similar to BI-RADS probablity scale based on the probability of malignancy for each technique. There is moderate variability in published results for some techniques. A conservative approach was used to develop this table. As more standardized methodology is used it is expected the table will be revised.

## 9.2 Areas for Further Research

### 9.2.1 Elastography–Pathology Correlation

There are several elastography findings that are unique to the breast. The size change observed in SE in both benign (smaller) and malignant lesions (larger) appears to occur only in breast. Desmoplastic reaction has been suggested as a possible cause for malignancies appearing larger on SE. However, this does not explain why benign lesions appear smaller. The size changes noted in the breast are not identified in phantom studies. It is not know if surgical specimens have similar size changes studied in vitro as noted in vivo. Further correlative studies with surgical pathology are needed to determine if the actual size of a malignant tumor is better defined by the elastographic size as opposed to the B-mode size. More detailed elastography pathology correlative studies are needed to determine the exact nature of the stiffness identified on both SE and SWE surrounding malignancies. These studies would be helpful in determining if the elastographic size should be used in surgical planning. We know that B-mode ultrasound and mammography often underestimate the size of malignancies compared to surgical pathology.

### 9.2.2 Tumor Grade Assessment

Preliminary work has demonstrated that the elastogram/B-mode (E/B) ratio is predictive of tumor grade. Low-grade malignancies such as ductal carcinoma in situ (DCIS) and mucinous or colloid cancers have E/B ratios of near 1. Invasive ductal cancers have higher E/B ratios, and the ratio appears to have some correlation with tumor grade.[28] Similar results have been found with SWE. Evans et al[193] reported that breast cancers with higher mean stiffness values at SWE had poorer prognostic features. They found that high histologic grade, large invasive size, lymph node involvement, tumor type, and vascular invasion all showed statistically significant positive association with high stiffness values. Further investigations are needed to determine if this information will prove clinically useful.

## 9.2.3 Poor Shear Wave Propagation in Cancers

Preliminary work suggests that shear wave generation or propagation is problematic in breast malignancies. This does not appear to occur in other organs. This can lead to false-negative results. This phenomenon occurs with both SWE systems and is most likely a fundamental problem of breast pathology and not with ultrasound SWE. This phenomenon leads to non–color coding of the malignancy or a poor-quality measure. Initial SWE algorithms did not fully account for this problem. Now that this phenomenon is known the addition of a quality measure or improved algorithms not color coding areas of poor-quality shear waves are being developed to solve this problem and limit the number of false-negative results.[65] The result is that in many breast cancers the shear wave velocity (Vs) cannot be determined. In some cancers the high Vs in the periphery of the lesion will allow for a true-positive result. But many breast cancers will not have elevated Vs in or around the lesion, with the areas of malignancy not color coded or having a poor-quality measure. In most cases if the lesion is solid and it does not color code the lesion has a high probability of being a malignancy.[65] In all of these cases SE documents these breast malignancies as true-positives. The combination of SE and SWE results will increase the diagnostic confidence in these cases.

## 9.2.4 Improved Understanding for Specific Pathologies

There have been very few studies of the elastographic features of individual pathologies. This book has presented the range of elastographic features for individual pathologies, mostly based on our experience, given the lack of published results. For example, fibroadenomas can have a wide range of elastographic findings from very soft to very stiff, from an E/B ratio of < 1 to > 1. We do not know if elastographic data will provide clinically useful information on a given pathology. Do stiff fibroadenomas with an E/B ratio > 1 have a higher probability of continued or rapid growth? Can this be used to select patients who could benefit from surgical removal? Can elastography be used to monitor large-duct papillomas and predict if they are progressing to atypia or malignancy? Some work as been done on using elastographic data to characterize malignancies. The E/B ratio and Vs max have been shown to correlate with tumor grade on preliminary studies.

## 9.2.5 Correlation between Semiquantitative and Quantitative Measurements

Very few studies have been performed where several measurements using different techniques are performed in the same patient. Is there a correlation between the Vs max and the elasticity/imaging (E/I) ratio? How do the E/I ratio and strain ratio (lesion to fat ratio) relate to each other? Our limited results suggest that the E/I ratio and strain ratio may not be significantly correlated. The E/I ratio measures a phenomenon that we do not understand but relates to the tumor interaction with adjacent tissue elasticity, whereas the strain ratio is a measure of stiffness. It appears a lesion can have low malignant strain ratio but have a large malignant E/B ratio. The strain ratio is more likely to correlate with the Vs max on SWE.

## 9.3 Future Developments

Elastography is still early in its development. Improvements in existing techniques as well as new techniques are certain to be developed. Elastography is an area of very active research not only for the breast but also for many other organs.[194]

### 9.3.1 Three-Dimensional Screening

The present two-dimensional (2D) technology limits elastography for breast cancer screening. Screening with SE will most likely be problematic for some time due to its relative nature. Both 2D SE and 2D SWE are limited in screening due to the long amount of time needed to screen the breasts with these techniques. Both techniques cannot be used in a scanning mode. At each location where an elastogram is obtained the probe must be stationary for at least several seconds.

The development of a three-dimensional (3D) shear wave technique would allow for breast screening in a reasonable amount of time. Works in progress of both SE (▶ Fig. 9.1) and SWE (▶ Fig. 9.2) have been reported. The present 3D probes scan a relatively small area, and evaluating both breasts for screening takes a prohibitive amount of time. The development of a 3D SWE probe that can evaluate a larger field of view (FOV) is needed to allow for routine screening with SWE.

The development of 3D elastography may help to improve lesion characterization and allow for evaluation of larger areas of breast tissue in a time-efficient manner. Evaluation with elastography in the coronal plane with the use of an opacity feature is presently being investigated. With only one acquisition the tumor volume can be interrogated for spiculation, extent of invasion, desmoplastic reaction, and Vs values throughout the volume. This may lead to improved presurgical planning and assessment of effectiveness of chemotherapy.

### 9.3.2 Added to BI-RADS

Addition of elastography to the BI-RADS lexicon is expected in the future. Given the excellent results of elastography in initial studies the addition of this technique to the BI-RADS ultrasound lexicon will most likely occur. The addition of elastography to the BI-RADS classification may be the ability to upgrade or downgrade BI-RADS category 3 or BI-RADS category 4A lesions, selecting patients more appropriate for biopsy. Further work is needed to determine if elastography will be able to downgrade BI-RADS 4B, 4C, or 5 lesions. With sensitivities of > 98% in several large studies using the E/B ratio in SE, lesions with an E/B ratio should be considered BI-RADS category 5 regardless of the conventional ultrasound findings. Using this technique the Positive Predictive Value (PPV) is 99%. Thus an E/I ratio value of < 1 has a < 2% probability of malignancy, suggesting the lesions with this finding fall into a maximum BI-RADS category 3 regardless of the BI-RADS category score on conventional ultrasound. Further studies need to be performed to determine if this is an appropriate approach.

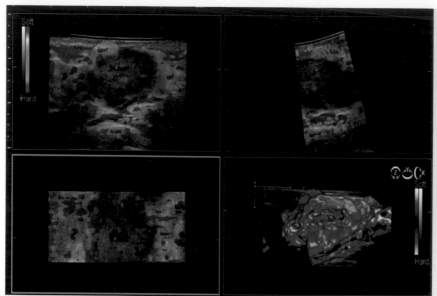

**Fig. 9.1** The three-dimensional (3D) strain elastogram of an invasive ductal cancer obtained on a Hitachi system (Hitachi Aloka America, Wallingford, CT) displayed as a 3D rendering. In addition to 3D rendering, imaging can be presented as slices that can be displayed in any plane. (Courtesy of Hitachi Aloka Medical, press release dated February 7, 2011)

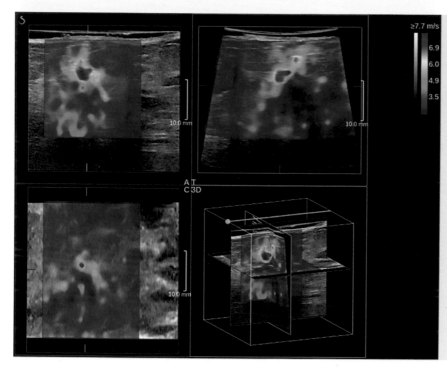

**Fig. 9.2** The three-dimensional images from an invasive ductal cancer obtained with a SuperSonic Imagine system (Bethel, WA). The axis can be moved to visualize a two-dimensional image from any plane. The data can also be displayed as multiple slices through the field of view slices in any plane. (Courtesy of Supersonic Imagine, press release dated March 8, 2011)

## 9.3.3 Standardization of Protocols

There are significant differences in results with strain ratio. This is partially due to some studies using subcutaneous fat as a reference, whereas others use fat at a similar depth to the lesion and still others use both fat and glandular tissue as the reference. Precompression will also affect the strain ratio because the stiffness of fat will be affected more than that of other lesions, leading to a lower strain ratio. There is also no convention as to where the regions of interest (ROIs) should be placed—whether they should include the entire lesion or the region with greatest stiffness. There is often artifactual soft signal adjacent to lesions that should not be used to calculate the strain ratio because this will artificially elevate the strain ratio (see Case 6.17).

The cutoff value for SWE varies from a maximum value of Vs of 4.1 m/s (50 kPa) to 5.2 m/s (80 kPa) in various studies. Precompression was not controlled in these studies, although they were performed with "a light touch." The effect of precompression can easily account for an elevated cutoff value of this range. Further studies that are well controlled for precompression are needed. A ring of high Vs surrounding a lesion has also been suggested as a diagnostic feature of malignancy. Care must be taken because precompression will cause the ring to form, even in benign lesions. This ring may be due to interaction of the acoustic radiation force impulse (ARFI) with the boundary effects when an interface of soft to hard tissue is present.[195]

## 9.3.4 Reporting

No guidelines have been developed for the reporting of SE or SWE results. We document all the elastographic parameters obtained on the images and store the images in our Picture Archiving and Communication System (PACS). We usually report the elastographic findings within the report as suggestive of benign or suggestive of a malignant lesion. If the elastographic findings change management from the BI-RADS score resulting from conventional ultrasound the report includes a more detailed discussion of the elastographic findings.

We use ► Fig. 5.2 to guide our interpretations. Until there is more standardization of protocols it is unlikely that a standard universal guideline for reporting will be agreed upon.

## 9.3.5 New Technology

There is a trend for both SE and SWE to be available on one ultrasound system. This allows a "toolbox" of elastography techniques. The elastographic examination can then be tailored to the needs of the patient. The ability to use multiple techniques will also increase diagnostic confidence if their results are concordant. Cases with nonconcordant results should raise suspicion of an unsuspected finding, such as two lesions adjacent to each other.

On SWE one system now provides four different maps that display the shear wave data. These include the velocity map, quality map, time map, and displacement map. For routine clinical use we evaluate the velocity map and the quality map. These two maps provide the information needed to accurately interpret the SWE results. The time and displacement maps are currently used for research and can be confusing to the novice. In general the quality map is most helpful when the shear wave velocities are low, suggestive of a benign lesion. In this case a high (good, green) quality map will increase the probability that the lesion is truly benign. If the quality map is poor on a lesion with low Vs the possibility of a false-negative result could be considered.[65] The other SWE vendor has incorporated the quality map with the velocity map, not color coding the image where the shear wave quality is poor. The algorithms on early systems did not adequately evaluate the shear wave quality for breast applications due to unexpected shear wave propagation in breast cancers. Newer algorithms are correcting this problem, and continued improvement in accuracy can be expected as these are developed.

New elastographic techniques are in development. With increasing precompression a ring of high Vs occurs at interfaces between soft and stiff tissues.[195] This may be secondary to reflection of the ARFI pulse at the interface. This appears to occur at lower levels of precompression in malignant lesions than in benign lesions. The possibility of a graded compression technique may lead to another method of characterizing breast masses and lead to improved definition of lesion borders.

## 9.4 Conclusions

Elastography, both SE and SWE, has high sensitivities and specificities in characterization of breast masses. The incorporation of elastography into the standard ultrasound breast exam is occurring. International guidelines have been published for the use of elastography, both SE and SWE, in characterization of breast pathology. Despite guidelines additional studies are under way to standardize the techniques, interpretation, and reporting of elastographic results. Within the next few years breast elastography will be more standardized.

Both SE and SWE have been shown to have high reproducibility, sensitivity, and specificity for characterization of breast lesions. Each has its advantages and disadvantages. The use of both techniques can increase diagnostic confidence when results are concordant.

Elastographic systems and the applications themselves continue to evolve, and new tools and new evidence will likely emerge. We anticipate that the direction of development, imaging methods, and diagnostic approaches will change and fragment in the future. It appears that elastography has already become an essential medical tool in the field of breast imaging.

# References

[1] Jellins J, Kossoff G, Reeve TS. Detection and classification of liquid-filled masses in the breast by gray scale echography. Radiology 1977; 125: 205–212

[2] Hilton SV, Leopold GR, Olson LK, Willson SA. Real-time breast sonography: application in 300 consecutive patients. AJR Am J Roentgenol 1986; 147: 479–486

[3] Stavros AT, Thickman D, Rapp CL, Dennis MA, Parker SH, Sisney GA. Solid breast nodules: use of sonography to distinguish between benign and malignant lesions. Radiology 1995; 196: 123–134

[4] American College of Radiology (ACR). American College of Radiology Breast Imaging Reporting and Data System (BI-RADS) Ultrasound. 4th ed. Reston VA: American College of Radiology; 2003

[5] Tanter M, Bercoff J, Athanasiou A, et al. Quantitative assessment of breast lesion viscoelasticity: initial clinical results using supersonic shear imaging. Ultrasound Med Biol 2008; 34: 1373–1386

[6] Ophir J, Céspedes I, Ponnekanti H, Yazdi Y, Li X. Elastography: a quantitative method for imaging the elasticity of biological tissues. Ultrason Imaging 1991; 13: 111–134

[7] Samani A, Zubovits J, Plewes D. Elastic moduli of normal and pathological human breast tissues: an inversion-technique-based investigation of 169 samples. Phys Med Biol 2007; 52: 1565–1576

[8] Frey H. [Realtime elastography. A new ultrasound procedure for the reconstruction of tissue elasticity] Radiologe 2003; 43: 850–855

[9] Krouskop TA, Wheeler TM, Kallel F, Garra BS, Hall T. Elastic moduli of breast and prostate tissues under compression. Ultrason Imaging 1998; 20: 260–274

[10] Hall TJ, Zhu Y, Spalding CS. In vivo real-time freehand palpation imaging. Ultrasound Med Biol 2003; 29: 427–435

[11] Bluemke DA, Gatsonis CA, Chen MH, et al. Magnetic resonance imaging of the breast prior to biopsy. JAMA 2004; 292: 2735–2742

[12] Morrow M. Magnetic resonance imaging in breast cancer: one step forward, two steps back? JAMA 2004; 292: 2779–2780

[13] Bamber J, Cosgrove D, Dietrich CF, et al. EFSUMB guidelines and recommendations on the clinical use of ultrasound elastography, I: Basic principles and technology. Ultraschall Med 2013; 34: 169–184

[14] Nakashima K, Shiina T, Sakurai M, et al. JSUM ultrasound elastography practice guidelines: breast. J Med Ultrason 2013; 40: 359–391

[15] Cosgrove D, Piscaglia F, Bamber J, et al. EFSUMB. EFSUMB guidelines and recommendations on the clinical use of ultrasound elastography, II: Clinical applications. Ultraschall Med 2013; 34: 238–253

[16] Barr RG, Nakashima K, Amy D, et al. WFUMB Guidelines and Recommendations on the Clinical Use of Ultrasound Elastography: Part 2; Breast. Ultrasound in Medicine and Biology, in press

[17] Emerson K. Diseases of the breast. In: Wintrobe MM, Adams RD, et al, eds. Harrison's Principals of Internal Medicine. 7th ed. New York, NY: McGraw-Hill; 1974 :582–587

[18] Barr RG. Sonographic breast elastography: a primer. J Ultrasound Med 2012; 31: 773–783

[19] Barr RG, Zhang Z. Effects of precompression on elasticity imaging of the breast: development of a clinically useful semiquantitative method of pre-compression assessment. J Ultrasound Med 2012; 31: 895–902

[20] Nightingale K, Soo MS, Nightingale R, Trahey G. Acoustic radiation force impulse imaging: in vivo demonstration of clinical feasibility. Ultrasound Med Biol 2002; 28: 227–235

[21] Fahey BJ, Nightingale KR, Nelson RC, Palmeri ML, Trahey GE. Acoustic radiation force impulse imaging of the abdomen: demonstration of feasibility and utility. Ultrasound Med Biol 2005; 31: 1185–1198

[22] Rouze NC, Wang MH, Palmeri ML, Nightingale KR. Robust estimation of time-of-flight shear wave speed using a radon sum transformation. IEEE Trans Ultrason Ferroelectr Freq Control 2010; 57: 2662–2670

[23] www.AIUM.org, "Breast Elastography in Routine Clinical Practice." Richard G. Barr, AIUM/SDMS Webinar

[24] Barr RG. Real-time ultrasound elasticity of the breast: initial clinical results. Ultrasound Q 2010; 26: 61–66

[25] Barr RG, Destounis S, Lackey LB, II, Svensson WE, Balleyguier C, Smith C. Evaluation of breast lesions using sonographic elasticity imaging: a multicenter trial. J Ultrasound Med 2012; 31: 281–287

[26] Destounis S, Arieno A, Morgan R, et al. Clinical experience with elasticity imaging in a community-based breast center. J Ultrasound Med 2013; 32: 297–302

[27] Barr R. Breast. In: Calliada F, Canapari M, Ferraioli G, Filice C, eds. Sono-Elastography Main Clinical Applications. Pavia, Italy: Edizioni Medico Scientifiche; 2012:49–68

[28] Grajo JRB, Barr RG. Strain elastography for prediction of breast cancer tumor grades. J Ultrasound Med 2014; 33: 129–134

[29] Ueno EIA. Diagnosis of breast cancer by elasticity imaging. Eizo Joho Medical 2004; 36: 2–6

[30] Itoh A, Ueno E, Tohno E, et al. Breast disease: clinical application of US elastography for diagnosis. Radiology 2006; 239: 341–350

[31] Park JSM. W.K. Inter and intraobserver agreement in the interpretation of ultrasound elastography of breast lesions. In: Radiological Society of North America 93rd Scientific Assembly and Annual Meeting; 2007; Chicago, IL. November 25–30, 2007

[32] Chiorean A, Duma M, Dudea S, et al. Short analysis on elastographic images of benign and malignant breast lesions based on color and hue parameters. Ultraschall Med 2008; 29: OP_2_13

[33] Duma M, Chiorean A, Dudea S, et al. Breast Lesions: correlations between ultrasound BI-RADS classification and UENO-ITOH elastography score. Ultraschall Med 2008; 29: OP_2_12

[34] Zhi H, Xiao XY, Yang HY, et al. Semi-quantitating stiffness of breast solid lesions in ultrasonic elastography. Acad Radiol 2008; 15: 1347–1353

[35] Zhu QL, Jiang YX, Liu JB, et al. Real-time ultrasound elastography: its potential role in assessment of breast lesions. Ultrasound Med Biol 2008; 34: 1232–1238

[36] Tan SM, Teh HS, Mancer JF, Poh WT. Improving B mode ultrasound evaluation of breast lesions with real-time ultrasound elastography—a clinical approach. Breast 2008; 17: 252–257

[37] Scaperrotta G, Ferranti C, Costa C, et al. Role of sonoelastography in non-palpable breast lesions. Eur Radiol 2008; 18: 2381–2389

[38] Cho N, Moon WK, Park JS, Cha JH, Jang M, Seong MH. Nonpalpable breast masses: evaluation by US elastography. Korean J Radiol 2008; 9: 111–118

[39] Chiorean AD, Duma MM, Dudea SM, et al. Real-time ultrasound elastography of the breast: state of the art. Medical Ultrasonography 2008; 10: 73–82

[40] Raza S, Odulate A, Ong EM, Chikarmane S, Harston CW. Using real-time tissue elastography for breast lesion evaluation: our initial experience. J Ultrasound Med 2010; 29: 551–563

[41] Chang JM, Moon WK, Cho N, Kim SJ. Breast mass evaluation: factors influencing the quality of US elastography. Radiology 2011; 259: 59–64

[42] Ueno E, Umenoto T, Matsumura T, Bando H, Tohno E, Waki K. New quantitative method in breast elastography: fat lesion ratio (FLR). Paper presented at: Radiological Society of North America 93rd Scientific Assembly and Annual Meeting; November 25–30, 2007; Chicago, IL. November 27, 2007.

[43] Thomas A, Degenhardt F, Farrokh A, Wojcinski S, Slowinski T, Fischer T. Significant differentiation of focal breast lesions: calculation of strain ratio in breast sonoelastography. Acad Radiol 2010; 17: 558–563

[44] Farrokh A, Wojcinski S, Degenhardt F. [Diagnostic value of strain ratio measurement in the differentiation of malignant and benign breast lesions] Ultraschall Med 2011; 32: 400–405

[45] Zhi H, Xiao XY, Yang HY, Ou B, Wen YL, Luo BM. Ultrasonic elastography in breast cancer diagnosis: strain ratio vs 5-point scale. Acad Radiol 2010; 17: 1227–1233

[46] Alhabshi SM, Rahmat K, Abdul Halim N, et al. Semi-quantitative and qualitative assessment of breast ultrasound elastography in differentiating between malignant and benign lesions. Ultrasound Med Biol 2013; 39: 568–578

[47] Stachs A, Hartmann S, Stubert J, et al. Differentiating between malignant and benign breast masses: factors limiting sonoelastographic strain ratio. Ultraschall Med 2013; 34: 131–136

[48] Barr RG, Lackey AE. The utility of the "bull's-eye" artifact on breast elasticity imaging in reducing breast lesion biopsy rate. Ultrasound Q 2011; 27: 151–155

[49] Nakashima K, Moriya T. Comprehensive ultrasound diagnosis for intraductal spread of primary breast cancer. Breast Cancer 2013; 20: 3–12

[50] Sarvazyan AP, Rudenko OV, Swanson SD, Fowlkes JB, Emelianov SY. Shear wave elasticity imaging: a new ultrasonic technology of medical diagnostics. Ultrasound Med Biol 1998; 24: 1419–1435

[51] Bercoff J, Tanter M, Fink M. Supersonic shear imaging: a new technique for soft tissue elasticity mapping. IEEE Trans Ultrason Ferroelectr Freq Control 2004; 51: 396–409

[52] Nightingale K, McAleavey S, Trahey G. Shear-wave generation using acoustic radiation force: in vivo and ex vivo results. Ultrasound Med Biol 2003; 29: 1715–1723

[53] Parker KJ, Lerner RM. Sonoelasticity of organs: shear waves ring a bell. J Ultrasound Med 1992; 11: 387–392

[54] Chang JM, Moon WK, Cho N, et al. Clinical application of shear wave elastography (SWE) in the diagnosis of benign and malignant breast diseases. Breast Cancer Res Treat 2011; 129: 89–97

[55] Athanasiou A, Tardivon A, Tanter M, et al. Breast lesions: quantitative elastography with supersonic shear imaging—preliminary results. Radiology 2010; 256: 297–303

[56] Evans A, Whelehan P, Thomson K, et al. Quantitative shear wave ultrasound elastography: initial experience in solid breast masses. Breast Cancer Res 2010; 12: R104

[57] Tozaki M, Isobe S, Sakamoto M. Combination of elastography and tissue quantification using the acoustic radiation force impulse (ARFI) technology for differential diagnosis of breast masses. Jpn J Radiol 2012; 30: 659–670

[58] Berg WA, Cosgrove DO, Doré CJ, et al. BE1 Investigators. Shear-wave elastography improves the specificity of breast US: the BE1 multinational study of 939 masses. Radiology 2012; 262: 435–449

[59] Schäfer FK, Hooley RJ, Ohlinger R, et al. ShearWave Elastography BE1 multinational breast study: additional SWE features support potential to downgrade BI-RADS-3 lesions. Ultraschall Med 2013; 34: 254–259

[60] Cosgrove DO, Berg WA, Doré CJ, et al. BE1 Study Group. Shear wave elastography for breast masses is highly reproducible. Eur Radiol 2012; 22: 1023–1032

[61] Lee SH, Chang JM, Kim WH, et al. Differentiation of benign from malignant solid breast masses: comparison of two-dimensional and three-dimensional shear-wave elastography. Eur Radiol 2013; 23: 1015–1026

[62] Youk JH, Gweon HM, Son EJ, Chung J, Kim JA, Kim EK. Three-dimensional shear-wave elastography for differentiating benign and malignant breast lesions: comparison with two-dimensional shear-wave elastography. Eur Radiol 2013; 23: 1519–1527

[63] Barr RG. Shear wave imaging of the breast: still on the learning curve. J Ultrasound Med 2012; 31: 347–350

[64] Bai M, Du L, Gu J, Li F, Jia X. Virtual touch tissue quantification using acoustic radiation force impulse technology: initial clinical experience with solid breast masses. J Ultrasound Med 2012; 31: 289–294

[65] Barr RG, Zheng Z. Shear wave elastography of the breast: value of a quality measure and comparison to strain elastography. Radiology; in press

[66] Barr RG, Zhang Z, Cormack JB, Mendelson EB, Berg WA. Probably benign lesions at screening breast US in a population with elevated risk: prevalence and rate of malignancy in the ACRIN 6666 trial. Radiology 2013; 269: 701–712

[67] Berg WA. Sonographically depicted breast clustered microcysts: is follow-up appropriate? AJR Am J Roentgenol 2005; 185: 952–959

[68] Berg WA, Campassi CI, Ioffe OB. Cystic lesions of the breast: sonographic-pathologic correlation. Radiology 2003; 227: 183–191

[69] Doshi DJ, March DE, Crisi GM, Coughlin BF. Complex cystic breast masses: diagnostic approach and imaging-pathologic correlation. Radiographics 2007; 27 Suppl 1: S53–S64

[70] Chen JH, Nalcioglu O, Su MY. Fibrocystic change of the breast presenting as a focal lesion mimicking breast cancer in MR imaging. J Magn Reson Imaging 2008; 28: 1499–1505

[71] Shetty MK, Shah YP. Sonographic findings in focal fibrocystic changes of the breast. Ultrasound Q 2002; 18: 35–40

[72] Hanson CA, Snover DC, Dehner LP. Fibroadenomatosis (fibroadenomatoid mastopathy): a benign breast lesion with composite pathologic features. Pathology 1987; 19: 393–396

[73] Kamal M, Evans AJ, Denley H, Pinder SE, Ellis IO. Fibroadenomatoid hyperplasia: a cause of suspicious microcalcification on mammographic screening. AJR Am J Roentgenol 1998; 171: 1331–1334

[74] Poulton TB, de Paredes ES, Baldwin M. Sclerosing lobular hyperplasia of the breast: imaging features in 15 cases. AJR Am J Roentgenol 1995; 165: 291–294

[75] Hoda SA, Brogi E, Koerner FC, et al. Rosen's Breast Pathology. 4th ed. Philadelphia: Lippincott Wilkins & Williams. 2014

[76] Gordon PB, Gagnon FA, Lanzkowsky L. Solid breast masses diagnosed as fibroadenoma at fine-needle aspiration biopsy: acceptable rates of growth at long-term follow-up. Radiology 2003; 229: 233–238

[77] Yang WT, Suen M, Metreweli C. Sonographic features of benign papillary neoplasms of the breast: review of 22 patients. J Ultrasound Med 1997; 16: 161–168

[78] Cardenosa G, Eklund GW. Benign papillary neoplasms of the breast: mammographic findings. Radiology 1991; 181: 751–755

[79] Daniel BL, Gardner RW, Birdwell RL, Nowels KW, Johnson D. Magnetic resonance imaging of intraductal papilloma of the breast. Magn Reson Imaging 2003; 21: 887–892

[80] Kim TH, Kang DK, Kim SY, Lee EJ, Jung YS, Yim H. Sonographic differentiation of benign and malignant papillary lesions of the breast. J Ultrasound Med 2008; 27: 75–82

[81] Han BK, Choe YH, Ko YH, Yang JH, Nam SJ. Benign papillary lesions of the breast: sonographic-pathologic correlation. J Ultrasound Med 1999; 18: 217–223

[82] Jakate K, De Brot M, Goldberg F, Muradali D, O'Malley FP, Mulligan AM. Papillary lesions of the breast: impact of breast pathology subspecialization on core biopsy and excision diagnoses. Am J Surg Pathol 2012; 36: 544–551

[83] Muttarak M, Lerttumnongtum P, Chaiwun B, Peh WC. Spectrum of papillary lesions of the breast: clinical, imaging, and pathologic correlation. AJR Am J Roentgenol 2008; 191: 700–707

[84] Mulligan AM, O'Malley FP. Papillary lesions of the breast: a review. Adv Anat Pathol 2007; 14: 108–119

[85] Lewis JT, Hartmann LC, Vierkant RA, et al. An analysis of breast cancer risk in women with single, multiple, and atypical papilloma. Am J Surg Pathol 2006; 30: 665–672

[86] Jagmohan P, Pool FJ, Putti TC, Wong J. Papillary lesions of the breast: imaging findings and diagnostic challenges. Diagn Interv Radiol 2013; 19: 471–478

[87] Jacklin RK, Ridgway PF, Ziprin P, Healy V, Hadjiminas D, Darzi A. Optimising preoperative diagnosis in phyllodes tumour of the breast. J Clin Pathol 2006; 59: 454–459

[88] Ridgway PF, Jacklin RK, Ziprin P, et al. Perioperative diagnosis of cystosarcoma phyllodes of the breast may be enhanced by MIB-1 index. J Surg Res 2004; 122: 83–88

[89] Bandyopadhyay R, Nag D, Mondal SK, Mukhopadhyay S, Roy S, Sinha SK. Distinction of phyllodes tumor from fibroadenoma: Cytologists' perspective. J Cytol 2010; 27: 59–62

[90] The American Cancer Society, www.cancer.org [accessed November 2014]

[91] Lifshitz OH, Whitman GJ, Sahin AA, Yang WT. Radiologic-pathologic conferences of the University of Texas M.D. Anderson Cancer Center. Phyllodes tumor of the breast. AJR Am J Roentgenol 2003; 180: 332

[92] Tan H, Zhang S, Liu H, et al. Imaging findings in phyllodes tumors of the breast. Eur J Radiol 2012; 81: e62–e69

[93] Oprić S, Oprić D, Gugić D, Granić M. Phyllodes tumors and fibroadenoma common beginning and different ending. Coll Antropol 2012; 36: 235–241

[94] Stavros AT. Breast Ultrasound. Philadelphia, PA: Lippincott Williams and Wilkins; 2004

[95] Seo HR, Na KY, Yim HE, et al. Differential diagnosis in idiopathic granulomatous mastitis and tuberculous mastitis. J Breast Cancer 2012; 15: 111–118

[96] Hines N, Slanetz PJ, Eisenberg RL. Cystic masses of the breast. AJR Am J Roentgenol 2010; 194: W122–33

[97] Son EJ, Oh KK, Kim EK. Pregnancy-associated breast disease: radiologic features and diagnostic dilemmas. Yonsei Med J 2006; 47: 34–42

[98] Magno S, Terribile D, Franceschini G, et al. Early onset lactating adenoma and the role of breast MRI: a case report. J Med Case Reports 2009; 3: 43

[99] Dialani V, Baum J, Mehta TS. Sonographic features of gynecomastia. J Ultrasound Med 2010; 29: 539–547

[100] Crichlow RW, Galt SW. Male breast cancer. Surg Clin North Am 1990; 70: 1165–1177

[101] Heruti RJ, Dankner R, Berezin M, Zeilig G, Ohry A. Gynecomastia following spinal cord disorder. Arch Phys Med Rehabil 1997; 78: 534–537

[102] Mathew J, Perkins GH, Stephens T, Middleton LP, Yang WT. Primary breast cancer in men: clinical, imaging, and pathologic findings in 57 patients. AJR Am J Roentgenol 2008; 191: 1631–1639

[103] Dershaw DD, Borgen PI, Deutch BM, Liberman L. Mammographic findings in men with breast cancer. AJR Am J Roentgenol 1993; 160: 267–270

[104] Lever WF, Schaumburg-Lever G. Tumors and cysts of the skin. In: Lever WF, Schaumburg-Lever G, eds. Histopathology of the Skin, 7th ed. Philadelphia: Lippincott-Raven. 1990; 535–536

[105] Giess CS, Raza S, Birdwell RL. Distinguishing breast skin lesions from superficial breast parenchymal lesions: diagnostic criteria, imaging characteristics, and pitfalls. Radiographics 2011; 31: 1959–1972

[106] Lee HS, Joo KB, Song HT, et al. Relationship between sonographic and pathologic findings in epidermal inclusion cysts. J Clin Ultrasound 2001; 29: 374–383

[107] Srivastava V, Basu S, Shukla VK. Seroma formation after breast cancer surgery: what we have learned in the last two decades. J Breast Cancer 2012; 15: 373–380

[108] Gaspari R, Blehar D, Mendoza M, Montoya A, Moon C, Polan D. Use of ultrasound elastography for skin and subcutaneous abscesses. J Ultrasound Med 2009; 28: 855–860

[109] Radiological Society of North America. Special ultrasound accurately identifies skin cancer. ScienceDaily, December 2, 2009. Retrieved November 26, 2013. http://www.sciencedaily.com%C2%AD /releases/2009/12/091201084103.htm

[110] Kennedy M, Masterson AV, Kerin M, Flanagan F. Pathology and clinical relevance of radial scars: a review. J Clin Pathol 2003; 56: 721–724

[111] Tabar L, Dean PB. Teaching Atlas of Mammography. Stuttgart: Thieme; 1985

[112] Andersen JA, Gram JB. Radial scar in the female breast: a long-term follow-up study of 32 cases. Cancer 1984; 53: 2557–2560

[113] Anderson TJ, Battersby S. Radial scars of benign and malignant breasts: comparative features and significance. J Pathol 1985; 147: 23–32

[114] Cohen MA, Sferlazza SJ. Role of sonography in evaluation of radial scars of the breast. AJR Am J Roentgenol 2000; 174: 1075–1078

[115] Morgan C, Shah ZA, Hamilton R, et al. The radial scar of the breast diagnosed at core needle biopsy. Proc (Bayl Univ Med Cent) 2012; 25: 3–5

[116] Dupont WD, Page DL. Risk factors for breast cancer in women with proliferative breast disease. N Engl J Med 1985; 312: 146–151

[117] Kohr JR, Eby PR, Allison KH, et al. Risk of upgrade of atypical ductal hyperplasia after stereotactic breast biopsy: effects of number of foci and complete removal of calcifications. Radiology 2010; 255: 723–730

[118] An YKSH, Kang BJ, Lee AW, Song BJ. Atypical ductal hyperplasia (ADH): Can the sonoelastography predict the upgrade of ADH to malignancy? J Korean Soc Radiol 2011; 64: 383–388

[119] Welch HG, Woloshin S, Schwartz LM. The sea of uncertainty surrounding ductal carcinoma in situ—the price of screening mammography. J Natl Cancer Inst 2008; 100: 228–229

[120] Ernster VL, Ballard-Barbash R, Barlow WE, et al. Detection of ductal carcinoma in situ in women undergoing screening mammography. J Natl Cancer Inst 2002; 94: 1546–1554

[121] Kerlikowske K, Molinaro AM, Gauthier ML, et al. Biomarker expression and risk of subsequent tumors after initial ductal carcinoma in situ diagnosis. J Natl Cancer Inst 2010; 102: 627–637

[122] Witkiewicz AK, Dasgupta A, Nguyen KH, et al. Stromal caveolin-1 levels predict early DCIS progression to invasive breast cancer. Cancer Biol Ther 2009; 8: 1071–1079

[123] Evans A. Ductal carcinoma in situ (DCIS): are we overdetecting it? Breast Cancer Res 2004; 6 Suppl 1: 23

[124] Orel SG, Mendonca MH, Reynolds C, Schnall MD, Solin LJ, Sullivan DC. MR imaging of ductal carcinoma in situ. Radiology 1997; 202: 413–420

[125] Stomper PC, Connolly JL, Meyer JE, Harris JR. Clinically occult ductal carcinoma in situ detected with mammography: analysis of 100 cases with radiologic-pathologic correlation. Radiology 1989; 172: 235–241

[126] Dershaw DD, Abramson A, Kinne DW. Ductal carcinoma in situ: mammographic findings and clinical implications. Radiology 1989; 170: 411–415

[127] Izumori A, Takebe K, Sato A. Ultrasound findings and histological features of ductal carcinoma in situ detected by ultrasound examination alone. Breast Cancer 2010; 17: 136–141

[128] Diaz NM, Palmer JO, McDivitt RW. Carcinoma arising within fibroadenomas of the breast. A clinicopathologic study of 105 patients. Am J Clin Pathol 1991; 95: 614–622

[129] Dupont WD, Page DL, Parl FF, et al. Long-term risk of breast cancer in women with fibroadenoma. N Engl J Med 1994; 331: 10–15

[130] Pick PW, Iossifides IA. Occurrence of breast carcinoma within a fibroadenoma. A review. Arch Pathol Lab Med 1984; 108: 590–594

[131] Deschênes L, Jacob S, Fabia J, Christen A. Beware of breast fibroadenomas in middle-aged women. Can J Surg 1985; 28: 372–374

[132] Ozzello L, Gump FE. The management of patients with carcinomas in fibroadenomatous tumors of the breast. Surg Gynecol Obstet 1985; 160: 99–104

[133] Gashi-Luci LH, Limani RA, Kurshumliu FI. Invasive ductal carcinoma within fibroadenoma: a case report. Cases J 2009; 2: 174

[134] Rajakariar R, Walker RA. Pathological and biological features of mammographically detected invasive breast carcinomas. Br J Cancer 1995; 71: 150–154

[135] Perou CM, Sørlie T, Eisen MB, et al. Molecular portraits of human breast tumours. Nature 2000; 406: 747–752

[136] Sørlie T, Perou CM, Tibshirani R, et al. Gene expression patterns of breast carcinomas distinguish tumor subclasses with clinical implications. Proc Natl Acad Sci U S A 2001; 98: 10869–10874

[137] Sørlie T, Tibshirani R, Parker J, et al. Repeated observation of breast tumor subtypes in independent gene expression data sets. Proc Natl Acad Sci USA 2003; 100: 8418–8423

[138] Brenton JD, Carey LA, Ahmed AA, Caldas C. Molecular classification and molecular forecasting of breast cancer: ready for clinical application? J Clin Oncol 2005; 23: 7350–7360

[139] Carey LA, Dees EC, Sawyer L, et al. The triple negative paradox: primary tumor chemosensitivity of breast cancer subtypes. Clin Cancer Res 2007; 13: 2329–2334

[140] Carey LA, Perou CM, Livasy CA, et al. Race, breast cancer subtypes, and survival in the Carolina Breast Cancer Study. JAMA 2006; 295: 2492–2502

[141] Cheang MC, Voduc D, Bajdik C, et al. Basal-like breast cancer defined by five biomarkers has superior prognostic value than triple-negative phenotype. Clin Cancer Res 2008; 14: 1368–1376

[142] Bland KI, Copeland EM, III, eds. The Breast: Comprehensive Management of Benign and Malignant Disorders. 4th ed. Philadelphia, PA: Saunders Elsevier; 2009

[143] Hilleren DJ, Andersson IT, Lindholm K, Linnell FS. Invasive lobular carcinoma: mammographic findings in a 10-year experience. Radiology 1991; 178: 149–154

[144] Berg JW, Hutter RV. Breast cancer. Cancer 1995; 75 Suppl: 257–269

[145] Krecke KN, Gisvold JJ. Invasive lobular carcinoma of the breast: mammographic findings and extent of disease at diagnosis in 184 patients. AJR Am J Roentgenol 1993; 161: 957–960

[146] Berg WA, Gutierrez L, NessAiver MS, et al. Diagnostic accuracy of mammography, clinical examination, US, and MR imaging in preoperative assessment of breast cancer. Radiology 2004; 233: 830–849

[147] Yeatman TJ, Cantor AB, Smith TJ, et al. Tumor biology of infiltrating lobular carcinoma. Implications for management. Ann Surg 1995; 222: 549–559, discussion 559–561

[148] Harvey JA. Unusual breast cancers: useful clues to expanding the differential diagnosis. Radiology 2007; 242: 683–694

[149] Newstead GM, Baute PB, Toth HK. Invasive lobular and ductal carcinoma: mammographic findings and stage at diagnosis. Radiology 1992; 184: 623–627

[150] Le Gal M, Ollivier L, Asselain B, et al. Mammographic features of 455 invasive lobular carcinomas. Radiology 1992; 185: 705–708

[151] Winston CB, Hadar O, Teitcher JB, et al. Metastatic lobular carcinoma of the breast: patterns of spread in the chest, abdomen, and pelvis on CT. AJR Am J Roentgenol 2000; 175: 795–800

[152] Harake MD, Maxwell AJ, Sukumar SA. Primary and metastatic lobular carcinoma of the breast. Clin Radiol 2001; 56: 621–630

[153] Evans WP, Warren Burhenne LJ, Laurie L, O'Shaughnessy KF, Castellino RA. Invasive lobular carcinoma of the breast: mammographic characteristics and computer-aided detection. Radiology 2002; 225: 182–189

[154] Harvey JA, Fechner RE, Moore MM. Apparent ipsilateral decrease in breast size at mammography: a sign of infiltrating lobular carcinoma. Radiology 2000; 214: 883–889

[155] Farshid G, Rush G. Assessment of 142 stellate lesions with imaging features suggestive of radial scar discovered during population-based screening for breast cancer. Am J Surg Pathol 2004; 28: 1626–1631

[156] Moore MM, Borossa G, Imbrie JZ, et al. Association of infiltrating lobular carcinoma with positive surgical margins after breast-conservation therapy. Ann Surg 2000; 231: 877–882

[157] Weinstein SP, Orel SG, Heller R, et al. MR imaging of the breast in patients with invasive lobular carcinoma. AJR Am J Roentgenol 2001; 176: 399–406

[158] Qayyum A, Birdwell RL, Daniel BL, et al. MR imaging features of infiltrating lobular carcinoma of the breast: histopathologic correlation. AJR Am J Roentgenol 2002; 178: 1227–1232

[159] Liberman L, Feng TL, Susnik B. Case 35: intracystic papillary carcinoma with invasion. Radiology 2001; 219: 781–784

[160] Wagner AE, Middleton LP, Whitman GJ. Intracystic papillary carcinoma of the breast with invasion. AJR Am J Roentgenol 2004; 183: 1516

[161] Lam WW, Chu WC, Tse GM, Ma TK. Sonographic appearance of mucinous carcinoma of the breast. AJR Am J Roentgenol 2004; 182: 1069–1074

[162] Cardenosa G, Doudna C, Eklund GW. Mucinous (colloid) breast cancer: clinical and mammographic findings in 10 patients. AJR Am J Roentgenol 1994; 162: 1077–1079

[163] Ishikawa T, Hamaguchi Y, Ichikawa Y, et al. Locally advanced mucinous carcinoma of the breast with sudden growth acceleration: a case report. Jpn J Clin Oncol 2002; 32: 64–67

[164] Wilson TE, Helvie MA, Oberman HA, Joynt LK. Pure and mixed mucinous carcinoma of the breast: pathologic basis for differences in mammographic appearance. AJR Am J Roentgenol 1995; 165: 285–289

[165] Kawashima M, Tamaki Y, Nonaka T, et al. MR imaging of mucinous carcinoma of the breast. AJR Am J Roentgenol 2002; 179: 179–183

[166] Chang S, Parker SL, Pham T, Buzdar AU, Hursting SD. Inflammatory breast carcinoma incidence and survival: the surveillance, epidemiology, and end results program of the National Cancer Institute, 1975–1992. Cancer 1998; 82: 2366–2372

[167] Robertson FM, Bondy M, Yang W, et al. Inflammatory breast cancer: the disease, the biology, the treatment [published correction appears in CA Cancer J Clin. 2011 Mar–Apr;61(2):134]. CA Cancer J Clin 2010; 60: 351–375

[168] Dawood S, Merajver SD, Viens P, et al. International expert panel on inflammatory breast cancer: consensus statement for standardized diagnosis and treatment. Ann Oncol 2011; 22: 515–523

[169] Walsh R, Kornguth PJ, Soo MS, Bentley R, DeLong DM. Axillary lymph nodes: mammographic, pathologic, and clinical correlation. AJR Am J Roentgenol 1997; 168: 33–38

[170] Yang WT, Suen M, Metreweli C. Mammographic, sonographic and histopathological correlation of benign axillary masses. Clin Radiol 1997; 52: 130–135

[171] Lee CH, Giurescu ME, Philpotts LE, Horvath LJ, Tocino I. Clinical importance of unilaterally enlarging lymph nodes on otherwise normal mammograms. Radiology 1997; 203: 329–334

[172] Yang WT, Chang J, Metreweli C. Patients with breast cancer: differences in color Doppler flow and gray-scale US features of benign and malignant axillary lymph nodes. Radiology 2000; 215: 568–573

[173] Abe H, Schmidt RA, Kulkarni K, Sennett CA, Mueller JS, Newstead GM. Axillary lymph nodes suspicious for breast cancer metastasis: sampling with US-guided 14-gauge core-needle biopsy—clinical experience in 100 patients. Radiology 2009; 250: 41–49

[174] Nori J, Bazzocchi M, Boeri C, et al. Role of axillary lymph node ultrasound and large core biopsy in the preoperative assessment of patients selected for sentinel node biopsy. Radiol Med (Torino) 2005; 109: 330–344

[175] Siegel R, Ward E, Brawley O, Jemal A. Cancer statistics, 2011: the impact of eliminating socioeconomic and racial disparities on premature cancer deaths. CA Cancer J Clin 2011; 61: 212–236

[176] Georgiannos SN, Chin J, Goode AW, Sheaff M. Secondary neoplasms of the breast: a survey of the 20th Century. Cancer 2001; 92: 2259–2266

[177] Klingen TA, Klaasen H, Aas H, Chen Y, Akslen LA. Secondary breast cancer: a 5-year population-based study with review of the literature. APMIS 2009; 117: 762–767

[178] Talwalkar SS, Miranda RN, Valbuena JR, et al. Lymphomas involving the breast: a study of 106 cases comparing localize and disseminated neoplasms Am J Surg Pathol 2008; 32: 1299–1309

[179] Zack JR, Trevisan SG, Gupta M. Primary breast lymphoma originating in a benign intramammary lymph node. AJR Am J Roentgenol 2001; 177: 177–178

[180] Yang WT, Lane DL, Le-Petross HT, Abruzzo LV, Macapinlac HA. Breast lymphoma: imaging findings of 32 tumors in 27 patients. Radiology 2007; 245: 692–702

[181] Ha KY, Wang JC, Gill JI. Lymphoma in the breast. Proc (Bayl Univ Med Cent) 2013; 26: 146–148

[182] Adrada B, Wu Y, Yang W. Hyperechoic lesions of the breast: radiologic-histo-pathologic correlation. AJR Am J Roentgenol 2013; 200: W518–30

[183] Linda A, Zuiani C, Lorenzon M, et al. Hyperechoic lesions of the breast: not always benign. AJR Am J Roentgenol 2011; 196: 1219–1224

[184] Sanguinetti A, Puma F, Lucchini R, et al. Breast metastasis from a pulmonary adenocarcinoma: Case report and review of the literature. Oncol Lett 2013; 5: 328–332

[185] Sousaris N, Mendelsohn G, Barr RG. Lung cancer metastatic to breast: case report and review of the literature. Ultrasound Q 2013; 29: 205–209

[186] Ji FF, Gao P, Wang JG, Zhao J, Zhao P. Contralateral breast metastasis from pulmonary adenocarcinoma: two cases report and literature review. J Thorac Dis 2012; 4: 384–389

[187] Williams SA, Ehlers RA, II, Hunt KK, et al. Metastases to the breast from non-breast solid neoplasms: presentation and determinants of survival. Cancer 2007; 110: 731–737

[188] Chung SY, Oh KK. Imaging findings of metastatic disease to the breast. Yonsei Med J 2001; 42: 497–502

[189] Sneige N, Zachariah S, Fanning TV, Dekmezian RH, Ordóñez NG. Fine-needle aspiration cytology of metastatic neoplasms in the breast. Am J Clin Pathol 1989; 92: 27–35

[190] Yang M, Nonaka D. A study of immunohistochemical differential expression in pulmonary and mammary carcinomas. Mod Pathol 2010; 23: 654–661

[191] Zamecnik J, Kodel R. Value of thyroid transcription factor-1 and surfactant apoprotein A in the differential diagnosis of pulmonary carcinomas: a study of 109 cases. Virchows Arch 2002; 440: 353–361

[192] Dennis JL, Hvidsten TR, Wit EC, et al. Markers of adenocarcinoma characteristic of the site of origin: development of a diagnostic algorithm. Clin Cancer Res 2005; 11: 3766–3772

[193] Evans A, Whelehan P, Thomson K, et al. Invasive breast cancer: relationship between shear-wave elastographic findings and histologic prognostic factors. Radiology 2012; 263: 673–677

[194] Barr RG. US elastography: applications in tumors. In: Luna JC, Hygino da Cruz LC, Jr, Rossi SE, eds. Functional Imaging in Oncology. New York, NY: Springer Heidelberg; 2014 :459–490

[195] Rouze NC, Wang MH, Palmeri ML, Nightingale KR. Parameters affecting the resolution and accuracy of 2-D quantitative shear wave images. IEEE Trans Ultrason Ferroelectr Freq Control 2012; 59: 1729–1740

# Index

Note: Page numbers set **bold** or *italic* indicate headings or figures, respectively.